INVISIBLE CAREGIVERS

INVISIBLE CAREGIVERS

Older Adults Raising Children in the Wake of HIV/AIDS

Edited by

Daphne Joslin

COLUMBIA UNIVERSITY PRESS

NEW YORK

COLUMBIA UNIVERSITY PRESS
Publishers Since 1893
New York   Chichester, West Sussex

Library of Congress Cataloging-in-Publication Data
Invisible caregivers : older adults raising children in the
wake of HIV/AIDS / edited by Daphne Joslin.
      p.   cm.
      Includes bibliographical references and index.
      ISBN 0–231–11936–4 (cloth : alk. paper) —
ISBN 0–231–11937–2 (pbk. : alk. paper)
      1. AIDS (Disease) in children—Social aspects.
2. AIDS (Disease) in children—Patients—Family
relationships. 3. AIDS (Disease) in children—Patients—
Services for. 4. Health education. I. Joslin, Daphne.
  RJ387 .A25 I484 2002
  362.1'98929792—dc21
                                2001047013

Columbia University Press books are printed on
permanent and durable acid-free paper.
Printed in the United States of America

c 10 9 8 7 6 5 4 3 2 1
p 10 9 8 7 6 5 4 3 2 1

To grandparents and all caregivers and families affected by the HIV/AIDS epidemic, especially Jeanne, Pat, Jose, and Aurea

and

To the memory of my grandmothers, Kate Helena Joslin and Gina Signorelli

Contents

The last two decades of the twentieth century witnessed unprecedented numbers of children eighteen years and younger in the United States residing in homes headed by a grandparent. Of the nearly four million children living in grandparent-headed households in 1997, 1.5 million had neither parent present (Lugaila 1998). "Skip-generation parenting" includes thousands of grandparents and older relatives such as great-grandparents and great-aunts who are raising children and adolescents because HIV disease has killed or disabled the parents. Where custodial responsibility has been documented, grandmothers are most often the surrogate parents to children of HIV-infected parents (Schuster et al. 2000; Draimin 1995; Schable et al. 1995; Cohen and Nehring 1994). The AIDS epidemic in the United States was projected to have orphaned more than 150,000 children by the year 2000 (Michaels and Levine 1992), leaving as many as 40,000 older adults as surrogate parents. Thousands more are now caring for children whose parents are infected but living with HIV disease. By 2010, hundreds of thousands of grandparents and other family elders will be raising children in the wake of HIV/AIDS around the globe. Despite this unprecedented caregiving responsibility, the older adults themselves are relatively invisible, hidden in the shadows of HIV care and the demands of raising a child.

Although surrogate parents in the HIV epidemic face problems shared with those raising children of incarcerated or drug-addicted mothers, HIV disease poses unique problems for both child and caregiver. To which friends and family members can a grandmother disclose the reason for her daughter's death? Should she also tell them of her four-year-old grandson's seropositive status? How does a seventy-six-year-old widowed grandmother handle the rage of her infected sixteen-year-old grandson who had watched his mother die from the disease seven years earlier? A fifty-three-year-old grandfather with primary responsibility for five young grandsons of a drug-using, infected mother has a bleeding ulcer that has already hospitalized him. Where can he find childcare, transportation, and health insurance so that he can seek medical attention? To whom does a sixty-four-year-old grandmother turn for guidance in discussing safer sex when her fifteen-year-old infected granddaughter begins dating?

Although older adults find comfort, satisfaction, and meaning in surrogate parenting in the wake of HIV/AIDS, caregiving imposes harsh and persistent threats to their own well-being. A grandmother in her thirties or forties defies classification as "older." However, the typical parental surrogate to HIV-affected children is a woman or couple in the mid- to late fifties, with some grandparents, great-grandparents, and great-aunts in their late seventies or early eighties. Parental surrogacy is thrust upon the elder generation when age-related chronic health problems surface and financial, emotional, and physical resources must be stretched to meet this new family responsibility. Given an extended period of child rearing for eighteen years or more, financial strain, social isolation, emotional stress, and neglected health problems may increase an older caregiver's risk of poor health, disability and dependency as he or she continues to age. From the vantage point of parental surrogacy, threats to a caregiver's physical and psychological well-being affect his or her capacity to serve as the primary parent until the child reaches maturity.

The implications of older adults raising children orphaned and affected by HIV disease are profound and complex, not only for individual caregivers and their families but also for professionals across a wide range of disciplines and service sectors. Entire communities and societies also feel the impact as their elder generation assumes the parental role of a generation lost to HIV/AIDS. Over the coming decade, HIV-determined parental surrogacy will have important implications for public policy, health and family service agencies, the "aging network," child welfare, and legal and educational systems. Service professionals, administrators, clergy, and educators will continue to meet caregivers in a variety of settings: as they escort infected family members to clinic appointments, apply for public benefits, learn from home-care staff how to adjust intravenous morphine injections and suction tracheal tubes, visit ill and dying children and grandchildren in hospitals, bury loved ones, and cope with children's behavioral and academic problems.

Caregivers, of course, are not the intended focus or identified patients of HIV and social-service programs. In most situations where elder parental surrogates are visible, it is only in their role as a child's caregiver. The mission of a pediatric AIDS clinic or Head Start Program, for example, is to serve the child, not the older caregiver. Older adults raising orphaned and affected children exist in the background, and in their commitment to care for the children they are reluctant to make their own needs known. Because most communities lack a service-delivery system designed to assist older parental surrogates, professional staff are often unable to identify caregiver needs, especially in HIV-affected families.

Multiple systemic barriers to case management and other services frustrate professionals who attempt to link caregivers to available resources. Barriers include professional ignorance about or denial that HIV disease affects older adults, eligibility restrictions on services funded through the Ryan White Comprehensive AIDS Resources Emergency Act of 1990 (CARE), limited funding and age restrictions of Older Americans Act (OAA)-funded services, and a fragmented health and human service system. The needs of elder HIV-affected surrogate parents are overlooked by public policies for HIV-infected persons and for older adults.

At the community and societal level, the implications of a lost generation of parents are unprecedented, yet this is the demographic profile of countries and communities hardest hit by the HIV pandemic—largely poor communities and nations of color. In policy reports and the popular press, the magnitude of this crisis at the community, national, and global level has been cast in terms of only orphaned and affected children, not the generation of elder caregivers. How communities will be affected by a generation of elders whose financial, social, and emotional resources are diminished by parental surrogacy and who have lost the caregivers for their own later lives remains to be seen. What national and global policy initiatives and strategies will be needed to address the greater vulnerability of these older adults? Two decades into the pandemic, these questions still have not been asked.

Nearly invisible, HIV-affected surrogate parents are a distinct group within two other groups that have received scholarly attention: those providing help to an HIV-ill family member or partner and those grandparents who are acting as parents. Although nearly 11 percent of grandparents in the United States report having assumed primary child-rearing responsibility for at least six months (Fuller-Thomson, Minkler, and Driver 1997), the number that has done so because of parental HIV disease is unknown. To date, there are no book-length studies of older adults raising children in the wake of HIV/AIDS, despite attention to AIDS orphaned children (New Jersey AIDS Partnership 1997; Boyd-Franklin, Steiner, and Boland 1995; Geballe, Gruendel, and Andiman 1995). This collection is intended to address an area virtually ignored by current policy and programs and to fill a vacuum in the practitioner-oriented and academically oriented literature on families and caregiving.

Because the issues affecting elder caregivers extend beyond a single area, this collection assembles a group of contributors with expertise in aging, HIV services, community health, child welfare, mental health, education, and public policy. The authors' professional disciplines include social work, nursing, medicine, health administration, gerontology, special education, and counseling. The book's primary goal is to generate, support, and guide program and policy initiatives that can address the complex issues embedded in the daily experience of these families and the professionals who work with them. Some readers may want to consider clinical and other "practice" issues with caregivers and families, others program design and service delivery, including outreach, staff training, and interagency coordination. Public policy professionals and attorneys will find the collection helpful in advocating the cause of their clients and in effecting systemic reforms. It is hoped that students and scholars will consider how academic resources can be harnessed through applied research to support these invisible caregivers and their families so that raising children in the wake of HIV/AIDS does not continue to compromise the older generation's well-being as it ages.

In the early 1990s the concept of "secondary survivor" was introduced to underscore the intergenerational impact of HIV/AIDS, notably in poorer African countries where "these survivors [bear] the full weight of sustaining a decimated, confused and demoralized community. . . . The surviving responsible person in the family is likely to be drawn from the older generation" (Beer, Rose, and Trout 1988). More than a decade later, "secondary survivors" reflect the global impact of HIV/AIDS and the transformation of orphaning "into a long-term, chronic problem" (Hunter and Williamson 2000:4) for the twenty-first century. In sub-Saharan African, Southeast Asian, Latin American, and Caribbean countries and U.S. urban areas hardest hit by the epidemic, the loss of the young adult and mid-life generation imposes harsh burdens on elderly caregivers. Yet, as the world's nations begin to cope with the estimated thirty million AIDS-orphaned children and the millions more who are living with infected parents (Hunter and Williamson 2000), the older parental surrogates may be further neglected. The aim of this book is to bring them out of the shadows and, in making them visible, contribute to their well-being and empowerment.

References

Beer, C., A. Rose, and A. Trout. 1988. AIDS: The grandmother's burden. In A. F. Fleming, M. Carballo, D. W. Fitzsimmons, M. R. Bailey, and J. Mann, eds., *The Global Impact of AIDS*, pp. 171–174. New York: Alan Liss.

Cohen, F. L., and W. L. Nehring. 1994. Foster care of HIV-positive children in the United States. *Public Health Reports* 109:60–67.

Draimin, B. 1995. A second family? Placement and custody decisions. In S. Geballe, J. Gruendel, and W. Andiman, eds., *Forgotten Children of the AIDS Epidemic*, pp. 125–139. New Haven: Yale University Press.

Fuller-Thomson, E., M. Minkler, and D. Driver. 1997. A profile of grandparents raising grandchildren in the United States. *The Gerontologist* 37:406–411.

Geballe, S., J. Gruendel, and W. Andiman, eds. *Forgotten Children of the AIDS Epidemic.* New Haven: Yale University Press.

Hunter, S., and J. Williamson. 2000. *Children on the Brink: Strategies to Support Children Isolated by HIV/AIDS.* Washington, D.C.: U.S. Agency for International Development.

Lugaila, T. 1998. *Marital Status and Living Arrangements: March 1997.* Washington, D.C.: U.S. Bureau of the Census.

Michaels, D., and C. Levine. 1992. Estimates of the number of motherless youth orphaned by AIDS in the United States. *Journal of the American Medical Association* 268: 3456–3461.

Minkler, M., and K. Roe. 1993. *Grandmothers as Caregivers: Raising Children of the Crack Cocaine Epidemic.* Thousand Oaks, Calif.: Sage.

Schable, B., T. Diaz, S. Chu, M. B. Caldwell, L. Conti, et al. 1995. Who are the primary caretakers of children born to HIV-infected mothers? Results from a multi-state surveillance project. *Pediatrics* 95:511–515.

Schuster, M. A., D. E. Kanouse, S. C. Morton, S. A. Bozzette, A. Miu, G. B. Scott, and M. F. Shapiro. 2000. HIV-infected parents and their children in the United States. *American Journal of Public Health* 90 (7): 1074–1081.

Acknowledgments

This book reflects collaboration and support by many people. My thanks to the contributors for their professional expertise and commitment to serve families affected by the HIV/AIDS epidemic. Their hard work and cooperation enabled this book to be realized. I am very grateful to John Michel at Columbia University Press for his encouragement and good humor, and to Gregory McNamee for copyediting with precision and calmness. I would especially like to thank Bernadette Capelle for her belief in the value of this collection.

The vision for this collection was inspired by my participation in the Coalition on AIDS of Passaic County (CAPCO), New Jersey. Special thanks go to Carol DeGraw, Carol Mevi-Triano, the Rev. Melynn Murphy, Nancy Begin, Shauna Haggar, Elizabeth Paskas, and John McCausland for sharing my belief that older caregivers in the HIV/AIDS epidemic should be made visible and their needs addressed through advocacy, programs, and public policy. Without their support of my research and advocacy, this book would never have been conceived or realized.

My own chapters in this book reflect interviews I conducted with grandparents raising HIV-affected and HIV-orphaned children. My debt to these caregivers is great. By sharing their stories they gave me the gift of being a witness to their lives. I hope that this book will extend my pledge of advocacy on their behalf.

I am especially grateful to friends and colleagues for their consistent and generous support. Nan Bauer-Maglin, Peter Stein, and Donna Perry gave patiently of their time during all phases of this book's production. Andrea Ades Vasquez and Jerry Markowitz were unfailing in their encouragement and love. Thanks also to Neill Rosenfeld for his calm and helpful responses. Peter Ford's hospitality was matched by his editing skills. I express special gratitude to Livia McGinnis for her wisdom, strength, and counsel.

I also thank my colleagues in the Department of Community Health at William Paterson University for their humor, patience, and kindness during this book's production. Thanks to Richard Blonna for advice, Merle Miller for clerical help, and Debra Singer for research assistance. I would like to honor the memory of Grace Galindo, who transcribed several interviews and assisted in Spanish translation, and who died before the book's completion. I gratefully acknowledge the support received through a grant from the William Paterson University Center for Research.

The devotion of families is at the heart of this book. To my daughters, Emily and Sophia Joslin-Roher, your pride in and appreciation of my work gave me sustenance and joy. Thanks also to Sophie for her organizational assistance and computer savvy. Being a witness to another's life and her work is a project of love. From cups of tea and healthy meals to endless hours of editing and proofing, my life partner, the Rev. Patricia Ackerman, nourished me in this book's creation. I am grateful for her friendship and honor her own commitment to social justice. Finally, this book honors the legacies of my parents, Vera Signorelli Joslin, R.N., and Doyle Joslin, M.D., for their dedication to public health and research in the service of healing.

Jerome Brown, CSW, worked for five years as a family specialist and family specialist supervisor at The Family Center in New York City. In these roles he was involved in the direct delivery and supervision of permanency planning services to families affected by AIDS. He currently works at the New York State AIDS Institute.

Wendy C. Budin received her Ph.D. from New York University in 1996. She is an associate professor in the Graduate Nursing Department at Seton Hall University. She is an expert in maternal child nursing and computer applications in nursing and has published widely in these areas, as well as in nursing research and patient care.

Gloria Caliandro received her Ed.D. in nursing from Columbia University in 1970. She is an expert in community health and is the primary author and editor of *Primary Nursing Care* (Scott Foresman, 1994). Before her retirement, she was associate dean and associate professor in the College of Nursing at Seton Hall University.

Mathilda Braceros Catarina is associate professor and director of the graduate program in counseling services at William Paterson University of New Jersey. She received her Ph.D. in urban school psychology from Fordham University and completed postgraduate training at the Family Therapy Institute of the State University of New York Health Science Center at Brooklyn. In addition to her research on children with HIV/AIDS, her interests and work include cross-cultural psychology, issues of race and gender, and prevention and re-duction of violence in our schools and communities.

Rachel Davis received her B.S. and R.N. degrees from Long Beach City Col-lege. She is a research nurse in the Division of Community Pediatrics of the University of Texas Health Science Center at San Antonio. She has been the clinic coordinator for the South Texas Family AIDS Network since 1996, co-ordinating the medical care for children, youth, and families living with HIV and AIDS.

Carol E. DeGraw, LCSW, received her MSW from Rutgers University in 1988. The former executive director of the Coalition on AIDS in Passaic County, New Jersey, she conducts workshops on HIV, case management, and senior issues on the local, state, and national levels.

Terence I. Doran, Ph.D., M.D., is associate professor in community pediatrics at the University of Texas Health Science Center at San Antonio. He has been the medical director for the South Texas Family AIDS Network since 1991, providing direct medical services for children and their families living with HIV and AIDS in South Texas. He is principal investigator for La Fron-tera project, a HRSA funded special project. His published research includes topics related to HIV as it affects families, children, and migrant seasonal farm workers in South Texas.

Barbara Draimin, DSW, is the founding executive director of the Family Center, which serves families throughout New York City by supporting parents, their children, and future caregivers in the transitions resulting from serious illness. Before creating this agency in 1993, Draimin was di-rector of planning at the New York Department of Social Services AIDS Division and associate to the commissioner of the New York Department for the Aging.

Jenny Grosz, CSW, a member of the faculty at the Albert Einstein College of Medicine, has worked in the field of pediatric AIDS since the mid-1980s. As codirector of the Developmental and Family Services Unit, an interdis-ciplinary team at the Children's Evaluation and Rehabilitation Center in the Bronx, she has developed an array of services for perinatally HIV-in-fected and -affected children. She has presented at regional, national, and international conferences and has written several articles and contributed chapters to major works on the psychosocial implications of growing up with HIV infection.

Phyllis Shanley Hansell received her Ed.D. from Columbia University in 1981. She is dean and professor of the College of Nursing at Seton Hall University. Previously she held the position of director of nursing research at Memorial Sloan-Kettering Cancer Center. An NIH-funded researcher, she served as principal investigator on a study that tested an intervention to boost social support in caregivers of children with HIV/AIDS. She is widely published in the area of care of seriously ill children and their families.

Ruth Harrison received her Ph.D. in nursing research and theory development from New York University. She is associate professor of nursing at William Paterson University of New Jersey. Her areas of research include health promotion among HIV-infected persons and spirituality and health.

Bruce Hartman received his Ph.D. in psychology from the Indiana University in 1981. He is professor of professional psychology in the College of Education and Human Services at Seton Hall University. An expert in tests and measurement, he has published widely in the area of research instrument evaluation.

Bert Hayslip Jr. received his Ph.D. in experimental developmental psychology from the University of Akron in 1975. He is regents professor of psychology at the University of North Texas. Dr. Hayslip is a fellow of the American Psychological Association, the Gerontological Society of America, and the Association for Gerontology in Higher Education. He is associate editor of *Experimental Aging Research,* editor of *The International Journal of Aging and Human Development,* and coauthor of *Hospice Care* (Sage, 1992), *Psychology and Aging: An Annotated Bibliography* (Greenwood Press, 1995), and *Grandparents Raising Grandchildren: Theoretical, Empirical, and Clinical Perspectives* (Springer Publishing, 2000).

Jan Hudis, MPH, is a co-founder and director of special projects at The Family Center in New York City. She has been involved in the design, implementation, and evaluation of services for families affected by AIDS for more than ten years.

Cynthia B. Hughes received her Ed.D. in nursing from Columbia University in 1980. She is a pediatric nurse practitioner and professor of nursing at California State University, Los Angeles. She is widely published in the area of parent/child nursing.

Daphne Joslin received her Ph.D. from New York University and her M.P.H. from Columbia University. Her research and advocacy in the area of HIV/AIDS and older adults began in 1990 while working at the New York City Department of Aging. She is currently associate professor of community health and director of the Institute for Creative Aging at William Paterson University of New Jersey. She has published articles on grandparents raising grandchildren, older adults affected and infected by HIV/AIDS, and employed caregivers. As an advocate, she co-founded the New York Association on HIV Over Fifty, the HIV/AIDS and Aging Committee of the Coalition on AIDS in Passaic County (CAPCO), and the Grandparents as Parents Task Force of Passaic County.

Joan Levine-Perkell, MSW, ACSW, is a clinical social worker and psychotherapist working at the Peninsula Counseling Center in New York. She has served as co-chair of the National Associations for HIV Over 50 and as a member of the New York City AIDS and Aging Task Force.

Nathan L. Linsk is professor at the Jane Addams College of Social Work at the University of Illinois at Chicago. He is the principal investigator for two federally funded education and advocacy centers, the Midwest AIDS Training and Education Center and the Great Lakes Addictions Technology Transfer Center. Linsk is currently principal investigator on a quality assurance and evaluation project assessing Title I Ryan White CARE services for the city of Chicago. His research about older adults, caregiving, case management and HIV includes numerous articles and three books, including *Wages for Caring: Compensating Home Care for the Elderly* (with S. Keigher, S. England, and L. Simon-Rusinowitz; Greenwood Press, 1992). He is founder and co-chair of the National Association on HIV Over Fifty.

Howard Lune received his Ph.D. in sociology from New York University in 1998. His work explores the organization of collective action, relations between state and civil society, and relations among community-based nonprofit organizations. He is now assistant professor of sociology at William Paterson University.

Sally Mason received her Ph.D. from the Jane Addams College of Social Work at the University of Illinois at Chicago. She is currently on the faculty of the Institute for Juvenile Research, Department of Psychiatry, University of Illinois. Her research and scholarly work focuses on families affected by HIV, specifically permanency planning with HIV-infected parents and relative caregivers of HIV-affected children.

Lockhart McKelvy, MSW, is clinical support supervisor for the Family Center in New York City. He served as coordinator of the Children in AIDS Families Project at Beth Israel Medical Center. He has written several journal articles and book chapters on HIV/AIDS and its effect on families.

Carol Mevi-Triano earned her Ed.D. from Rutgers University. She is the assistant director of community medicine at a large urban New Jersey medical center. In this capacity she oversees all outpatient HIV programs for children, adolescents, adults, and their families.

Namposya Nampanya-Serpell received her Ph.D. in policy sciences from the University of Maryland in 1998. Her professional experience includes work as an economist in the Zambian government and as a UNICEF program officer. She has also worked as a technical advisor to many organizations, including Save the Children Federation, UNAIDS, Family Health International, and Project Support International.

Elizabeth C. Paskas, R.N., received her bachelor of science from William Paterson University. She worked as a treatment care manager in Passaic County, New Jersey, where she developed programs to assist people with HIV to adhere to their treatment regimens. She now works at the Hackensack University Medical Center. She continues her efforts to educate the community on the issues surrounding people with HIV and their families.

Cynthia Cannon Poindexter, MSW, Ph.D., is an assistant professor at the Boston University Graduate School of Social Work. She was one of the first ten national John A. Hartford Geriatric Social Work Scholars, receiving a grant to study HIV-affected older caregivers.

Phyllis Russo received her Ed.D. in administration in higher education in 1996 from Seton Hall University, where she is an associate professor in the Undergraduate Nursing Department. She is a coauthor of *Oncology Nursing: Pathophysiology and Assessment* (Macmillan, 1997).

INVISIBLE CAREGIVERS

Introduction

DAPHNE JOSLIN

At the age of sixty-three, Ella McIntyre[1] buried her thirty-seven-year-old daughter and three-and-a-half-year-old granddaughter within three months, both dead of AIDS. Despite glaucoma, arthritis, osteoporosis, and chest and back pain, she has not been to a physician in more than four years, except for a fractured ankle. When she quit her job three years ago so that she could care for her daughter and granddaughter full time, she lost all health benefits. A widow living on Social Security, she cannot afford private health insurance, is too young for Medicare, and has an income that exceeds Medicaid eligibility limits. "I can't afford to be hospitalized and I can't go for a checkup," she says. Uncertain of how to move forward with her life, she stays away from home as much as she can, running errands, window shopping, and looking for craft projects so that she can keep busy. Her house has too many memories, and the depression she thought would lift after the Christmas holidays has continued into the early spring. "Sometimes I think I am crazy," she says, lighting another cigarette. She does not know how to find a job at her age and doubts that anyone would hire her.

Like Ella McIntyre, Rose Crimeri has felt the crushing impact of AIDS on her family. Also widowed, she is the sole caregiver for her eight-year-old granddaughter, Julia. After Mrs. Crimeri's thirty-three-year-old daughter died of AIDS in Florida the year before, Julia moved to live with her sixty-seven-year-old grandmother in a northeastern suburb. Conflict abounds between Mrs. Crimeri and Julia's father's family. He, too, died of AIDS, and although none of his sisters want primary responsibility for Julia, they expect Mrs. Crimeri to bring her to visit each week, regardless of homework or after-school activities. Mrs. Crimeri would like to adopt her granddaughter, but one aunt told her, "You can't adopt. You're too old."

Julia's grief and fears related to her mother's death are among her grandmother's major concerns. Julia watched the ambulance take her dying mother away. The child then threatened to jump off her loft bed. "I was able to get her to go to a children's art therapy program given by a hospice program here. I talk with my minister when I'm upset or to a close friend. But my sister is a cold person and not sympathetic."

Extremely agitated during the interview, Mrs. Crimeri does not know whether Julia is infected. "I am afraid to have her tested. I don't want to upset her. What would be said to her about the test? Does the school tell the child? Would I have to inform the school [if she tested positive]? I don't even know what I should tell her about her mother's death. I don't know if I want to know [if she is infected]." Although Mrs. Crimeri is financially secure, the unanticipated responsibility of parental surrogacy contributes to her anxiety. "I have no health insurance for her and I don't know how long I can do this. I am healthy now, but . . ." Her voice trails off as she shrugs hopelessly. "I have to live until she's eighteen."

Unwilling to be interviewed in her apartment, Thelma Davis talks about her experience as we sip coffee at a local diner. Employed as a caseworker at a group home for adolescent girls, Ms. Davis is divorced and lives with her infected four-year-old granddaughter Alana, whom she has been raising since birth because of her daughter's drug addiction. A twenty-six-year-old daughter also lives in the household and helps with some of Alana's care. Alana's mother is dying of AIDS and has been living in a residence for infected women. "I am always running—between the hospital [where her thirty-two-year-old daughter is dying of AIDS], home, and work. I never have time for myself. I'm tired and depressed from having lost my father last year."

Ms. Davis enjoys talking about her granddaughter, although she feels overwhelmed by the responsibility of caring for her. "She is so bright. I can't keep up with her questions. And I enjoy her company. But I feel like a prisoner. I try hard not to be resentful. I had my kids young and thought I would be free. It feels like she's been with me forever. I have no time to myself. I can't just go home and say "I've put my eight hours in, now I can rest." It's story time, bath time, dinner time. My other daughter and son help out, but it's on their good will. They won't cancel their plans. And Alana's health is always on my mind, even though she is in excellent health now."

Ms. Davis's emotional stress profile[2] shows high levels of depression and anxiety. Sleep problems, an ulcer, back pain, and tension are among her physical stress symptoms. "Alana's four-year-old active mind and my fifty-seven-year-old tired body just don't go together. I am thankful [given her HIV status] that she has so much energy. She's doing what a normal four-year-old should do, but I'm doing what a fifty-seven-year-old should not have to do. I know she should be in a regular daycare center. But my sister keeps her, and that gives me peace of mind, especially if I am running late at work." Managing the disclosure of her granddaughter's HIV status is stressful. "If I start to look for a regular day care—and I know I have to when she starts school—it means that I have to tell them she's infected. I don't want to."

As these personal narratives illustrate, older adults become surrogate parents to HIV-affected and orphaned children under complex and painful circumstances. Research on African American grandmothers raising children of the crack cocaine epidemic found three patterns by which they assumed parental surrogacy: sudden, negotiated, or inevitable assumption. Whether they assumed responsibility without warning, in tandem with the mother's parental care, or after a protracted period of maternal behavioral decline, grandmothers felt a profound sense of loss (Roe, Minkler, and Barnwell 1994). Similar patterns and a sense of loss describe the assumption of parental surrogacy for HIV-affected children. Some, like Rose Crimeri, not having known the parent's HIV status, become the caregiver suddenly when the child's parent dies. Others offer intermittent household help, HIV care, or childcare over a protracted course of HIV disease. Some, like Thelma Davis, begin caregiving because of parental drug addiction, becoming the primary parent as HIV disease progresses or as addiction disables the mother's parental capacity. Still others, like Ella McIntyre, quickly assume parental surrogacy because of rapid and progressive physical decline of the infected parent. In each pattern, minor children may be infected, and at different disease stages.

Chapter Overview

HIV disease imposes unique and complex circumstances of surrogate parenting determined by the trajectory of HIV disease, medical treatment and family care, AIDS stigma, isolation, death, and loss. This chapter outlines key issues that will be discussed in later chapters. Because most HIV-affected surrogate parents are grandparents and, for some period of time, care for a family member with HIV disease, usually an adult child of grandchild, I will summarize here the relevant literature pertaining to "grandparents as parents"[3] and HIV caregivers. The extent and patterns of HIV-affected surrogate parenting over the coming decades will be shaped by many factors. I will also review trends in female HIV infection and mortality and access and adherence to new antiretroviral therapies by infected women, especially mothers.

In chapter 2, "Caregiving Profiles," Carol Mevi-Triano and Elizabeth Paskas present the personal narratives of three women who are raising HIV-affected or orphaned children. In her own voice, each describes how she came to be raising her grandchildren, her fears and frustrations, and sources of support and comfort. Prominent in each caregiver's profile is a strong spirituality. In chapter 3, "Stigma, Isolation, and Support," Cynthia Cannon Poindexter describes the nature of the toxic social and interpersonal environment created by AIDS stigma and discusses how health and human service practitioners can address caregiver isolation and reluctance to seek support. The complexity of HIV-related death and grief is the focus of chapter 4, "Death, Loss, and Bereavement," by Joan Levine-Perkell and Bert Hayslip Jr. They examine bereavement in older adults and children, the impact of multiple family deaths, disenfranchised grief, and cultural determinants of grief and bereavement. In chapter 5, "Caregiver Physical Health and Emotional Well-Being," Ruth Harrison and I use the concept of the "hidden patient" as a framework to describe caregivers' chronic and stress-related health problems. Health-promotion needs of older surrogate parents are examined in relation to self-care, help-seeking, and access to medical care.

In chapter 6, "Stress and Social Support in Older Caregivers of Children with HIV/AIDS: An Intervention Model," Phyllis Shanley Hansell, Cynthia Hughes, Wendy Budin, Phyllis Russo, Gloria Caliandro, Bruce Hartman, and Olga Hernandez describe the role of social support in buffering caregiver stress. The chapter presents findings from an innovative model to improve coping strategies through enhanced social support. The HIV-infected child and adolescent are the focus of chapter 7, "Caring for the Infected Child," by Jenny Grosz. She examines how pediatric HIV disease and medical treatment affect children's psychosocial needs and behavior, using cases from a caregiver support group at a pediatric mental health program for infected children. In chapter 8, "Their Second Chance: Grandparents Caring for Their Grandchildren," Lockhart McKelvy and Barbara Draimin use case experiences from a social service program to describe areas of family conflict as well as caregiver resilience. The chapter offers strategies of family intervention. Chapter 9,

"Custody and Permanency Planning," by Jan Hudis and Jerome Brown, examines custodial and legal issues related to infected parents' need to plan for the future care of their children. They present legal options including guardianship, adoption, and foster care with case examples, illustrating the complex permanency planning process. Drawing from a model supportive service program for older HIV-affected parental surrogates, Carol DeGraw describes caregiver case management needs in chapter 10, "Case Management Challenges and Strategies." She discusses supportive service arrangements, barriers to client outreach and recruitment, and client and system advocacy strategies. In chapter 11, "Caregivers and the Educational System," Matilda Catarina discusses the school-related impact of HIV/AIDS on infected and affected children. Strengthening children's academic performance and psychosocial development, she argues, calls for supportive program and informed response by teachers, administrators, and counselors.

As a global epidemic, HIV disease affects families across national boundaries. With growing rates of HIV infection among women of childbearing age worldwide and rising tides of immigration fueled by war, persecution, and globalization, older caregivers may be recent immigrants who have left their country of origin to care for an adult child and/or her surviving offspring in another country. Terence Doran, Howard Lune, and Rachel Davis use case histories from Mexican families in the South Texas border region to discuss late-life surrogate parenting in the context of migration and immigration in chapter 12, "Immigrant and Migrant Families." Policies and programs related to child welfare, health insurance, aging, HIV/AIDS care, and welfare reform are examined in chapter 13, "Policy Implications for HIV-Affected Older Relative Caregivers," by Nathan Linsk, Cynthia Cannon Poindexter, and Sally Mason. The authors discuss how program eligibility, benefits, payment mechanisms, and policy assumptions affect older surrogate parents and their families. Broadening the book's focus beyond the United States, in chapter 14, "The Global Implications," Namposya Nampanya-Serpell draws attention to the pandemic's catastrophic impact on families in sub-Saharan Africa, South and Southeast Asia, and the Caribbean. Nampanya-Serpell presents initiatives at the community level with recommendations for national and international strategies to support the elder generation of caregivers. In the concluding chapter, I propose a framework of elder, family, and community empowerment to guide program and policy initiatives that are designed to support older HIV-affected surrogate parents. Strategies to enhance caregiver well-being, I argue, must promote not only greater personal efficacy but also social justice, reducing disparities in wealth and income that are concentrating HIV disease and late-life surrogate parenting among impoverished and marginalized communities.

Grandparents as Parents

In part, the strains faced by HIV-affected surrogate parents are no different from those of caregivers who serve because of parental neglect, abuse, drug use, incarceration, abandonment, or non-HIV deaths. By the 1990 census, the dramatic increase in grandchildren living with grandparents or other relatives reflected an unprecedented number of grandparents who were "parents of last resort." Capturing this national trend in changing household composition and parenting roles, 1997 census data showed 3.7 million grandparents in the United States who were raising minor children below the age of eighteen (Lugalia 1998). Earlier reports found that in one-third of these households the children's parents are absent (Saluter 1992). More than one in ten grandparents raise grandchildren for at least six months, with many shouldering the responsibility for at least three years (Fuller-Thomson, Minkler, and Driver 1997). Despite many satisfactions, custodial grandparents face overwhelming physical, economic, and emotional demands reflected in greater psychological distress (Kelley 1993), depression (Fuller-Thomson, Minkler, and Driver 1997), neglected physical health (Rogers 1996; Joslin and Brouard 1995; Burton 1993; Minkler, Roe, and Price 1992) and poorer self-reported health (Marx and Solomon 2000). For many, custodial grandparenting continues a pattern of heavy life burdens, family distress, and economic strain (Burnette 1997; Strawbridge et al. 1997).

Parental surrogacy imposes a financial burden on the vast majority of older caregivers. Fixed incomes are insufficient to meet the needs of an expanded household and growing children. Employed grandparents who reduce work to part-time or withdraw entirely from the labor force lose income, health insurance, and other benefits (Odulana, Camblin, and White 1996; Simon-Rusinowitz et al. 1996). Exclusion of grandchildren or other minors from health insurance policies imposes yet another financial strain. African American and Latino surrogate parents are more likely to assume this additional familial responsibility with low incomes (Fuller-Thomson, Minkler, and Driver 1997). The economic vulnerability of custodial grandparents was documented by an AARP study finding that 56 percent of grandparent-headed households had incomes below $20,000 in 1992 (Chalfie 1994) and that nearly 25 percent of custodial grandparents were living below the poverty line (Fuller-Thomson, Minkler, and Driver 1997). In the absence of comprehensive policies to assist older surrogate parents, those needing financial support face inadequate and means-tested programs such as the Personal Responsibility and Work Opportunities Act of 1996 (PRA) (Mullen 2000).

Financial strain, inadequate housing, and anxiety over children's developmental, medical, and psychological needs create enormous stress. While resenting the loss of personal time, privacy, and money, grandparents may also feel guilty and inadequate because of their adult child's failure to fulfill the parental role (Musil, Schrader, and Mutikani 2000). Normal childrearing problems are magnified for those raising children with behavioral needs associated with maternal drug use, parental neglect, and child abuse. Grandparents with drug-abusing adult children contend with theft, physical threats, erratic behavior, and household disruption (Minkler and Roe 1993).

Poorer self-reported health among custodial grandparents cannot be attributed to surrogate parenting alone. Yet consistent findings from small nonrandom and large random samples mark older surrogate parents as a high health-risk population, with poorer self-rated health, greater risk of functional disabilities interfering with mobility, and somatic stress symptoms such as back or stomach pain (Minkler and Roe 1993). Poorer health is especially noted among residents of poor communities and those of color (Dowdell 1995; Joslin and Brouard 1995; Burton 1992; Minkler, Roe, and Price 1992), and those raising children alone (Marx and Solomon 2000). Lack of time, physical exhaustion, anxiety, and depression cause grandparents to neglect their own health (Joslin and Harrison 1998; Jendrek 1996; Joslin and Brouard 1995; Burton 1992; Minkler, Roe, and Price 1992), resulting in missed medical appointments and exacerbation of chronic conditions (Grant 1997; Miller 1991).

HIV-Affected Surrogate Parenting:
Convergence of Stigma, Stress, and Loss

HIV disease compounds the stress experienced by older surrogate parents, imposing a *convergence* of HIV-determined issues related to diagnosis, disclosure, stigma, disease progression, symptom and treatment management, dying, and bereavement. The portraits that open this chapter capture some of the problems older surrogate parents face: neglected physical health, social isolation, depression, AIDS stigma, family conflict, financial strain, and the children's grief and their own. Those raising infected children have organized their entire lives around the disease and its associated anxieties and responsibilities.

"I sometimes worry about which one of us will die first. Either is more than I can bear to think about," said Anita Marrone, who is raising her thirteen-year-old infected granddaughter. New antiviral therapies require constant vigilance and fail to abate anxiety. "It's like being under a cloud. You never know when they could fail. . . . She's healthy now, but you have to watch every little thing. She's been complaining of headaches and being tired for weeks. She had bronchitis this winter. You look at everything and wonder . . ."

Stigma and Social Isolation

Exacerbating caregivers' social isolation because of HIV care, childrearing, and housekeeping, the toxic social environment created by AIDS phobia and stigma erodes emotional and practical social support, leading to social withdrawal by both infected and uninfected (Crawford 1996). AIDS stigma extends beyond the infected person to caregivers and other uninfected family members (Poindexter and Linsk 1998, 1999; McGinn 1996; Fair, Spencer, and Winer 1995; Lesar, Gerber, and Semmel 1995–1996; Christ and Wiener 1994; Roth, Siegel, and Black 1994; Herek and Capitanio 1993; Powell-Cope and Brown 1992). In the face of real or anticipated rejection, caregivers become both socially isolated from family, friends, neighbors and religious institutions (Poindexter and Linsk 1999; Roth, Siegel, and Black 1994; Powell-Cope and Brown 1992), and are reluctant to seek assistance from formal agencies (Lesar, Gerber, and Semmel 1995–1996; Powell-Cope and Brown 1992; Cates et al. 1990).

Ella McIntyre's world shrank when she become the sole caregiver to her daughter and granddaughter, both with AIDS. "I don't go out much any more. I'm only relating to doctors, nurses, and family, so I don't see other people. I don't have the money to go out and I don't have many people that I trust." Support groups for HIV-affected families may be inaccessible to those raising infants and young children, or also caring for an ill or dying adult. At the same time, older adults may be reluctant to attend a support group, having been raised in a generation that maintains the privacy of family issues and speaks less in terms of personal feelings. Cultural values may also prohibit sharing "family business' outside of the family. Knowing that HIV is a disease largely of the young, older adults may be reluctant to join support groups where they feel they might be out of place.

Even in families where children are not infected, HIV stigma, internalized shame, and social isolation haunt young and older generations. "My grandsons were teased. "Your mother has AIDS." They didn't want to play outside. They were getting into fights. I told them to just let it go." Mae Hawkins's eyes fill with tears as she talks about her three adolescent grandsons.

Given the fear and reality of social rejection, surrogate parents must often maintain the secrecy of HIV diagnosis even within a close circle of family and friends. In a pristine metropolitan area suburb, I complete an interview with a seventy-two-year-old grandmother who, in a difficult informal arrangement with her former son-in-law, is a co-parent to her six-year-old uninfected grandson. She and I sit in her living room; her sister visiting from California and a neighbor sit across the room, curious about a study on grandparents raising children. Oddly, Evelyn Connor is comfortable continuing the interview in the same room with them, although she lowers her voice to a whisper when discussing her daughter's death from AIDS. "They don't know," she said, gesturing toward her sister and neighbor. Only my niece in New York knows why Ann died."

Adult children's reluctance to disclose their own HIV status can impose the burden of disclosing both the parent's and child's infection on the surrogate parent (Tasker 1992). Anita Marrone recalls, "My daughter Angela didn't want anyone to know [she had AIDS] so I couldn't say anything to anyone. She wouldn't even let me call any agencies to get help or let me tell Jessie [her granddaughter]. So after her mother died, I had to tell [her granddaughter] that she died from AIDS. And I was the one who told her that she was HIV positive." Compounding the shame of a stigmatized disease, caregivers may feel responsible for what has befallen their family, wondering, as a forty-nine-year-old grandmother did who had buried her daughter and an infant grandson, "What did I do wrong? My other kids turned out fine . . ."

HIV/AIDS Caregiving and Stress

HIV disease intensifies the normal strains of family care of the chronically ill (Pearlin, Aneshensel, and LeBlanc 1997; Walker et al. 1996; Wardlaw 1994), becoming the caregiver's all-consuming focus. Coordinating medication regimens and medical appointments, managing treatment side effects and disease symptoms, contending with the ill person's emotional needs, and providing hands-on personal care and housekeeping assistance impose overwhelming physical and emotional demands on the caregiver. Many older surrogate parents are serial caregivers for several infected relatives, often as they assume responsibility for young children, who may also be infected. Letitia Williams, raising a three-year-old infected granddaughter, had also cared for a daughter and infant grandson, both of whom died of AIDS. Typically, the infected adult is a daughter, daughter-in-law, or son, with many elders facing the infection, illness, and deaths of multiple members of the same generation. Caregiving patterns for infected women in the United States are not well known, although a recent study of HIV-infected parents and their children in that country found that grandmothers were the predominant caregivers (Schuster et al. 2000). Studying infected adults in Thailand, researchers have found that almost two-thirds of those who died of AIDS had been cared for by a parent (Knodel et al. 2000).

Chronic fatigue and physical exhaustion (Turner and Pearlin 1989), somatic physical and psychological symptoms (Trice 1988; LeBlanc, London, and Aneshensel 1997), emotional exhaustion (Turner, Catania, and Gagnon 1994) and depression (LeBlanc, Aneshensel, and Wight 1995) are common among HIV caregivers. A catastrophic illness with an unpredictable course, HIV disease has been termed a "physiological and emotional time bomb" (Roth, Siegel, and Black 1994). Minor health problems of childhood—colds, ear infections, flu, headaches—assume different proportions in families where the child is infected, which explains Anita Marrone's constant vigilance. Parental surrogates must learn to cope with infected babies and children who may have difficulty swallowing and eating (Marder and Linsk 1995). Caregivers can feel overwhelmed in trying to disinfect the environment to protect the infected family member(s) and in handling blood and bodily wastes to reduce transmission risk to themselves and others (Goicoechea-Balbona 1998; Levine-Perkell 1996). How new combination therapies are transforming family care of HIV-infected children and adult has not been studied. Recent research suggests that as HIV becomes more of a chronic condition, the intensity and length of caregiving may shift (Theis et al. 1997), with family members assuming responsibility for long term care (Cates et al. 1990). Older parental surrogates are likely to be providing HIV-related care to infected adults and children over a prolonged and unpredictable period that includes acute infections, severe symptoms, and treatment side effects. Caregivers are called on to administer medications and treatments and to observe the infected person's response to treatment (Baker 1999; Baker, Sudit, and Litwak 1998; Freeman, Rodriguez, and French 1996).

Employed caregivers of infected family members worry about taking time off from work when a child is ill or for medical and other appointments. "My boss doesn't understand my responsibilities for these [seven] grandchildren. She thinks I am just the grandmother. I'm afraid I will lose my job." Caring for her daughter with AIDS meant that Mae Hawkins had to reduce her job to part time. Like Ella McIntyre, she lost medical benefits when she assumed dual roles of HIV care and surrogate parenting. With the loss of income, Ms. Hawkins worries about how she will pay for medical and dental care for her grandsons, who are ineligible for Medicaid because they are uninfected. Stress and shame are compounded for those seeking financial assistance for infected family members or their surviving uninfected children when they encounter a hostile and demeaning public assistance system (Cates et al. 1990).

Death and Dying

Historically, death has been the most common reason for grandparents assuming parental responsibility for children. Today, HIV/AIDS has "come to rival or surpass other important causes of death taking the lives of mothers of young children" (Michaels and Levine 1992). Older caregivers to HIV-affected and orphaned children often suffer the emotional trauma of an adult child's death, usually a daughter. Parental loss of a child of any age produces unparalleled and prolonged grief (Levine-Perkell 1996; de Vries and Lana 1994; Gorer 1965). As they assume parental responsibility for a grandchild or other young relative, these older adults confront the loss of the caregiver for their own later years.

Caregiver bereavement over the loss of a daughter or daughter-in-law may be suspended in order to focus on children's grief, fear or rage at death's intrusion into their lives. Moreover, as the opening vignette of Ella McIntyre describes, it is not uncommon for HIV-affected families, particularly those of infected women, to face the deaths of multiple family members within a short time (Honey 1988). Grieving for one family member is interrupted by another death. Where HIV has infected multiple members of young families, grandparents and other third- and fourth-generation caregivers face an endless shadow of death. Fearing personal rejection and ostracism, many AIDS caregivers and other affected family members hide the cause of death. "Disenfranchised" grief, spawned by the stigma of AIDS, disrupts the grieving process by isolating the bereaved from potential social supports (Doka 1989). When the tragic circumstances under which surrogate parenting was assumed cannot be shared, death's impact as a major cause of stress in one's life is amplified.

The Epidemic's Course:
New HIV Therapies and Demographic Trends

Treatment advances have transformed HIV disease from a fatal illness to a chronic illness that can be stabilized for many years. Highly active retroviral therapy (HAART) can reduce and maintain the HIV viral load, the amount of HIV virus in the blood, to undetectable levels. Infected persons gain extended symptom-free periods and overall improved quality of life. But HAART requires rigid adherence to complex combinations of antiviral agents and prophylactic medications to prevent further damage to the immune system, viral replication, and development of opportunistic infections. Complex therapies may fail, produce drug resistance, and have powerful side effects. Adherence is complicated because multiple drugs must be maintained at the proper temperature, taken at exactly the right time and in relationship to food consumption and digestion. Medication regimens may include as many as four different antiretroviral medications on a daily basis—as many as twenty to twenty-five pills a day—with conflicting dosage schedules (e.g., with or without food) and interrupted sleep. Infected persons must engage in active problem-solving in order to organize personal and family schedules around dosing and medical care, cope with severity and frequency of side effects (dizziness, nausea, vomiting, diarrhea, peripheral neuropathy, and disfigurement ["protease paunch"]), maintain medication refrigeration, get prescriptions refilled, and manage general stress (Erlen and Mellors 1999; Proctor, Tesfa, and Tompkins 1999). In order to minimize disabling side effects and reduce the risk of drug resistance, frequent medical visits are needed for viral-load monitoring and medication readjustment (Linsk and Keigher 1997). Medication regimens can disorder daily life, with a resulting adherence rate ranging from 20 percent to 80 percent (Holsemer et al. 1999).

Media images of the end of AIDS are appealing, particularly at a time of political belt-tightening for social programs that appear to cater to the morally weak and socially marginal, as the HIV-infected are often portrayed. The management of the epidemic appears reducible to the right combination of medications, vigorous medical management, and self-care. Yet as public health and HIV/AIDS communities know well, success stories associated with the new combination therapies do not tell the whole story (Altman 1997, 1998). Drug resistance and cross resistance to combination therapies result in failure rates as high as 30 percent to 50 percent. In a study of almost three thousand infected U.S. residents, nearly a third who were receiving antiretroviral therapy were noncompliant. Because the sample included only those receiving care over a two-year period, those less adherent to medical regimens and with greater limitations in accessing care may have even greater deficiencies in medical monitoring and antiretroviral therapy (Shapiro et al. 1999). By 1998, the 42 percent decline in AIDS mortality from 1996 to 1997 had dropped to 20 percent for 1997 to 1998. Although the smaller decrease still reflects successful early and aggressive combination therapies, viral drug resistance and adherence barriers are making a mortality rate plateau likely (Fleming et al. 2000).

Early testing, access to expensive therapies, and dedicated, single-minded attention to drug adherence is greatly limited by poverty and family responsibility. Once an epidemic primarily of white, gay men, infected individuals or those at risk are increasingly poor, female, and people of color. In the United States, the majority of new AIDS cases are African American or Latino/a, populations that tend to lack regular medical care and encounter multiple access barriers to testing and treatment (Levi and Kates 2000). Recent data show that infected African Americans and Latinos are tested at a later stage of disease (Fleming et al. 2000) and are less likely to receive HIV care (Shapiro et al. 1999). Between 800,000 and 900,000 individuals in the United States were living with HIV as the new century began (Centers for Disease Control and Prevention 2000), with nearly 300,000 of those women, men and children diagnosed with AIDS (Centers for Disease Control and Prevention 1999).

HIV Disease and Women

Female HIV infections represent 30 percent of approximately 40,000 new infections each year (CDC 2000). New infections among women occur at a more rapid rate than among males (Stein et al. 2000; Wortley and Fleming 1997), making women one of the fastest-growing infected groups in the United States. Twenty-three percent of new AIDS cases are female (Levi and Kates 2000), reflecting a steady increase. African Americans and Latinas show consistently higher AIDS rates than do white women (Wortley and Fleming 1997). AIDS continues to be a leading cause of death for women of reproductive age in the United States and elsewhere around the globe. Although female AIDS deaths have declined in recent years, the decline has been less pronounced than for men. Again, the burden of disparity is borne by African Americans and Latina/os.

The course of HIV disease among infected women cannot be separated from socioeconomic and familial circumstances, inasmuch as the majority of infected women are low-income mothers or women of child-bearing age (Sowell, Moneyham, and Aranda-Naranjo 1999). Compared with 18 percent of infected men in the United States, 60 percent of infected women have children, more than three-quarters of whom live with their children (Stein et al. 2000). Because others' needs take priority over theirs—caregiving responsibilities for children, and often for an infected male partner as well—infected women delay seeking medical care for themselves (Stein et al. 2000; Sowell, Moneyham, and Aranda-Naranjo 1999; Linsk and Keigher 1997). Infected women often neglect their own health because they focus attention on their children, fulfilling their own psychosocial needs in the face of their and their infected children's mortality. S. N. Broun (1999) describes psychotherapy clients who lacked the energy or strength to eat yet prepared dinner for their husbands. Women may refuse medications to avoid family questions and schedule medical appointments around family obligations and the need to maintain secrecy in the family (Hackl et al. 1997).

In families burdened by HIV and poverty, an older adult, usually the infected woman's mother or mother-in-law, is vital to sustaining familial and household organization and in providing social support to infected mothers. Among a national sample of infected adults, 30 percent of parents of minor children had AIDS and another 60 percent had symptomatic HIV disease. As further indicators of conditions that would interfere with parental capacity, 21 percent of these parents had been hospitalized during the prior six months, 18 percent had home health-care needs, 45 percent exhibited psychiatric symptoms, and 15 percent had drug or alcohol dependence (Stein et al. 2000). In a study of infected mothers of young children, more than 80 percent said their own mothers were aware of their HIV status, compared with only 20 percent of their fathers. More than two-thirds named their mothers as part of their support network, compared with only 17 percent of their fathers (Williams et al. 1997). Where children of infected females lived with another relative, grandmothers tend to be the predominant caregivers (Schuster et al. 2000). The grandmother or great-grandmother may be the only uninfected person capable of raising children and caring for infected adults.

Because the use of Zidovudine (AZT) has decreased perinatal transmission, there are fewer children infected with the virus. However, improved pediatric treatment means that prenatally and perinatally infected children are surviving into adolescence in families where parents may have died or are also living with HIV disease. In the latter case, mothers may also be substance abusers, living on the streets, or incarcerated—situations where grandmothers are likely to assume parental responsibility. Infected parents may be well enough to parent their children but with intermittent symptomatic periods of a life organized around treatment regimens and side effects. In families where the mother is living with HIV-infected, older adults may be co-parents, fulfilling permanent, temporary, or intermittent parental surrogacy. Practically, helping an infected mother means that the caregiver either shares a household with the younger generations or goes to their home almost on a daily basis. Mornings are especially difficult for someone living with HIV disease. Pain from peripheral neuropathy, chronic fatigue, interrupted sleep, wasting syndrome, strokelike symptoms, and chronic diarrhea make it difficult for a mother with young children to manage HIV symptoms, medication regimen, and side effects and also get children dressed, fed, and off to school. In addition to help with child care and housekeeping, the children's mother may need encouragement to eat, follow treatment regimens, and get to medical appointments. Loneliness, social isolation, and depression—common among infected women (Hackl et al. 1997; Kaplan, Marks, and Mertens 1997)—can further debilitate an infected mother, increasing her dependency upon an older relative for assistance and support.

Elder Caregivers to Affected and Orphaned Children:
A Persistent Need

In the early 1990s the AIDS epidemic was projected to orphan between 82,000 and 150,000 children in the United States by the year 2000 (Michaels and Levine 1992). New estimates that reflect the impact of new therapeutic strategies and continued increase in female infection have not been made, nor are there systematic data as to the number of older adults raising AIDS-orphaned children. However, using the estimated 150,000 orphaned minors, the number of older adults raising HIV orphaned children could reach more than 50,000 by 2010. Grandmothers are the surrogate parents in nearly two-thirds of documented custodial responsibility for HIV-affected children (Cohen and Nehring 1994; Draimin 1995; Schable et al. 1995) and are raising, on average, two children (Joslin, Mevi-Triano, and Berman 1997). Thousands of other grandparents will care for children whose parent is living with HIV disease yet disabled by the symptomatic periods, acute infections, and treatment side effects. The greatest share will be from poor, African American and Latino/a families, given the disproportionate female infection rate among from these populations. Not all caregivers will be elderly. Childbearing patterns in poor communities yield grandparents in their thirties. Yet where documented around the globe and in the United States, raising HIV-affected and infected children is a late-life generation task, primarily of grandmothers. In countries hardest hit by the pandemic, such as Zimbabwe, recent data show that 45 percent of caregivers of orphaned children were grandmothers, with one-third being sixty years or older (Foster et al. 1996). Data from two New Jersey projects documented caregiver ages from forty-seven to seventy-five and forty-six to seventy-nine, respectively, with mean ages of fifty-nine and fifty-seven (Joslin et al. 1997; Joslin and DeGraw 1998).

Invisible Caregivers

Paradoxically, rather than being *more* visible because their lives are so multiply burdened, older parental surrogates to HIV-affected and orphaned children and adolescents have been nearly invisible in research and program initiatives. Media vignettes are heart-wrenching and sentimental, but few identify caregiver needs and how community resources are responding to this group of older parental surrogates (Lee 1994). Most AIDS-care research has either focused on caregivers to gay men or has not identified the special issues related to older adults raising affected and infected children (LeBlanc, London, and Aneshensel 1997; Theis et al. 1997; LeBlanc, Aneshensel, and Wight 1995). Though valuable, the scant gerontological research on older adults as HIV caregivers (Poindexter and Linsk 1998, 1999; Hansell et al. 1998; Longman 1995; Brabant 1994; Dolan and Nokes 1992) has not focused on surrogate parents per se but rather on the strain associated with caring for a terminally ill adult child, AIDS stigma, and social isolation. One exception is a phenomenological study of grandmothers raising infected grandchildren (Caliandro and Hughes 1998) that identified common themes in caregivers' experiences, such as normalization of the infected child, spirituality as a coping mechanism, and diminishing resources. The consuming focus of HIV care, childrearing, social isolation, bereavement, reluctance to self-identify as a family affected by AIDS, and poverty's grip on family priorities may render older surrogate parents less accessible as a research population (Poindexter 1998; Joslin 1996).

The invisibility of HIV affected older parental surrogates in current gerontological and HIV/AIDS research is paralleled by benign neglect of community agencies, notably those serving HIV-infected persons and those serving older adults. Although nurses, social workers, case managers, and physicians in AIDS care may be aware of the stress experienced by caregivers, the catastrophic nature of HIV disease tends to focus professional time on medical management of infected persons and their psychosocial needs. Moreover, funding guidelines mandate professional attention to only the infected person. The caregiver is brought into focus only as she or he assists the infected person. The Ryan White Comprehensive Resources Emergency (CARE) Act, which is the basis of publicly funded HIV programs, restricts publicly funded services to infected persons or to family members in their caregiving capacity. Services must be terminated once the infected person dies. Comprehensive, family-centered systems of care established under CARE's Title IV include noninfected family members, but only from the vantage point of the infected person's needs. Access to case management, transportation, mental health, and psychosocial and family support services is determined by the care plan for the infected family member. Federal technical support documents from the Health Resources and Services Administration (HRSA) outline the Title IV goals as providing funds to "coordinate medical, psychological/social and social support services for women, children, youth and families' (Health Resources and Services Administration 1997). Yet the needs of caregivers are not specified, and publicly funded initiatives under CARE have not targeted the older caregivers in HIV-affected families.

Seeking to address the unmet needs of HIV-affected older surrogate parents, a countywide AIDS coalition in Passaic County, New Jersey, began its program initiative with a needs assessment conducted with staff of HIV/AIDS agencies. Case managers, social workers, nurses, and program administrators provided insight into the barriers older adults face in accessing supportive services. In particular, staff pointed to systemic issues that contribute to older caregivers' being overlooked, such as the lack of formal procedures for screening and assessing caregiver needs. As one social worker noted, "Because they aren't the focus of the agency, no one stops to assess what they need as they take on responsibility for the children." Another case manager observed, "We need an evaluation process that would identify at risk grandparents and let them know what services are available. Of course, that also means that we would have to have services in place to refer them to." The director of an adult HIV medical day program observed, "Most agencies can't help the grandparents because they don't have any place to send them for help. There is no central point of information or access for caregivers. Agency staff do not know what is available." Without programs designed to assist older surrogate parents and accessible to HIV-affected caregivers, staff are not able to offer referrals for supportive services and information. Ironically, as an illustration of these barriers, during one interview a social worker received a telephone call from a grandmother in her mid-fifties who was raising three uninfected grandchildren, ages two, six, and eight. Their mother, an agency client, had died earlier in the year. After reducing her employment to part-time in order to care for the children, the grandmother could not pay a $2,000 utility bill. Because no one in the household was infected, the family was ineligible for both emergency financial assistance and case management under Ryan White funding. HIV diagnosis of a household member confers service benefits that are terminated when the infected person dies. Not only are financial and housing benefits lost, but caregivers and uninfected children are also cast into a "no service zone" where they disappear from the HIV service delivery system, no longer eligible for case management assistance.

Benign ageism and lack of gerontological education also contribute to caregivers' programmatic neglect. Several staff noted that knowledge of community resources and public benefits for older adults were beyond the training and experience of many professionals in HIV/AIDS care. Even outside the HIV service system, when seeking services from age-integrated programs, older adults are often ignored, losing out in competition with younger age groups for professional attention and assistance (Monk 1990).

Although eligibility for supportive services funded under the Older Americans Act is not dependent on disease diagnosis, chronological age restricts in-home and community services to those sixty and older. Yet, even where older surrogates would qualify for age-restricted in-home and community supportive services, such as case management, housekeeping, respite, and transportation, the AIDS stigma and ignorance prevents many aging network programs from conducting outreach or program development to assist such caregivers. Although collaboration between HIV/AIDS and aging programs has occurred in New York City, San Francisco, northern New Jersey, and southern Florida (Joslin and Nazon 1996), AIDS-phobia in the larger society infects the aging network as well (Lloyd 1989). Implementing a case-management program for older surrogate parents, a local AIDS coalition's outreach efforts to a county office on aging were met with, "There's no AIDS here" or "It doesn't affect seniors' (Joslin and DeGraw 1997).

Vision and Purpose

We live in a time of intense concentration on the part of the media on the bizarre and the tragic. Daytime talk shows glitter with refugees from family turmoil. Ironically, as public and political support for social programs for the economically disadvantaged has diminished, public appetite for stories of personal tragedy has seemingly become insatiable. To focus on older surrogates to HIV-affected and orphaned children runs the risk of sensationalizing yet another group of individuals cast adrift in hopeless circumstances. However, without informed and systematic attention by community programs, practitioners, and policy makers, older HIV-affected parental surrogates will continue to absorb the burden of care with tremendous costs to themselves and their families. The professional practice, political advocacy, and academic research that inform this book express the hope that this written forum will stimulate public advocacy, program development, staff training, and service coordination. Through its relevance to those who work with older surrogate parents, or on behalf of HIV-affected and orphaned children and their families, this book seeks to support those individuals in health and human services, education, public policy, and academia whose commitment is to serve those on the margins of society, living in the shadows without a voice. Produced in a climate of "welfare reform" and in the absence of political debate about national health insurance, the book's authors affirm collaboration across professional disciplines and service systems. The isolation that compromises caregivers' well-being is paralleled by our professional isolation within and across disciplines and programs, an isolation that weakens our capacity to be truly effective advocates and innovators.

Notes

1. The names of caregivers have been changed to protect their privacy.

2. The cases described here are drawn from an exploratory study conducted in 1996 in northern New Jersey whose purpose was to gather descriptive information about older surrogate parents of HIV-affected and orphaned children. Study objectives, methodology, and findings will be reported in greater detail in chapter 5, "Physical Health and Emotional Well-Being."

3. Not all older surrogate parents to HIV-affected and orphaned children are grandparents. Great-grandmothers and great-aunts also assume this role. Yet because case records from HIV service programs indicate that most older parental surrogates are grandmothers, the relevant literature on these "parents of last resort" provides a framework for understanding the issues faced by third- and fourth-generation family members raising children.

References

Altman, L. K. 1997. With AIDS advance, more disappointment. *New York Times,* January 19, 1997: A3, A14.

——. 1998. Troubling side effects are linked to effective AIDS drug therapy. *New York Times,* July 7, 1998, F7.

Baker, S. 1999. Home care: Addressing the needs of people living with AIDS and their caregivers. *Nursing Clinics of North America* 1:201–212.

Baker, S., M. Sudit, and E. Litwak. 1998. Caregiver burden and coping strategies used by informal caregivers of minority women living with HIV/AIDS. *Journal of Cultural Diversity* 5:11–16.

Brabant, S. 1994. An overlooked AIDS affected population: The elderly parent as caregiver. *Journal of Gerontological Social Work* 22:131–145.

Broun, S. N. 1991. Psychosocial issues of women with HIV/AIDS. *AIDS Patient Care and STDs* 13:119–126.

Burnette, D. 1997. Grandmother caregivers in inner-city Latino families: A descriptive profile and informal supports. *Journal of Multi Cultural Social Work* 5:121–138.

Burton, L. M. 1992. Black grandparents rearing grandchildren of drug-addicted parents: Stressors, outcomes and social service needs. *The Gerontologist* 32:744–751.

Calindro, G., and C. Hughes. 1998. The experience of being a grandmother who is the primary caregiver for her HIV-positive child. *Nursing Research* 47:107–113.

Cates, J. A., L. L. Graham, D. Boeglin, and S. Tiekler. 1990. The effect of AIDS on the family system. *Families in Society: The Journal of Contemporary Human Services* 71:195–201.

Centers for Disease Control and Prevention. 1997. *HIV/AIDS Surveillance Report* 9 (2).

——. 1999. *HIV/AIDS Surveillance Report* 11.

——. 2000. *CDC Update: A Glance at the Epidemic.* Atlanta: Centers for Disease Control and Prevention.

Chalfie, D. 1994. *Going It Alone: A Closer Look at Grandparents Parenting Grandchildren.* Washington, D.C.: American Association of Retired Persons.

Christ, G. H., and L. S. Wiener. 1994. Psychosocial issues in AIDS. In V. T. Devita, ed., *AIDS: Etiology Diagnosis and Treatment and Prevention,* pp. 275–297. Philadelphia: Lippincott.

Cohen, F. L., and W. L. Nehring. 1994. Foster care of HIV positive children in the United States. *Public Health Reports* 109:60–67.

Connor, E., R. Sperling, P. Kiselev, G. Scott, M. O'Sullivan, R. Van Dyke, et al. 1994. Reduction of maternal-infant transmission of human immunodeficiency virus type 1 with zidovudine treatment. *New England Journal of Medicine* 331:1173–1180.

Crawford, A. M. 1996. Stigma associated with AIDS: A meta-analysis. *Journal of Applied Social Psychology* 26:398–416.

de Vries, B., and R. D. Lana. 1994. Parental bereavement over the life course: A theoretical intersection and empirical review. *Omega* 29:47–69.

Doka, J. D. 1989. *Disenfranchised Grief: Recognizing Hidden Sorrow.* New York: Lexington Press.

Dolan, M., and K. Nokes. 1992. Experiences of New York Puerto Rican family members living with AIDS. *The Journal of the Association of Nurses in AIDS Care* 3:23–28.

Dowdell, E. B. 1995. Caregiver burden: Grandmothers raising their high risk grandchildren. *Journal of Psychosocial Nursing* 33 (3): 27–30.

Draimin, B. 1995. A second family? Placement and custody decisions. In S. Geballe, J. Gruendel, and W. Andiman, eds., *Forgotten Children of the AIDS Epidemic,* pp. 125–139. New Haven: Yale University Press.

Erlen, J. A., and M. P. Mellors. 1999. Adherence to combination therapy in persons living with HIV: Balancing the hardships and the blessings. *Journal of the Association of Nurses in AIDS Care* 10:75–84.

Fair, C. D., E. D. Spence, and L. Wiener. 1995. Healthy children in families affected by AIDS: Epidemiological and psychosocial considerations. *Child and Adolescent Social Work Journal* 12:165–181.

Fleming, P. L., P. M. Wortley, J. M. Karon, K. M. DeCock, and R. S. Janssen. 2000. Tracking the HIV epidemic: Current issues, future challenges. *American Journal of Public Health* 90 (7): 1037–1041.

Foster, G., C. Makufa, R. Drew, S. Kambeu, and K. Saurombe. 1996. Supporting children in need through a community-based orphan visiting program. *AIDS Care* 8: 389–403.

Freeman, R., G. Rodriguez, and J. French. 1996. Compliance with AZT treatment regimen of HIV seropositive injection drug users: a neglected issue. *AIDS Education and Prevention* 8:58–63.

Fuller Thomson, E., M. Minkler, and D. Driver. 1997. A profile of grandparents raising grandchildren in the United States. *The Gerontologist* 37:406–411.

Geballe, S., J. Gruendel, and W. Andiman, eds. 1995. *Forgotten Children of the AIDS Epidemic.* New Haven: Yale University Press.

Goicoechea-Balbona, A. 1998. Children with HIV/AIDS and the families: A successful social work intervention based on the culturally specific health care model. *Health and Social Work* 23 (1): 61–69.

Gorer, G. 1965. *Death, Grief and Mourning.* London: Cresset Press.

Grant, R. 1997. The health status of grandparent caregivers. Paper presented at the Annual Scientific Meeting of the Gerontological Society of America, Cincinnati, Ohio.

Hackl, K. L., A. M. Somlai, J. A. Kelly, and S. C. Kalichman. 1997. Women living with

HIV/AIDS: The dual challenge of being a patient and caregiver. *Health and Social Work* 22:53–62.

Hansell, P. S., C. B. Huges, G. Caliandro, P. Russo, W. C. Budin, B. Hartman, and O. Hernandez. 1998. The effect of a social support boosting intervention on stress, coping and social support in caregivers of children with HIV/AIDS. *Nursing Research* 47: 79–86.

Health Resources and Services Administration. 1997. CARE Act Overview: The Title IV Program. *CARE Notes,* special issue.

Herek, G. M., and J. P. Capitanio. 1993. Public reactions to AIDS in the United States: A second decade of stigma. *American Journal of Public Health* 83:574–577.

Holsemer, W. L., I. B. Corless, K. M. Nokes, J. G. Turner, M. Brown, G. Powell-Cope, J. Inouye, S. B. Henry, P. K. Nicholas, and C. J. Portillo. 1999. Predictors of self-reported adherence in persons living with HIV disease. *AIDS Patient Care and STDs* 13:185–197.

Honey, E. 1988. AIDS and the inner city: Critical issues. *Social Casework: The Journal of Contemporary Social Work* 69 (6): 365–370.

Jendrek, M. P. 1996. Grandparents who parent their grandchildren: Effects on lifestyle. In J. Quadagno and D. Street, eds., *Aging for the Twenty-First Century: Readings in Social Gerontology,* pp. 286–305. New York: St. Martin's.

Joslin, D. 1995. Older adults as caregivers in the HIV/AIDS epidemic. *CAPCO Capsules* 2 (4): 3–7.

——. Needs assessment of Passaic County AIDS service providers. Unpublished report. Wayne, N.J.: William Paterson University.

Joslin, D., and A. Brouard. 1995. The prevalence of grandmothers as primary caregivers in a poor pediatric population. *Journal of Community Health* 20:383–402.

Joslin, D., and C. DeGraw. 1997. *OASIS Project Final Report.* Paterson, N.J.: Coalition on AIDS in Passaic County.

Joslin, D., and R. Harrison. 1998. "The hidden patient": Older relatives raising children orphaned by HIV disease. *Journal of the American Women's Medical Association* 53 (2): 65–71, 76.

Joslin, D., C. Mevi-Triano, and J. Berman. 1997. Grandparents raising children orphaned by HIV/AIDS: Health risks and service needs. Paper presented at the 50th Annual Scientific Meeting of the Gerontological Society of America, Cincinnati, Ohio.

Joslin, D., and M. Nazon. 1996. HIV/AIDS and aging networks. In K. Nokes, ed., *HIV/AIDS and the Older Adult,* pp. 129–140. Washington, D.C.: Taylor and Francis.

Kaplan, M. S., G. Marks, and S. Mertens. 1997. Distress and coping among women with HIV infection. *American Journal of Orthopsychiatry* 67:80–91.

Kelley, S. J. 1993. Care giver stress in grandparents raising grandchildren. *IMAGE: Journal of Nursing Scholarship* 25 (4):331–337.

Kelley, S. J., and E. G. Damato. 1995. Grandparents as primary caregivers. *Maternal Child Nursing* 20:326–332.

Kennedy, J. F., and V. T. Keeney. 1988. The extended family re-visited: Grandparents raising grandchildren. *Child Psychiatry & Human Development* 19:26–35.

Klevens, R. M., T. Diaz, P. L. Fleming, M. A. Mays, and R. Frey. 1999. Trends in AIDS among Hispanics in the United States, 1991–1996. *American Journal of Public Health* 89 (7): 1104–1106.

Knodel, J. E., M. Van Landingham, C. Saengtienchai, and W. Im-em. 2000. Older people and AIDS: Quantitative evidence of the impact in Thailand. PSC Research Report 00-448. Population Studies Center, University of Michigan.

LeBlanc, A. J., C. Aneshensel, and R. G. Wight. (1995) Psychotherapy use and depression among AIDS caregivers. *Journal of Community Psychology* 23:127–142.

LeBlanc, A. J., A. S. London, and C. S. Aneshensel. 1997. The physical costs of AIDS care giving. *Social Science and Medicine* 45:915–923.

Lee, F. R. 1994. AIDS toll on the elderly: Dying grandchildren. *New York Times,* November 21, 1994, A1, B6.

Lesar, S., M. M. Gerber, and M. I. Semmel. 1995–1996. HIV infection in children: Family stress, social support and adaptation. *Exceptional Children* 62 (3): 224–236.

Levi, J., and J. Kates. 2000. HIV: Challenging the health care delivery system. *American Journal of Public Health* 90:1033–1036.

Levine-Perkell, J. 1996. Caregiving issues. In K. Nokes, ed., *HIV/AIDS and the Older Adult,* pp. 115–128. Washington, D.C.: Taylor & Francis.

Linsk, N. L., and S. M. Keigher. 1997. Of magic bullets and social justice: Emerging challenges of recent advances in AIDS treatment. *Health and Social Work* 22 (1): 71–74.

Lloyd, G. 1989. AIDS and elders: Advocacy, activism and coalitions. *Generations* 13 (4): 32–35.

Longman, A. J. 1995. Connecting and disconnecting: Bereavement experiences of six mothers whose sons died of AIDS. *International Health Care for Women* 16 (1): 85–95.

Lugalia, T. *Marital Status and Living Arrangements: March 1997.* Current Population Reports, Series P-29, No. 560. Washington, D.C.: U.S. Bureau of the Census, 1998.

Marder, R., and N. Linsk. 1995. Addressing AIDS long-term care issues through education and advocacy. *Health and Social Work* 20:75–80.

Marx, J., and J. C. Solomon. 2000. Physical health of custodial grandparents. In C. Cox, ed., *To Grandmother's House We Go and Stay: Perspectives on Custodial Grandparents,* pp. 37–55. New York: Springer.

McGinn, F. 1996. The plight of rural parents caring for adult children with HIV. *Families in Society* 77:269–278.

Michaels, D., and C. Levine. 1992. Estimates of the number of motherless youth orphaned by AIDS in the United States. *Journal of the American Medical Association* 268:3456–3461.

Miller, D. 1991. The "Grandparents Who Care" support project of San Francisco. Paper presented at the Annual Scientific Meeting of the Gerontological Society of America, San Francisco.

Minkler, M., and E. Fuller-Thomson. 1999. The health of grandparents raising grandchildren: Results of a national study. *American Journal of Public Health* 89:1384–1389.

Minkler, M., and K. Roe. 1993. *Grandmothers as Caregivers: Raising Children of the Crack Cocaine Epidemic.* Thousand Oaks, Calif.: Sage.

Minkler, M., K. Roe, and M. Price. 1992. The physical and emotional health of grandmothers raising children in the crack cocaine epidemic. *The Gerontologist* 32:752–761.

Monk, A. 1990. *Handbook of Gerontological Social Services.* 2d ed. New York: Columbia University Press.

Mullen, F. 2000. Grandparents and welfare reform. In C. Cox, ed., *To Grandmother's House We Go and Stay: Perspectives on Custodial Grandparents,* pp. 113–131. New York: Springer.

Musil, C. M., S. Schrader, and J. Mutikani. 2000. Social support, stress and special coping tasks of grandmother caregivers. In C. Cox, ed., *To Grandmother's House We Go and Stay: Perspectives on Custodial Grandparents,* pp. 56–70. New York: Springer.

Odulana, J. A., L. D. Camblin, and P. White. 1996. Cultural roles and health status of contemporary African American young grandmothers. *The Journal of Multicultural Nursing and Holistic Health* 2:28–35.

O'Hara, M. J. 1995. Care of children with HIV infection. In P. Kelly, S. Holman, R. Rothenberg, and S. P. Holzemer, eds., *Primary Care of Women and Children with HIV Infection,* pp. 103–131. Boston: Jones and Bartlett.

Pearlin, L. I., C. S. Aneshensel, and A. J. LeBlanc. 1997. The forms and mechanisms of stress proliferation: The case of AIDS care givers. *Journal of Health and Social Behavior* 38 (3): 223–236.

Pearlin, L. I., I. Semple, and H. Turner. 1988. Stress of AIDS care giving: A preliminary review of the issues. *Death Studies* 12:501–517.

Poindexter, C. C., and N. Linsk. 1998. The sources of social support in a sample of HIV-affected older minority caregivers. *Families in Society* (Sept.–Oct.): 491–503.

———. 1999. HIV-related stigma in the lives of a sample of HIV-affected older minority caregivers. *Social Work* 4:46–61.

Powell-Cope, G. M., and M. A. Brown. 1992. Going public as an AIDS family care giver. *Social Science and Medicine* 34 (5): 571–580.

Proctor, V. E., A. Tesfa, and D. C. Tompkins. 1999. Barriers to adherence to highly active antiretroviral therapy as expressed by people living with HIV/AIDS. *AIDS Patient Care and STDS* 13 (9): 535–544.

Roe, K., M. Minkler, and R. Barnwell. 1994. The assumption of caregiving: Grandmothers raising the children of the crack cocaine epidemic. *Qualitative Health Research* 4 (3): 281–303.

Roth, J., R. Siegal, and S. Black. 1994. Identifying the mental health needs of children living in families with AIDS or HIV infection. *Community Mental Health Journal* 30 (6): 581–592.

Saluter, A. F. 1992. *Marital Status and Living Arrangements: March 1991.* Current Population Reports, Series P-20, No. 461. Washington, D.C.: U.S. Bureau of the Census.

Sanders, C. M. 1989. Comparison of adult bereavement in the death of a spouse, child and parent. *Omega* 10:303–322.

Schable, B., T. Diaz, S. Chu, M. B. Caldwell, L. Conti, et al. 1995. Who are the primary caregivers of children born to HIV infected mothers? Results from a multi-state surveillance project. *Pediatrics* 95:511–515.

Schiller, N. G. 1993. The invisible women: Caregiving and the construction of AIDS health services. *Culture, Medicine and Psychiatry* 17:487–512.

Schultz, R., and G. M. Williamson. 1991. A 2-year longitudinal study of depression among Alzheimer's caregivers. *Psychology and Aging* 6:569–578.

Schultz, R, P. Visintainer, and G. M. Williamson. 1990. Psychiatric and physical morbidity effects of caregivers. *Journal of Gerontology* 45:181–191.

Schuster, M. A., D. E. Kanouse, S. C. Morton, S. A. Bozzette, A. Miu, G. B. Scott, and M. F. Shapiro. 2000. HIV-infected parents and their children in the United States. *American Journal of Public Health* 90:1074–1081.

Shapiro, M. F., S. C. Morton, D. F. McCaffrey, J. W. Senterfit, J. A. Fleishman, J. F. Perlman, L. A. Athey, J. W. Keesey, D. P. Goldman, S. H. Berry, and S. A. Bozzette. 1999. Variations in the care of HIV-infected adults in the United States: Results from the HIV cost and service utilization study. *Journal of the American Medical Association* 281 (24): 2305–2315.

Siminoff, L. A., J. A. Erlen, and C. W. Lidz. 1991. Stigma, AIDS and quality of nursing care: State of the science. *Journal of Advanced Nursing* 16:262–269.

Simon-Rusinowitz, L., C. A. Krach, L. N. Marks, D. Piktalis, and L. B. Wilson. 1996. Grandparents in the workplace: The effects of economic and labor trends. *Generations* 20:41–43.

Sowell, R. L., L. Moneyham, and B. Aranda-Naranjo. 1999. The care of women with AIDS. *Nursing Clinics of North America* 34 (1): 179–199.

Stein, M. D., S. Crystal, W. E. Cunningham, A. Ananthanarayanan, R. Andersen, B. J. Turner, S. Zierler, S. Morton, M. H. Katz, S. A. Bozzette, M. F. Shapiro, and M. A. Schuster. 2000. Delays in seeking HIV care due to competing caregiving responsibilities. *American Journal of Public Health* 90:1138–1140.

Strawbridge, W. J., M. I. Wallhagen, S. J. Shema, and G. A. Kaplan. 1997. New burdens or more of the same? Comparing grandparent, spouse and adult-child caregivers. *The Gerontologist* 37 (4): 505–510.

Szinovacz, M., S. DeViney, and M. Atkinson. 1997. Effects of surrogate parenting on grandparents' depression and self-esteem: A panel analysis. Paper presented at the 50th Annual Scientific Meeting of the Gerontological Society of America, Cincinnati.

Tasker, M. 1992. *How Can I Tell You? Secrecy and Disclosure with Children when a Family Member Has AIDS*. Bethesda, Md.: Association for the Care of Children's Health.

Theis, S. L., F. L. Cohen, J. Forrest, and M. Zelewsky. 1997. Needs assessment of caregivers of people with HIV/AIDS. *Journal of the Association of Nurses in AIDS Care* 8:76–84.

Trice, A. D. 1988. Post-traumatic stress syndrome-like symptoms among AIDS caregivers. *Psychological Review* 63:656–658.

Turner, H. A., and L. I. Pearlin. 1989. Issues of age, stress and caregiving. *Generations* 13:56–59.

Turner, H. A., J. A. Catania, and J. Gagnon. 1994. The prevalence of informal caregiving to persons with AIDS in the United States: Caregiver characteristics and their implications. *Social Science and Medicine* 38:1543–1552.

U. S. Bureau of the Census. 1991. *Marital Status and Living Arrangements: March 1990*. Current Population Reports, Series P-20, No. 450. Washington, D.C. U.S. Bureau of the Census.

———. 1994. *Marital Status and Living Arrangements: March 1993*.

Walker, R. J., E. C. Pomeroy, J. S. McNeil, and C. Franklin. 1996. Anticipatory grief and AIDS: Strategies for intervening with care giver. *Health and Social Work* 21 (1): 49–58.

Wardlaw, L. A. 1994. Sustaining informal care givers for persons with AIDS. *Families in Society* June, 373–384.

Weiler, Jane. 1995. Respite care for HIV-affected families. *Social Work in Health Care* 21 (1): 55–67.

Williams, A. B., A. Shahryarinejad, S. Andrews, and P. Alcabes. 1997. Social support of HIV infected mothers: Relationship to HIV care seeking. *Journal of the Association of Nurses in AIDS Care* 8 (1): 91–98.

Worden, W. J. 1991. Grieving a loss from AIDS. In *AIDS and the Hospice Community,* pp. 143–150. New York: Hawthorne Press.

Wortley, P. M., and P. L. Fleming. 1997. AIDS in women in the United States. *Journal of the American Medical Association* 278:911–916.

Wright, L. K., E. S. Clipp, and L. K. George. 1993. Health consequences of caregiver stress. *Medicine, Exercise, Nutrition and Health* 2:181–195.

2

Caregiving Profiles

CAROL MEVI-TRIANO AND ELIZABETH C. PASKAS

Caregivers' own voices seldom are heard except insofar as they call attention to the needs of their families. This chapter, comprising three narratives that have been constructed from interviews with three grandmothers who are raising infected and affected grandchildren, offers the voices of caregivers themselves. The grandchildren or adult children of the grandmothers have been clients of a regional HIV treatment center in the northeastern United States. Two of the grandmothers are African American and one is Puerto Rican. They are all urban caregivers whose narratives reflect not only the impact of HIV disease but also the assaults of substance abuse, violence, incarceration, and poverty on family life. Despite overwhelming circumstances, the grandmothers have maintained stable homes for their grandchildren while coping with the unpredictability of HIV disease, the loss of their children, and the stigma of AIDS.

Four broad questions guided these interviews:

1. Under what circumstances did they come to raise their grandchildren?
2. What it is like to be raising a grandchild because of HIV disease?
3. How has their caregiving role affected their own lives?
4. What enables them to cope?

Mrs. B.

Betty, as "Mrs. B."[1] likes to be called, is a grandmother raising her ten-year-old grandson, Mitchell. They live in a two-family house that they share with

Betty's cousin, a woman in her late fifties, a few years older than Betty. They also share in the care of Mitchell, a child who was infected through the perinatal transmission of HIV. These two African American women have been Mitchell's "parents" while he has grown up in an urban northern New Jersey community.

When we began, Betty described how she came to be raising Mitchell and reminisced about her daughter whose birthday was the next day. "Well, they had always been living with me. She wasn't married, and when the baby [Mitchell] was born they were always there. . . . Ever since she was fourteen every two years she was leaving, getting her own place. When she turned sixteen, she was leaving, getting her own place. . . . Every two years she would leave and get her own place." In fact, Betty's daughter never left, and there was a closeness between the three of them until her daughter's death eight years earlier, when Mitchell was two.

In a straightforward manner, Betty said, "When she passed, I just kept him. . . . It had to be done, I mean he had to be cared for." She believed that her daughter's death was the result of kidney failure and internal bleeding. Betty experienced the death as a great shock. "The doctors weren't able to ever tell me what was wrong with her. . . . They never knew what caused it or anything." There had been no mention of HIV/AIDS at all. The daughter's death occurred in the early 1990s, and it was not unusual then for someone to die from HIV/AIDS without receiving an accurate diagnosis.

"Two months after she passed, I had been taking Mitchell to the doctor because of sores in his mouth. . . . Everything we tried, he wouldn't clear up. He had ulcers and everything. . . . They started doing tests and everything and one of the doctors asked me would I sign for an HIV test, and I told him yes, go ahead, because she had been tested in the hospital twice for HIV, so I'm told. I had asked for the test and they said she came back negative. And so I told him, yes, go ahead and test him. Every time a test would come back it would come back negative. When they called for the last test they told me to come into the office—I knew then, you know, when he told me to come into the office, I knew that was what they would tell me." Betty was told that Mitchell was HIV-infected just two months after her daughter had died of essentially unknown causes. At the time, she felt "scared, angry, lost—lost as to what to do" for Mitchell and for herself.

She described the process of raising and coping with a grandchild who was HIV-infected, including the gradual process of disclosure as she told family members and friends of Mitchell's illness. "I think I only told my younger son [she has two sons] and he just told me to have hope, you know, as long as he lives there's hope, and for a year I didn't tell anyone else and it was, oh God, what a year, but Mitchell got very sick one time. . . . And then I said, I have to tell the rest of the family because if something happens, they're going to want to know. And when I did tell them, it was like a burden was lifted, like I lost a whole lot of weight. . . . They took it, you know, they started helping me care for him and everything. They were wondering why I had never told them before but there had been so many things said about this disease and everything and I didn't want—I thought maybe they would turn against him and he was so close to the family and they had taken him places and everything, I didn't want that to change." Initially family members felt "disbelief . . . and were scared he wouldn't live."

Betty poignantly described how she began to come to terms with Mitchell's diagnosis and accept help both from family members and from God. She already had experienced the death of her daughter and had taken on herself the care of her grandson, who at times was very ill. His father had not been "seen since my daughter passed. He was at the wake. . . . When something is going on at school and the kids' fathers come, he wants to know where his father is, how come he doesn't have a father, but we has cousins that take up time with him if he needs a male."

Both Betty and Mitchell have strong family support. Her youngest son lives in Washington, D.C., and in the beginning "he would come home on the weekends and help me out, take him places. . . . He usually takes him for a week every summer . . . and we visit, we go there. . . . The [son] in New York has two children of his own. . . . My granddaughter is eight and my granddaughter just turned six." Betty's cousin "lives downstairs, she takes care of him while I'm working. . . And then after we found about his diagnosis and everything, she makes, I mean, I make his appointments and she takes him to the appointments because she does housework and she doesn't work every day. . . . She takes him to school, picks him up from school, cares for him while I'm working."

Her cousin came to know of Mitchell's diagnosis through a situation that also expressed Betty's fear that her grandson might not live very long. "When I first found about his diagnosis I was working second shift and coming home around twelve or one o'clock. I used to come in the room and this is all I thought about while I was working, about him, was he all right. . . . My cousin at the time didn't know because I didn't want her calling home all the time, checking up on him or anything like that, worrying or so—and she make a remark one night and she said, you know Betty, you come home and stand over him and he's sleeping and you're looking at him like you could eat him up, and I'm saying to myself, I'm just so glad that he's alive when I walk in the door, but then after I told her she realized why I was doing this."

Fearing that Mitchell might not live very long, Betty constantly thinks about his health and well-being whether he is at school, at camp, or with relatives. When we discussed his first experience at a sleep-away camp for children who are HIV-infected, she acknowledged that she felt "a little anxious about it. I'm worried about his medications being given, but he loves being around kids—so—he's shy for about ten or fifteen minutes and then you want to send him home, but this is my only concern, about him being a little homesick. . . . I'm sure he will be well taken care of . . . but, you know, this is his first time being away from me and his medications being given by somebody other than myself and my babysitters."

Betty wants to keep Mitchell safe and unaware of his diagnosis, but Mitchell's time in school complicates her desire to protect him: "I don't think he is mature enough to know. And I had thought about—my son in Washington wants me to tell him. . . . He might be old enough in age but I don't think he's mature enough. So I said that I was going to tell him before he went to camp, then I said no, I better not, because he was having such a hard time in school this year. . . . He didn't pass, you know. The teacher said that there were four of them that picked on him because he was smaller than the other kids. . . . He had a rough year."

Betty acknowledged that it had been a rough year for herself as well. "The rough spots are when he's not feeling good, then it makes me feel not so good, and worrying about whether this is it, what do I do now. . . ." Her worry about Mitchell's health at times exacerbates her own health problems, which include diabetes and hypertension. "I manage until I think something is bothering me and then I just eat like I'm going crazy." When she starts to feel this way, she does not confide in those close to her, those who usually help with Mitchell such as her cousin. "Oh, they don't know. I don't show them because my cousin is very, I think she worries about him more than I do, if that's possible, but she shows it more, you know, if he gets hurt, then she's right there."

Her fear that Mitchell will die has changed over time, and now she experiences relief in the knowledge that God will take care of everything. "I don't know what made it change. I was sitting at my job one day and I went to the bathroom and I came out of the bathroom and my girlfriend that knows told me, you know, I don't know whether I had a talk with God or whether God talked to me, but I'm not worried any more because I realize now that it's not in my hands, it's up to God what's going to happen to him. All I can do is what the doctors tell me to do and give him my love and care, that's all I can do." Her need to protect Mitchell is very strong and although others are there to help her and she feels supported by God, the rough spots still come along. "I think it all goes down to having people around you, your support system. I think it is very important. I am not a devout Christian but I do believe in God. And I believe that he answers prayers, I know he works miracles, because my second child was a miracle because when he was nine years old he had Rocky Mountain spotted fever and when the doctors took him to Newark, they said he wouldn't make it through the night, but he did."

Given her life circumstances, Betty says, she has "everything I need. I don't have everything I want, but who does? But I'm comfortable." She agreed that she and Mitchell have a rhythm in their lives and that her sons and her cousin are always there to support them. The loss of her daughter is still with her, and the death continues to remain a mystery. My conversation with Betty reveals a sense of a deep devotion, love, and affection toward Mitchell. The necessity of her presence in his life clearly is articulated when she states, "What else would I do with my life now?"

Mrs. N.

Mrs. N is a sixty-four-year-old grandmother living in Paterson, New Jersey. She grew up in Puerto Rico with her grandmother, who raised her after her mother died. She never had the privilege of going to school because she had to help her grandmother with homemaking; therefore, she does not know how to read and write. The interview was conducted in Spanish.

Mrs. N. is married and is raising nine grandchildren who range in age from three to eighteen years. It had been very difficult to arrange for the interview. For the first interview appointment, Mrs. N. was not at home when I arrived. Her eighteen-year-old granddaughter Sandra explained, "She had to meet with someone regarding housing. She apologizes and will call to reschedule." Mrs. N. was in the process of looking for adequate housing that would accommodate the growing family. Other appointments were arranged but were interrupted either by unexpected visits or by her husband's unexpected presence in the home. Mrs. N. did not want her husband to be around when she discussed her personal situation because "he does not approve of strangers knowing their business."

After several attempts, we finally met one midmorning. Mrs. N and the children were in the living room watching cartoons when I arrived. Immediately she asked her granddaughter Silvia to entertain the children in the kitchen so she could sit and talk with me in the main bedroom. The small bedroom had one full-size bed, one twin-size bed, and a cot folded in the corner. Additionally, it was crowded with furniture, did not have a door, and opened into the living room, thereby providing no privacy. Mrs. N. apologized for the meeting conditions and explained that the bedroom was supposed to be a dining room but was used as a bedroom because of the large family. The bedroom overlooks the neighborhood street. The area is poverty-ridden and overcrowded, with many different people just "hanging out" in front of dilapidated houses.

Mrs. N. sat on the full-size bed in the main bedroom as she began to tell her story. "There are twelve people living in this apartment. My daughter, Nancy, and my nine grandchildren live with my husband and me. I am raising five granddaughters and four grandsons." She said that although her husband works he cannot help her much with money. However, he does help watch the children every now and then.

Mrs. N. tells how she assumed responsibility of her grandchildren. "My daughter, Nancy, who lives with me, is in and out a lot using drugs. She is always in and out of jail. Right now she is in jail. She is trying to get into a drug rehab program. . . . Nancy has two sons, Chris, eleven years old, and Javier, three years old. Mrs. N. points to Javier: "I have always been taking care of him but it has only been months since his mother gave custody of him to me. Chris was born premature. He was born slightly retarded with problems because of his mother's abuse with drugs.

"Several years ago, my daughter Lourdes died of AIDS. She has four children that I am raising. Her kids are Sandra, eighteen years old; John, seventeen years old; Silvia, sixteen years old; and Fred, ten years old and HIV-positive. While Lourdes was sick and abusing drugs, Sandra, John, and Silvia were living with their father. Their stepmother used to abuse them so DYFS [Division for Youth and Family Services] took them away from their father. Fred, who has a different father, was living with his mother in the streets. When Lourdes died, there was no one else to watch her children, so they [DYFS] handed them over to me. Currently, John is not living with me. He is an in-patient at a drug rehab program. Sometimes he comes over on the weekends to visit.

"I have another son who died, my son José. He killed himself with a double dose of a poisoned drug. But, one day I was looking through his papers and my daughter Nancy found a paper which said he was infected with AIDS. He died of AIDS! Jose and his girlfriend, who also has AIDS, have a fourteen-year-old daughter, Rose. Rose's mother is on drugs and very sick, that is why I also have Rose to care for." Mrs. N. lowered her head and said sadly, "This affects me a lot because my son and daughter did not listen to my advice that they were going to die, and they left me all alone.

"I am also caring for Ralph, thirteen years old; Jackie, twelve years old; and Marilyn, nine years old. My daughter Clara abandoned them a few years ago because her husband used to beat her. She could not take it anymore and feared for her life. One day she just picked up and left! But at least I know the kids are safe because they are with me."

Mrs. N relates how it is to care for a child living with HIV: "I have to have more care for him, give him his medicine, be more attentive. They are giving him [Fred] those pills over there." She points to corner where there is a tall dresser with several pill bottles. "I can't understand what the directions say in English. They are also giving him [as she points to Chris] pills for the liver. They are also giving them [Fred and Chris] pills because they are hyperactive." She continues, "Right now they want to take away the SSI [Social Security Insurance] I get for [Fred]. They did not send me the Medicare check for him this month because his teacher says he is fine. However, he is still going to a psychiatrist and the psychiatrist is giving him medicine. If they take away his Medicare, how am I going to be able to take him to the psychiatrist? With what money will I pay for all his medicines? Right now there are some people trying to help me with a lawyer to see if I can win this case. If I don't win it, then they will take away all [Fred's] benefits."

Mrs. N. continues to describe her difficulties in raising her grandchild living with HIV disease: "I take good care of him so that he doesn't cut himself and infect other children with his blood. I give him his food, his medicine and that is how I sustain him. I have to go to the doctor more times with him. More often, I have to take him to the clinic so they can draw blood. If not to the clinic, I take him to the hospital on the third floor for his check up. Other times, I take him to the dentist for a checkup. The [psychiatrist] sometimes comes to see [Fred and Chris]. He will come to see the children when they are not feeling well. You know? Now in school, with Fred, Fred was thrown out of school because he was a Latino child who only wanted to fight. He even wanted to hit the people around him, the teachers and the others. [The school] sent him home and had a teacher come to the house. The teacher would come two days and other times she would not come. She would be here for two hours, sometimes one hour, sometimes less than an hour and then she would leave. The last time she was supposed to come to give him class, she did not come. The other day, she did not come. That is what I have to tell you."

Mrs. N.'s voice conveyed the frustration she was feeling with the school. Unfortunately, she is naive about the school system and many other things in life. She thinks that she should accept what the school says because that is the way it is. Mrs. N. continues to vent her anger and frustration: "[The school] put Fred in an after-school program. What if he hurts himself? Then, this other child [the child Fred fought with] also had problems in school fighting with other kids. Well, then, you would suppose that if they are kids in a special school, they are supposed to give them more attention. You hear? If they are going to watch one of them, they have to watch them all so that they do not hit each other. [Fred] would sometimes start the fight and other times not."

Mrs. N's disappointment with the school with which she struggles daily is evident when she declares: "I have accepted their [the school's] help because . . . I do not know the reason why! Ever since they took him out of school, or rather they threw him out of school, they have not sent me any correspondence. Not even now, do I know what school he will be attending when classes start again. I know nothing; I don't know what they are going to do. However, he has to attend school because he has to go to school where he feels comfortable because that is what I want for him. You understand? Maybe treating him with love, because he is not treated with love. He comes home upset and I treat him with love and later, I start to cry. Then he tells me, "I'm sorry mama," and he comes over and kisses me. Then I tell him to behave, behave and then there is nothing else that needs to be said."

As to why Fred acts out in school, she says, "Maybe he gets it from his mother. Because when his mother died, he was already older. He was with her before he came to live with me. He would be up and down on the streets with her. He lived in that apartment with all those people and she had him up and down the streets with her. God knows! Sometimes she would bring him over early and leave him with me. She was at a bar with him one day and he started to play with the game machines, which they have at those places. They brought it to her attention because he could break it. So she hit him and he started to bleed through the nose."

Mrs. N. became upset and repeated, "He started to bleed! Later on around here, by the other place on River Street, they hit him and he also started to bleed. Then I guess those were the conditions he was being raised under before he came to live with me and he was already use to this. You understand? He thought everything was accomplished by hitting or starting fights. Now he is a bit more tranquil. But first [the school] had to call the police, the security. Fred wanted to hit the policeman. The policeman brought him home in cuffs. I don't think that was necessary. He is only a child! What he should have done was take him by the hand and bring him home to me. When I went to the school . . . this happened again, when I went to school after they called me, Fred was tied up. They had his hands tied like this [she crossed her arms at her back] in back of him so he would stay still. His one hand got loose and the principal threw him on the floor and put one foot like this [as she stomped on the floor] to hold his hand with force. That hurts the child. I did not say anything because since they are from the government, then the principal and the others will not do what I ask them. They will do what he [the principal] says. You understand?" Mrs. N. stated that Fred's behavior would not get any better. "I don't know what to do. But it is the school and the husbands [the mother] has had; she has exposed Fred to their behavior."

About the issue of confidentiality involved when raising a child who is living with HIV, Mrs. N said: "I have not told anyone. The only one that knows about it is the school nurse because if he should fall and get cut or if he fights with another child and blood is involved she needs to be aware of it. Right now the school nurse, his doctor, and no one else knows. I have not told Fred that he is HIV-positive because I don't want him to tell other children about it and then people will mistreat him."

Mrs. N. talked about issues she feels other grandparents, who are not raising their grandchildren, do not understand: "It is not the same to be raised by a blood relative which will not abuse them to being raised by someone not familiar to them that might abuse or beat them. The grandmother, no matter what, is a blood relative and has to treat them right. She can't beat them or anything like that. Those that are not relatives, I can't imagine how they would care for them. Now I have more work trying to care for my grandchildren. But, since I don't have my own children, who have died . . . at least I have my grandchildren. A little bit of happiness having them since I do not have their parents."

As a grandparent, Mrs. N. is at an age at which she should be enjoying her life by watching her grandchildren grow up with their own parents.

Instead, she is playing the role of parent all over again without the help of her children. "I do not leave my grandchildren home alone to go out. I watch them! I feed them at their scheduled times, I take them to the doctor when they are sick. I buy them their clothes, whatever they need. I don't know how other grandmothers are. I treat all my grandchildren the same. However, the one that has AIDS [Fred], I have to pay more attention to him. I have to care more for him. I have to take more care of him."

Throughout the interview, Mrs. N.'s attention was distracted by children screaming as they played. She constantly looked over her shoulder to ensure that the children were safe. The children would run in and out of the room, even though Mrs. N. had asked Silvia to try to keep them playing in the kitchen. Silvia had a hard time trying to keep watch over all the children. For the couple of hours that I was there, I was overwhelmed. I could only imagine what it is like for Mrs. N. day in and day out. I asked her, "How do you do it? Who helps you?" She replied, "I received very little help from life. The little that helps me is God. I ask God to give me strength. To keep me healthy so I can raise them until He comes for me. I ask God that He does not come for me at this moment, until they are able to take care of themselves better. That is the only thing I ask. Outside of that, I ask that the government give me assistance so that I am able to buy them what they need. That God keeps me healthy, gives me strength to do what I need to do, and keep them healthy as well. That is all that I expect. At least for the child that is sick. I ask God for help." She shrugs her shoulders and sighs, saying, "I ask God!"

Mrs. N does not talk very much about her husband. I asked her if he helped her at all and she responded, "Sometimes my daughter helps me. She gives me a hand so that I can buy them any little thing they may want, if not, my husband finds a way. You understand? That is how." As for other family members' or friends' support, Mrs. N comments, "There are some people that do not want me to watch them. If I do not have them, then someone else will. Other people may come to mistreat them. I do not know where they will end up so I do not listen to what they have to say. I take care of my grandchildren and that is all! When they are grown-ups . . . if they do not help me with them, then they should not tell me what is good or bad either. So, I know what is bad for them and what is not."

Diabetes and other health problems have taken their toll on Mrs. N.'s own health. She takes care of herself because she wants to be around as long as possible for her grandchildren. However, inasmuch as her life revolves around her grandchildren, it is about them that she always worries. Mrs. N.

concluded the interview on a loving, warm note: "I sometimes feel bad about all the problems they [the grandchildren] are facing at this young age. All the suffering that they are going through! Sometimes I start to cry and other times I wipe my tears and ask God to watch my children [grandchildren]. I also ask God to help me, too!"

Five months after the completion of the interview, Mrs. N. and her family moved into a public shelter. They could no longer live in substandard housing but were unable to obtain Section 8 housing because of a long waiting list.

Mrs. C.

At the time of the interview Mrs. C. was raising five grandchildren and two grandnieces and also had her daughter and her two children living with her. The grandchildren include two HIV-infected grandsons, aged eight and ten. An African American woman in her late fifties or early sixties, Mrs. C. has an engaging smile. Her devotion to her family is ever present as we discuss her life raising two HIV-infected grandsons. She does not work outside of the home and is dependent on public benefit programs for the material support of her entire family. Chronically ill with diabetes, hypertension, arthritis, and heart disease, Mrs. C. perseveres despite the daily demands on her life. This family's life in an urban area of northern New Jersey is overshadowed by poverty, substance abuse, and violence.

Mrs. C. described how she came to be raising all of these children and her two grandsons in particular. "My daughter was living with me at the time and then gave birth to the kids. . . . She started to get into a lot of problems and trouble and got sent away a couple of times. So I took the kids, so I have been having them since . . . For ten years, the oldest one is ten." Then, in summing up her daughter's life, Mrs. C. gave us a glimpse of her devotion and commitment to her grandchildren. "Well, she was kind of headstrong and she wanted the street life and she went into selling crack back and forth and got caught and went to jail. So they had nobody to take care of the kids and I took all of my grandkids, to keep them with me and not pass them out to other people."

In addition to these grandchildren, Mrs. C. has a twenty-year-old daughter and her children. Mrs. C. had this to say: "She has two. I have no problem with her, the only thing is her income . . . can't meet with her getting an apartment of her own so she stays with me off and on . . . and the two grand-nieces, their mother [Mrs. C.'s sister's daughter] went on crack too and her grandmother killed her grandfather so they put her in jail and gave me the kids. So I have them for ten years. She's on crack too."

She appears uncertain as to whether her daughter and son-in-law, the parents of the infected grandsons, were themselves infected with the virus. "Both of them say they're not because they've been incarcerated so many times, they say they're not, so I don't know." It was not until her grandsons became sick that Mrs. C. became aware of their infection. "Well, they're sick—I had them since birth . . . they get infections, and it kept turning into pneumonia, so when they got about four, one was four and the other about five, they were in the hospital with pneumonia and they tested them and she told me they had HIV. It was very hard at first, you know. All kinds of thoughts were entering my mind, everything. . . . You know what they used to say about HIV, you don't live long and all that, all that came to my mind. . . . Right now I'm a little afraid. . . . The youngest one stays sick a lot. After [the doctor] told me he went into the second stage. I was really frightened but the medicine they gave him helps him. He seems to be coping with it pretty good."

Mrs. C. then discusses some of the difficult times and how her grandsons came to know of their infection. "Both of them know because they go to this program . . . they go to group. . . . And they ask me would it be all right if [the staff] teach them what they have and talk about it, and I told them sure, so they mostly know what they got. They understand that." She relates that the oldest grandson, who is ten, "understands what is happening because I sit down and I tell him and I tell him why he has to take his medication and how it is important to him and if he's not taking the medication, I will tell the doctors, I will tell on him. . . . You have to tell him the medication is for his health and is good if he wants to live. That it's important for him. . . . He understands, he's very smart.

"Their father knows. I told him as soon as they told me. I don't like to hide things. I want them to know what's going on in the boys' lives." Other family members know and help out when Mrs. C. is in need. "I have three brothers and one sister. . . . My sister is wonderful. . . . She visits me during the day, if I have to get up during the night. I need a ride or anything, she's there for me. Take them back and forth to the hospital or doctor."

It is clear from her responses that she loves her grandsons. She affirms, "I do. I told them that's what's keeping me going. I'm sick too, but you know if I sit down and think how sick I am, what should I do, I should have done this, I should have done that, I have to take care of my grandkids and I'll be doing all right. . . . The doctor gets at me sometimes about taking my medication on time—every day. . . . Since I went to the doctor and got myself together with medications and stuff, I feel pretty good. . . . I used to be sickly but I go to the doctor regularly and I get regular checkups as well." Apparently Mrs. C.'s love for her grandchildren is the motivating force for her own care. "Well, like I said, my kids go and they need me, so I might as well try to get myself together so that I can take care of them because they're important to me and I know what they have is important, so I'm going to keep their life together so I can keep mine together. . . . I'm going to try to help them as much as I can."

Mrs. C. began to discuss in more detail her relationship with her family, and especially the death of her oldest daughter and some of the difficulties she encounters with her grandsons. "I understand because I had a child of my own die of AIDS and I knew what was going on, because she tried to hide stuff from me too, and after the doctor wrote me a note, I found out about her and every time she would get sick I would rush her up to the hospital and they would give me a mask and stuff and tell me I'm not allowed in the room. I told them I wasn't scared about catching nothing and I took care of her. . . . So this is not new to me. . . . She died in '95. . . . When she was dying I had to take care of her. She suffered and I took care of her until she passed . . . so I had to cope with the boys after taking care of her." Mrs. C. then reflected on her life: "So I had my grandkids so I'm pretty satisfied. When I was young I went out a lot—I had a good time when I was young, so I don't regret nothing now. . . . Life is what you make it." When she considered how her circumstances may differ from others, Mrs. C. noted, "I have a girlfriend but her [grandchildren] don't have AIDS, but she has to take care of them because her oldest daughter is on drugs and she has to take care of her kids like I do. . . . It's a shame some of the grandparents don't want to be bothered with their grandkids, they wouldn't take their grandkids for nothing. . . . I don't understand that. [They're] theirs from blood. How could they turn a kid down when a kid is in need? I would take in a stranger if I could and take care of them, if I had to take care of them I would. I love kids."

Mrs. C.'s philosophy of life involves a devotion to children: "Oh, around in the '80s I had eleven kids. . . . It was just like a whole big family. I loved them and whatever I could do for them, I would do it. I shared anything I had with them. I treated them all as one, they're the same, there's nothing different about them. . . . I used to collect people's kids, take care of people's kids when they would go away for a week. They'd still be there clean and healthy. I love kids."

Mrs. C. is supported by what she terms "strength, wisdom, and prayer." These inner resources are buttressed by "friends and family and a very special social worker, Sarah. . . . She's a miracle worker, she helps me with everything clothing, food and my bills and talking to people who have denied me checks and stuff. Their father was incarcerated for four years and he got out. He doesn't live too far from us. . . . He really has done an amazing job since he's been out of jail. He comes and sees the kids, he helps. . . . Their mother comes around every now and then too. . . . She's still on drugs. I tried to ask her if she's going to go to rehab somewhere and she says yeah, but I don't think she's really interested in going nowhere right now. It makes me feel bad because I always say, why don't you get your life together so you can be a mother again to your kids. I don't understand it. Then she gets these boyfriends on drugs. Naturally she's not going to get off drugs so I tried to talk to her but right now there's no talking. . . . But the father is the most help . . . and now he's paying child support. . . . He makes sure they get their medicine. If they don't want to take it from me they take it from him. . . . When I'm not able to go to the school, he goes to the school for me. He takes days off from his job to go to school. . . . He takes them to his house. He takes them to the park. He plays football and basketball, whatever they want. He buys whatever they want, so he's really been trying to be good to his kids. Well, he always has been. I had no trouble with him when the kids was born."

Despite the apparent support Mrs. C. has had with the children, she has "had quite a bit of problems with the oldest one in school. He's kind of moody in school and he fights with the kids, he doesn't want to listen to the teacher and everything and he wants to be the boss half the time. . . . I have to run back and forth to school. . . . The school helped, they usually sat and talked to him and calmed him down. . . . He likes sports and stuff. . . . If they think he's dying or sick they send him home. They give him a day to get himself together. They try to work with him." The younger grandson also experiences problems. "The boys picked on him. . . . He likes to go to Joan [his mental health counselor]. He sits down and she talks to him and I go in sometimes for the meeting and she talks with me." This time with the school counselor gives Mrs. C. a better understanding of what is happening with the boys.

For Mrs. C., the ultimate goal is "to stay well enough so I can help them with their medication and they stay well." The poverty, illness, violence, and deaths that have stalked the lives of Mrs. C. and her family only underscore her strength and her love for her grandchildren and grandnieces.

Shortly after the completion of this interview, Mrs. C.'s youngest grandson died from AIDS, followed by the death of Mrs. C.'s mother.

Notes

1. The names used in these narratives have been changed to protect their privacy.

3

Stigma, Isolation, and Support for HIV-Affected Elder Parental Surrogates

CYNTHIA CANNON POINDEXTER

Older surrogate parents raising HIV-affected[1] and HIV-infected children have all the stresses and challenges of other grandparent caregivers, with an added problematic factor: potent and pervasive HIV-related stigma, which can contribute to emotional stress and social isolation (Draimin 1993; Gutheil and Chichin 1991; Allers 1990). After almost two decades, HIV remains one of the most stigmatized circumstances in this country (Herek et al. 1998). HIV-related stigma decreases the chances that a family will disclose the diagnosis, which in turn lessens the possibility of obtaining relevant emotional and practical support during times of stress (Poindexter and Linsk 1998, 1999).

HIV stigma matters greatly in the lives of grandparent caregivers because it precipitates difficult decisions concerning stigma management and HIV disclosure, increased social isolation, and lack of social support due to restricted disclosure of the diagnosis, the unbuffered stress of providing child care and HIV care due to the stigma and isolation, and thwarted help seeking for their own physical and mental well-being. At a time when they expected to be free of childrearing responsibilities, they are caring for younger relatives who may become ill and/or die from a hidden, stigmatized disease without the social support that might help to buffer the intense stress.

This chapter will review literature concerning social support and stigma, explore these concepts in the context of HIV disease, discuss some of the consequences of HIV stigma through three case studies, and offer some implications for intervention.

Stigma

Stigma, the discrediting, blaming, or labeling someone pejoratively, has harmful social and psychological effects on the labeled person and on his or her associates (Goffman 1959, 1963). The effects of stigma have been documented for a wide variety of behaviors, situations, and biomedical conditions and were first labeled in the HIV field by Herek and Glunt (1988).

Three subsets of stigma have been identified: (1) associative stigma, (2) internalized stigma, and (3) stigma management. Associative (first called "courtesy") stigma is ascribed to persons who are attached as caregivers or acquaintances to persons who are stigmatized (Goffman 1963). HIV-related stigma has an impact on HIV-affected older caregivers, even when they are not themselves HIV-infected, because of their association with persons who are HIV-positive. Internalized stigma, the acceptance of society's discrediting of oneself, can occur without the presence of active discrimination and can lower a person's sense of self-esteem and prestige (Ainlay, Coleman, and Becker 1986; Schur 1983). Internalized stigma often has great influence on the way in which persons make decisions regarding HIV status disclosure, including HIV-affected caregivers (Poindexter and Linsk 1999). People who carry a stigma or an associative stigma are aware of the real or potential negative reactions of others and are uncertain about how they might be treated (Page 1984). This awareness can be associated with the stigmatized person's concealment, defensiveness, and isolation, as well as concerns about privacy, secrecy, visibility, and disclosure (Goffman 1963). Stigma management refers to how the stigmatized person considers disclosure decisions (Page 1984; Goffman 1963). When the condition is hidden or not obvious, then fear of exposure may become even more pronounced (Dubay 1987). People tend to "weigh" the costs and benefits of disclosure and to consider whether disclosure of a stigmatizing situation might enhance self-esteem, decrease isolation, improve relationships, solve or avoid problems, or further an activist goal (Cain 1991). HIV-affected older surrogate parents manage the effects of HIV-related stigma in a variety of ways, making decisions about disclosure based on the perceived costs and dangers.

Social Support

Receipt of emotional and practical support[2] has been linked to stress reduction and maintenance of physical and emotional health (Gottlieb 1985; Pearlin 1985;

Cohen 1983; Turner 1983). Social support has been shown to have positive emotional and physical effects for persons living with HIV (Nott, Vedhara, and Power 1995; Pakenham, Dadds, and Terry 1994; Green 1993; Linn et al. 1993; Hays, Turner, and Coates 1992; Lesserman, Perkins, and Evans 1992; Blaney et al. 1991) and for HIV-affected caregivers (Wardlaw 1994; McKinlay et al. 1993). It has also been shown to be a positive factor in aging (Cohen and Syme 1985) and a stress mediator among caregivers for frail elders (Rapp 1996; Minkler and Roe 1993). Seeking social support can be stymied, however, when the individual perceives the possibility of being stigmatized. Research on alcoholism, for example, suggests that a person's concerns about being negatively labeled or stigmatized can discourage him or her from seeking formal help (Cunningham et al. 1993; Sobell, Sobell, and Toneatto 1992; Klingeman 1991).

HIV-Related Stigma

HIV-infected persons and their support persons experience a particular and more intense type of discrimination and prejudice, identified as "AIDS-related stigma"[3] (Herek and Glunt 1988), for two reasons: HIV is associated with contagion, serious illness, and death; and HIV has been closely associated with groups that are already highly stigmatized, such as injecting drug users and men who have sex with men (Herek and Glunt 1988). Similar in many ways to cholera-related stigma in the early 1830s in this country, HIV stigma is at this time pervasive and potent (Herek 1999; Herek and Capitanio 1998). HIV stigma may be more severe and more powerful than other forms of stigma because it is so intricately related to social ostracism, personal vulnerability, death, fear of contagion, attribution of blame, and discrimination by association (Pryor and Reeder 1993). HIV-related stigma has been documented in the United States among the general public (Borcher and Rickabaugh 1995; Herek and Capitanio 1992, 1993; St. Lawrence et al. 1990; Blendon and Donelan 1988), physicians (Sherer and Goldberg 1994; Kelly et al. 1987), nurses (Peate 1995; Eliason 1993; Hall 1992; Siminoff, Erlen, and Lidz 1991; Denker 1990; Faugier and Wright 1990; Kelly et al. 1988), mental health practitioners (Knox and Clark 1993), and social workers (National Association of Social Workers 1995; Wiener and Siegel 1990). HIV-infected persons have reported that HIV-related stigma has negative effects socially (such as isolation because they are reluctant to ask for formal and informal support) and psychologically (such as lowered self-esteem and self-efficacy) (Moneyham et al. 1995; Laryea and Gien 1993; Macks 1993;

Crandall and Coleman 1992; Powell-Cope and Brown 1992; Lang 1991; Longo, Sposs, and Locke 1990).

ASSOCIATIVE HIV STIGMA AND CAREGIVING   HIV stigma is so pervasive that those who are associated with infected persons fear and experience the censure as well. A recent study of HIV volunteerism found that associative HIV stigma profoundly affects AIDS service volunteers at all stages of their volunteer experiences, often influencing decisions about whether to continue to provide support to persons with HIV (Snyder, Omoto, and Crain 1999). Family members providing HIV-related care frequently confront HIV stigma, which in turn affects diagnosis disclosure and is associated with isolation and social rejection (Lesar, Gerber, and Semmel 1995; Bor, Miller, and Goldman 1993; Brown and Powell-Cope 1991, 1993; McKinlay et al. 1993; Melvin and Sherr 1993; Matocha 1992). In a sample of fifty-two persons from twenty-five HIV-affected, predominantly minority urban families, many respondents reported feeling stressed by the secrecy and ostracism related to HIV stigma, shunned by health care and social service providers, and alienated from extended family due to HIV stigma (Mellins and Ehrhardt 1994).

INTERNALIZED HIV STIGMA AND CAREGIVING   People internalize HIV stigma through an awareness of the behavior and attitudes of others. Older surrogate parents of children with HIV are part of our society, a culture in which ubiquitous HIV stigma is witnessed, perceived, anticipated, and feared. Therefore, disclosure decisions are sometimes made based on perceived, feared, or anticipated reactions, whether or not there is actual discrimination or negative judgment (Green 1995; Crandall 1991). This means that caregivers sometimes keep the HIV secret because of the expectations about reactions, even if they have not actually experienced discrimination (Poindexter and Linsk 1999).

STIGMA MANAGEMENT AND HIV CAREGIVING   Because they are affected by associative and internalized HIV stigma, HIV-affected elder surrogate parents must find ways to manage the feared effects of HIV stigma in order to protect themselves, their families, and the children under their care. Decisions are made, usually carefully and deliberately, about who must know the diagnosis and who can be trusted not to mistreat the child and family and possibly to react with emotional support and acceptance. Powell-Cope and Brown (1992) highlighted a strategy of stigma management for the caregivers studied which involved disclosure in stages. People usually begin this process by deciding to tell family members and other people whom they trust will keep it a secret and not mistreat the HIV-infected or affected persons. The continuum of stigma management ends with "going public," the ultimate stage of disclosure (Powell-Cope and Brown 1992).

Two especially salient issues for grandparent caregivers are disclosure to the HIV-positive children and disclosure to school systems. Lipson (1994) points out that the oncology model—that is, the standard practice of telling children with cancer what their diagnoses and prognoses are—has not been universally applied for children with HIV, most likely due to HIV stigma, which is what makes HIV different from cancer. Parents, grandparents, and other caregivers may want to protect the infected child and his or her family from HIV stigma resulting from disclosure to others (Wiener, Battles, and Heilman 1998). In addition, persons parenting children with HIV have agonizing decisions to make about disclosure within the school system, feeling torn between wanting school authorities to know and feeling afraid of what the HIV-positive children might face if the secret is known. There are often twin fears: that the other children will ostracize the HIV-infected children and that parents and school-system employees will limit the child's opportunities (Poindexter 1997).

HIV STIGMA AND SOCIAL SUPPORT   HIV-related stigma is inversely related to obtaining and maintaining beneficial social support (Herek and Glunt 1988). Fear of rejection due to HIV stigma results in the loss of emotional and practical support both for persons with HIV (Lang 1991) and their caregivers (Poindexter and Linsk 1998; Jankowski, Videka-Sherman, and Laquidara-Dickinson 1996; Kreibick 1995; Lesar, Gerber, and Semmel 1995; Ogu and Wolfe 1994; Lippman, James, and Frierson 1993; Brown 1992; Reidy, Taggart, and Asselin 1991). HIV stigma may isolate caregivers because social support is more difficult to obtain or request when one is fearful of disclosing the whole truth about the family's situation (Poindexter and Linsk 1998; Green 1993; Brown and Powell-Cope 1992; Perreault et al. 1992; Gutheil and Chichin 1991; Septimus 1990), especially if it involves admitting to substance use or unacceptable sexual behavior (Brown, Mitchell, and Williams 1992; Cates et al. 1990). Older adults may have greater difficulty with HIV stigma because of this secondary disclosure (Solomon 1996; McKinlay et al. 1993; Perryman 1993; Gutheil and Chichin 1991; Allers 1990) and therefore may be more isolated than their younger counterparts (Baker 1992; Septimus 1990).

There is little empirical evidence regarding help-seeking or the use of HIV-specific service agencies by elder grandparent caregivers. However, it is likely that older persons are less likely to seek help from AIDS service organizations. In his analysis of service use, Emlet (1993) found that HIV-infected people over age fifty accessed support services (buddies) far less frequently than the individuals under age fifty. Reluctance to seek formal assistance may be related to older persons' perception that AIDS service organizations are more appropriate for the young. Moreover, fear of HIV stigma may be greater among this cohort of older adults.

Vignettes

Excerpts from research interviews illustrate the awareness and management of HIV stigma among HIV-affected grandparent caregivers. These three surrogate parents for minor HIV-infected grandchildren were a subset of a small sample (N = 7) of HIV-affected caregivers over the age of fifty in the Boston, Massachusetts area in 1998. This convenience sample was recruited through fliers posted in health care and social service facilities. Participants were paid $25 per interview and were interviewed twice in their homes, with approximately a week between interviews, for an hour and a half each session. The interviews were unstructured and open-ended; this exploratory study was designed to solicit the caregivers' experiences on a variety of topics, including HIV stigma. Audiotapes were transcribed and the transcriptions checked for accuracy; interviews were then coded for major themes.

Vignette 1. Coralee[4] is a seventy-two-year-old divorced African American woman who left her second husband and home in Georgia to come to Boston because of the birth of her grandchild Tyrone, who is now seven years old. Her daughter Carol called her from the hospital after giving birth to Tyrone, telling her that she had just tested HIV-positive. Coralee returned to Boston and cared for Carol until she died, and is now Tyrone's only caregiver. Tyrone, who developed symptomatic HIV shortly after birth, is on combination therapy. Coralee also raises another grandchild, an HIV-negative two-year-old named Dougie, who is hyperactive and developmentally delayed, possibly because his birth mother used substances during pregnancy. Dougie's father is Coralee's son. Coralee is struggling with some health problems; she has chronic diarrhea, fatigue, and mobility problems (especially with stairs and driving).

Vignette 2.   Victoria is a fifty-three-year-old widow who labels herself 'mixed race" because her mother was white and from Portugal and her father was African American. Victoria has been the primary caregiver for her adult HIV-positive son, Ronny, when he becomes ill. Ronny identifies himself as African American. Victoria lives in a high-rise residential program for persons with HIV; she lives in the apartment of her former daughter-in-law Susan (who is HIV-positive and who identifies herself as white) and twin four-year-old grandchildren: Cindy, who is HIV-positive, and Little Ronny, who is HIV-negative. Victoria helps care for the twins each day and provides personal care for Ronny, Susan, and Cindy during episodic HIV-related illnesses. Victoria feels very strongly about confronting HIV stigma and irrational fear of contagion when and where she finds it: she reported animated verbal arguments with a coworker, her boss, and with an agency-based housekeeper because she experienced their negative judgments of persons with HIV. Susan and Ronny have gone public as persons with HIV, a decision Victoria supports.

Vignette 3.   Peggy is a seventy-year-old widowed Caucasian woman who identifies herself as Irish-American Catholic. Her only child, her son Donny, has HIV disease and heroin addiction and is now in jail. She legally adopted her son's HIV-positive eleven-year-old daughter Monnie shortly after her birth, because both Monnie's parents were actively using illegal drugs. Monnie's mother Teresa is cocaine-addicted and incarcerated. At birth Monnie tested positive for cocaine; at eighteen months she tested positive for HIV. Monnie occasionally has HIV-related symptoms, but is able to attend school regularly. Peggy and Monnie now live in a small, substandard apartment and are struggling financially. Peggy spends much time and effort trying to be certified for a section 8 voucher so that she and Monnie can move to a better place. Peggy says that her major concern as a caregiver is how to raise a preadolescent girl "in this day and age" because things are so different from when she grew up and from when she raised Donny. Peggy has a heart condition; she has already had bypass surgery once and is scheduled for another operation.

HIV-Related Stigma

The power of HIV stigma, managing associative stigma, and making decisions about HIV disclosure were identified in these grandmothers' stories. Coralee watched as some people became uncomfortable around Carol after she was hospitalized with AIDS, and she was outraged by it:

There were people who avoided touching my daughter. My daughter was like a huggy-kissy kind of person . . . and the first thing that she did was kiss them. I could tell by the body language, you know, that isn't what they wanted. . . . It's a disease, you know. And if they got it from drugs, that's a disease, too. I don't know people who haven't had unsafe sex. I don't think anybody deserves to be treated badly because of HIV, absolutely not.

Coralee had also personally experienced stigma directly from some of her own family members and from a neighbor who ostracized Tyrone: "We had a couple of family members who reacted badly and I felt hurt, yes I felt hurt. . . . They were so ignorant, you know, that they felt like that. . . . A mother who lives right across the street . . . says he can't come over and play. So, he doesn't." One of Coralee's daughters-in-law acted uncomfortable about Tyrone's visiting his cousins, but Coralee did not blame her for her reaction: "I knew that she was anxious about it and I don't hold that against her. As a matter of fact, I commend her for what she's trying to do, protect the children."

Victoria explained that although she did not hesitate to be a caregiver to her family members with HIV, she knew that not everyone comes to that conclusion:

There are so many families, nobody realizes how many families there are affected or infected, it's like the families don't want to be bothered. They don't want to talk about it; it's like being in denial. . . . There's so many people, I've worked with a woman and her son same age as my son had it, she worked in a hospital and she denied him, totally denied him. I said how can you do that? . . . I never rejected either one of them, you know. . . . I don't do that, cause that's just me. . . . I took everybody in.

Peggy was also aware of HIV stigma but said that she did not hesitate to become the surrogate parent for her granddaughter: "Everybody is afraid of it but me. I'm not afraid of it. . . . DSS [Department of Social Services] has a problem putting children with any kind of HIV problem. . . . But that's not me."

Responses of these three respondents represented a continuum of stigma management, from privacy to visibility: Peggy did not disclose the HIV diagnosis at all, Coralee disclosed selectively and carefully, and Victoria's family went public. Peggy did not talk about being an HIV-affected surrogate parent with anyone outside of Monnie's medical care system; she explained when asked who she talked to about Monnie's having HIV that her stigma management consisted of nondisclosure: "[I talk] just to Children's Hospital. I know it sounds crazy, but there isn't anybody else who knows."

Coralee's strategy was to make careful decisions about whom to tell and under what circumstances, so she was less likely to have to confront negative reactions:

> All the people I don't think who don't need to know, I don't volunteer to tell them. . . . Most of the people who I deal with don't know. . . . And because of that . . . I haven't seen that [stigma] too much. I just don't think that it's something I need to discuss. . . . I wouldn't feel it necessary to just tell a casual acquaintance. It isn't something that you always know how a person is going to react to it, you know, so why introduce it if it's not necessary.

Victoria's stigma management was made easier because the family had gone public:

> These kids are poster kids. They have been put on the flyers. When they were six months old they were in the *Gazette,* a group of Girl Scouts made them a quilt, and their pictures were taken with the Girl Scouts. So they've done well. They've done videos. They were on the new flyer for CAP [Children's AIDS Project]. . . . They are pretty famous little kids. They are on a commercial for AIDS too.

Victoria supported the decision of her son and daughter-in-law to go public because she saw this as a service to others:

> If an interview or presentation, or any of that stuff is going to help, God bless it, whether it's in my family or somebody else's family. I won't say they don't care [about stigma], but they are being open with it cause they are involved in so much. I give them that much credit because . . . why hide it? If you are going to accept me then accept me for what I am and what I have. If you can't accept me for that, that's your problem, you know.

As discussed earlier, two of the difficult stigma management tasks for grand-parent caregivers are deciding whether to tell the child of the diagnosis, and deciding whether to tell the school. Two of the interviewees (Coralee and Peggy) are raising school-aged children who were old enough to understand the information. Both of these grandmothers paid attention to the timing of the disclosure to the HIV-positive child. Coralee has not yet told her seven-year-old grandson the name of his illness, but plans to when he is older and asks for the information: "I think at some point when he's older, it could get to the point where he says 'I want to know.'" She is a little concerned about what Tyrone might face when he is older and his peers learn of his diagnosis:

> I think he might have some problems, especially when he's old enough and other people that he knows and people that he would be associated with are old enough to understand and heard. . . . I think maybe ten or twelve, early teenagers might be a different story.

Peggy had only recently allowed the diagnosis to be disclosed to her grand-daughter Monnie; she explained that previously: "I never allowed it" because she did not think Monnie would be able to protect the secret. Recently she decided that Monnie was mature enough to hear the truth and manage dis-closure decisions. A letter that Monnie wrote on the day of her disclosure confirmed for Peggy that Monnie was indeed ready:

> A few days ago I found out the truth about myself. I was born with the scariest disease called HIV. HIV stands for Human Immune Deficiency Virus. Now I understand why I have so many blood tests to monitor my blood, and another reason I go to a special camp. That camp is for chil-dren with diseases like mine. The reason this was caught was because my father and mother had this deadly disease and they got it from sharing drug needles. And from what I heard, HIV can cause AIDS, which stands for Acquired Immune Deficiency Syndrome. When I found out that I had been sickly, I was quite shocked but wouldn't everyone be? I know that HIV causes death too, but I hope to live a long and happy life.

For the guardians of school-aged children, disclosure to school personnel is a difficult decision. Coralee has not yet told Tyrone's teachers, and was antici-pating disclosing soon and watching for their reactions:

We haven't gone to the teachers, which I want to do next week, I want to tell her so that she understands. I'm attentive to if it's going to make a difference in his teacher's attitude toward him. I don't think it will but I'm not positive.

Peggy also had not told any adults at Monnie's school why she was taking pills: "We just said it was medicine. . . . You don't have to know this, all you got to do is give her the medicine."

Social Isolation

Associative and internalized HIV stigma can restrict grandparent caregivers from disclosing the HIV diagnosis. When they cannot tell the truth about the stressful realities of their lives, they may not be able to solicit the formal and informal social support which can help buffer the stress of surrogate parenting and HIV caregiving. The resulting lack of emotional and practical support may increase their isolation from peers, neighbors, family members, and friends.

Elder surrogate parents to HIV-infected and affected children often face multiple and complex sources of stress. Each of these three caregivers spoke about struggling financially and needing help with transportation and housing. In addition to these monetary and logistical concerns, these grandmothers also spoke about many other sources of stress: their own diminished health and functioning; the emotional and physical strain associated with caring for a grandchild with a life threatening disease; feeling unsafe in the neighborhood; family conflicts over illegal drug use; lack of time for themselves and for maintaining social contacts; and worries about the children's future if the caregiver dies. Older caregivers also are in a situation that is developmentally unexpected; they probably did not plan to raise children again, as Coralee explains:

My life is quite different than what I wanted it to be. I had retired and . . . you know it isn't what I planned for. Like with my friend, she's my age . . . she's old and she goes back to her house and goes to bed and it's a whole different situation. And that's how it should be because she has worked and raised her children, they're grown and gone.

These grandmothers needed formal services and informal social support to buffer unusual stress, but they were not getting the level of support or care which they desired. This was partially due to the demands of full time HIV-related care and child raising, which made it difficult for them to maintain friendships, participate in church and other social activities, or seek assistance for their own needs. However, childrearing was not the sole reason for their not being supported socially. HIV stigma also contributed to their isolation.

The amount of isolation reported was directly related to their degree of comfort with disclosure of HIV diagnosis. Victoria, because the care recipients had gone public and she was living with them in a building designated for HIV-affected families and HIV-infected persons, did not feel as alone as did Coralee and Peggy. Victoria made it clear that she could ask for someone to listen to her if she needed to and if she trusts the listener: "I'll talk to anybody to a point . . . if I feel comfortable. . . . I don't care where it goes. I really don't." She was receiving emotional support for her HIV caregiving from the man she was dating, a close female friend, and a gay couple in the building to whom she had grown close, all of whom talked with her freely about the presence of HIV in the family and the unique stress associated with that. Coralee did not make it widely known that her daughter and grandson had AIDS, but she had disclosed those facts to church members, and therefore felt some emotional support from some of them, even though she was highly aware of the possibility of Tyrone's presence making some church members uneasy. Peggy, who had disclosed to no one except Monnie's doctors and social workers, reported that she was completely isolated, feeling both starved for adult companionship and worn out with childrearing. Peggy talked about not having confidants or anyone to do anything with:

> I know it sounds crazy, but there isn't anybody. . . . I'm alone . . . I have no friends, you know, like a woman friend? . . . Any place I go, Monnie and I go alone.

When asked what it would be like when Monnie was away for two weeks at a special camp, Peggy responded:

> I love it, because I've been doing this, taking care of Monnie, since she was an infant, a lot of trips to Children's Hospital, and I'm tired, I want some freedom. I have no relatives to have freedom. . . . I can't do it no more, it's the end of summer, I have to have freedom.

All three of these grandmothers said that they were currently getting no formal support for themselves, such as transportation, support group, help with finding or financing housing, or respite care. Coralee and Peggy spoke about lacking the means of transportation for running necessary errands and looking for housing; Coralee's vision and mobility problems made driving problematic and Peggy does not own a car and found it difficult to look for housing and to visit her son in jail. Victoria had earlier sought out a support group, but it disbanded before she was able to join; she has stopped looking for one because her family members' health is better now and she is less panicked about them. Peggy had attended one newly formed support group meeting, was the only attendee, and did not go back. All three were trying to qualify for subsidized housing and to move to a more suitable place: less expensive, safer, and without stairs (Coralee and Peggy) or with more space and privacy (Victoria).

Coralee was especially clear about the need for some relief from caregiving so she could socialize more: "I would like to have some time, even if it's just evenings, where I could go to meetings." She had tried numerous times to secure an appropriate and dependable respite worker from an agency, and had been repeatedly disappointed. Coralee provided an important insight into how HIV stigma can contribute to isolation and stress: as was shown in earlier quotes, she had been told by a neighbor and a daughter-in-law, both mothers of small children with whom Tyrone could have played, that he was not welcome because he is HIV-positive. Coralee was feeling trapped, not being able to have a break from caregiving. Another source of respite for her might be to leave Tyrone with a church group, but that possibility was closed to her because of her fear of Tyrone's infecting others as well as fear that Tyrone would be embarrassed or hurt:

> The brothers talk to you that you have to be aware that there are people there who are not as open as you are and there are some restrictions, not based on the Church, by the Kingdom Hall, but out of your own concern for other people, the rights of other people, consideration for them, there are certain kinds of things that you watch. He knows that he don't drink out of the water fountain because I tell him that it's forbidden . . . that way the people who drink don't have to be concerned about him, and he doesn't get his feelings hurt. . . . And I don't allow him to romp with the other kids. . . . You couldn't do that to fellow Christians, bring him in without them knowing, because that would be wrong, because if they feel frightened by it, if they're threatened by it, they need to know so they can protect them to whatever degree they want to. . . . I think that they have a right to know.

Implications

As these three HIV-affected older caregivers illustrated, when raising a minor grandchild who has HIV, one can manage one's internalized fear of censure by making decisions along a continuum of disclosure. The stage of disclosure in which the caregiver lives is strongly associated with the level of social support and isolation. Victoria was freer to talk about the daily struggles in her life as an HIV-affected caregiver because the family had gone public and she herself did not fear others' judgment; she therefore was feeling fairly supported and connected. Coralee, neither fully hidden nor public, was cautious and watchful about protecting the information in order to protect her grandson; she therefore was experiencing some support and some isolation. Peggy was completed hidden as an HIV caregiver and intensely isolated.

HIV stigma sets up a cycle: the experience and fear of stigma keeps people from disclosing the HIV diagnosis and seeking the support that could help them to face HIV and withstand the stigma. Friend, family, and church relationships can be strained and reduced with HIV stigma so substitute social support is necessary. It is up to health-care and social-service professionals to help these grandparents mediate the effects of HIV stigma. The compound problems in their lives may frustrate or baffle practitioners. Sometimes social-service and health-care professionals assume that someone else is working with the families. Regardless of these challenges, it is vital that professional helpers take more responsibility for the well-being of these heroic yet hidden caregivers.

HIV-affected older caregivers are invisible partially because of their own stigma management, but also in part because service providers do not see them. The first order of business is therefore for medical and social service providers to look for this population. Practitioners may need to increase their observation in places where perhaps they are not accustomed to looking for stressed older people: child day care centers, schools, pediatric clinics, HIV treatment centers, and drug treatment centers. Helpers also probably need to ask questions that they have not been accustomed to asking. HIV practitioners should ask persons with HIV, "Who takes care of you at home? Whom do you depend on?" Gerontological practitioners should strive to make it safe to talk about HIV, saying something like: "Sometimes grandparents find themselves raising grandchildren because of AIDS; I'm wondering if your family is affected by HIV and if you'd like to talk about that." It is imperative that the helping professions notice them.

The three grandmothers presented in this chapter said that the adults and children with HIV were connected to medical and social service organizations, but they reported no emotional support for themselves. Why is that? Perhaps grandparent caregivers are primarily focused on the persons with HIV and not thinking about their own needs; perhaps they are unaware that services might be available to them; or perhaps they fear rejections, ostracism, social isolation, or blame due to HIV stigma. When professionals identify households with HIV-affected grandparent caregivers, they should be prepared to offer individual counseling that can help them learn to manage stigma, make disclosure decisions, and possibly cope with hidden bereavement. Volunteer buddies and support groups can help to reduce caregiver isolation and burden by creating a safe place to vent, grieve, compare stories, and feel understood. The isolation, failure to seek help for oneself, and lack of social support should be addressed because the already intense stress of HIV caregiving could be mediated through services and connection; stress, in turn, can have a deleterious effect physical and mental health. Health care professionals must begin to serve them.

Practitioners can help their colleagues notice, understand, and serve HIV-affected grandparent caregivers. Gerontological specialists should look for opportunities to provide workshops and information on HIV to the aging network, include HIV in state and regional training plans, and address HIV as routinely as other diseases are addressed. HIV practitioners should strive to include older caregivers' issues in workshops and classes, raising these concerns when speaking to professionals, volunteers, and students. The national AIDS Education and Training Centers should offer programs that focus on older HIV-affected caregivers. Outreach and educational programs should focus on clergy, congregations, and faith-based organizations so that spiritual environments become safe places to talk about HIV caregiving. Professionals should help spread the word.

When aging and HIV occur together, there is a hybrid of ageism and HIV stigma. Although there have been much progress made, the HIV network has not yet adequately addressed its inherent ageism, and the aging network has not yet adequately addressed its HIV phobia. Grandparent caregivers may perceive the AIDS-service network as not being meant for HIV-negative caregivers, and the aging network as not being prepared to address HIV. Consequently, the service provision systems are discriminating against these hidden elder HIV-affected surrogate parents, and persons with needs related both to aging and to HIV remain invisible and neglected. HIV and aging service systems should coordinate their efforts so that both networks can forge ways to support HIV-affected grandparent caregivers. Legislative advocacy, joint sponsorship of services, and cosponsored professional training about the intersection of HIV and aging are a few of the possible tasks. The aging and HIV networks should bridge this gap.

Conclusion

HIV infection rates continue to increase. There is not yet a cure or vaccine for HIV, and it is not clear that the current therapies will work indefinitely, even if one receives early detection and treatment and adheres to the difficult protocols. Parents with end-stage HIV will therefore be likely to ask their elder parents to take on childrearing functions, and the older relatives will continue to do so (Mellins, and Ehrhardt 1994; Boland, Czamiecki, and Haiken 1992; Levine 1990).

Social support may decrease in older adulthood even without the presence of a stigmatizing illness like HIV (Minkler 1985). A lessening of social support may have serious ramifications for elders because it increases the likelihood that stress will have a deleterious effect (Sauer and Coward 1985). Caregivers such as the three in this chapter face not only decreasing social support and increasing stress due to aging but also HIV-care and HIV stigma. Because HIV continues to carry a stigma more intense than do other illnesses, HIV-affected individuals and families are isolated more often than others (Herek and Capitanio 1998). This isolation occurs during an extraordinarily stressful situation; instead of getting support for stress, the caregivers are in danger of intensified stress due to stigma.

HIV-affected grandparents and other elder caregivers exist in a challenging environment. First, taking care of adults and children with HIV is an emotionally stressful task because the illness is unpredictable and life threatening, and it is often a physically difficult task as well. Second, HIV-affected caregivers are often coping with concurrent stressors like poverty, substandard housing, their own health challenges, and the incarceration or drug use of adult children. Third, they are living with HIV-related stigma—a compound stigma, made up of fear of contagion and death, moral judgment, and its association with marginalized groups (Pryor and Reeder 1993). For grandparent caregivers, HIV-related stigma often occurs in the further stigmatized context of classism, racism, ageism, and sexism. As stigma piles on stigma, they become further isolated.

HIV-affected grandparents are providing emotionally and physically difficult care (even when they are aware of pervasive stigma); had not expected to be called on to parent again; and are facing many other environmental, familial, and personal stresses. It seems that our care system is content to rely on these hidden and isolated caregivers. It is true that this population demonstrates enormous strength and resilience. However, this fact should not excuse helpers from identifying them, seeking them out, and providing them practical and emotional support. Social-service professionals do not yet fully understand the mental and physical price that these caregivers pay for their valiant role. For the sake of both the HIV-affected caregivers and the HIV-affected children who depend on them, helpers must recognize them, respond to them, offer them services, help them manage stigma, and support them in their care struggles.

Notes

1. *HIV-affected* is commonly used to designate those associated with persons with HIV.

2. Social support can be informal (volunteers, friends, and/or family members), or formal (organized social and/or medical services).

3. I will refer to this concept as "HIV stigma" or "HIV-related stigma" because it is not confined to those who have received a diagnosis of AIDS, which is the symptomatic phase of HIV disease. Stigma is present for the entire spectrum of HIV illness.

4. All names of caregivers and care receivers are pseudonyms.

References

Ainlay, S. C., L. M. Coleman, and G. Becker. 1986. Stigma reconsidered. In S. C. Ainlay, G. Becker, and L. M. Coleman, eds., *The Dilemma of Difference: A Multidisciplinary View of Stigma*, pp. 1–16. New York: Plenum.

Allers, C. T. 1990. AIDS and the older adult. *The Gerontologist* 30 (3): 405–407.

Baker, L. S. 1992. The perspective of families. In M. L. Stuber, ed., *Children with AIDS*, pp. 45–67. Washington: American Psychiatric Press.

Blaney, N. T., K. Goodkin, R. O. Morgan, D. Feaster, C. Millon, J. Szapocznik, and C. Eisdorfer. 1991. A stress-moderator model of distress in early HIV-1 infection: Concurrent analysis of life events, hardiness and social support. *Journal of Psychosomatic Research* 35 (2–3): 297–305.

Blendon, R. J., and K. Donelan. 1988. Discrimination against people with AIDS. *New England Journal of Medicine* 319 (15): 1022–1026.

Boland, M. G., L. Czamiecki, and H. J. Haiken. 1992. Coordination care for children with HIV infection. In M. L. Stuber, ed., *Children with AIDS*, pp. 33–48. Washington: American Psychiatric Press.

Bor, R., R. Miller, and E. Goldman. 1993. HIV/AIDS and the family: A review of research in the first decade. *Journal of Family Therapy* 15 (2): 187–204.

Borcher, J., and C. A. Rickabaugh. 1995. When illness is perceived as controllable: The effects of gender and mode of transmission on AIDS-related stigma. *Sex Roles* 33 (9–10): 657–668.

Brown, G., J. Mitchell, and S. B. Williams. 1992. The African American community. In M. L. Stuber, ed., *Children with AIDS*, pp. 21–32. Washington: American Psychiatric Press.

Brown, M. A. (1992). Caregiver stress in families of persons with HIV/AIDS. In S. L. Feetham et al., eds., *The Nursing of Families: Theory/Research/Education/Practice*, pp. 211–223. Newbury Park, Calif.: Sage.

Brown, M. A., and G. M. Powell-Cope. 1991. AIDS family caregiving: transitions through uncertainty. *Nursing Residency* 40 (6): 338–345.

——. 1993. Themes of loss and dying in caring for a family member with AIDS. *Residential Nursing Health* 16 (3): 179–191.

Cain, R. 1991. Stigma management and gay identity development. *Social Work* 36 (1): 67–73.

Cates, J. A., L. L. Graham, D. Boeglin, and S. Tielker. 1990. The effect of AIDS on the family system. *Families in Society: The Journal of Contemporary Human Services* (April): 195–201.

Cohen, F. 1983. Stress, emotion, and illness. In L. Temoshok, C. Van Dyke, and L. S. Zegans, eds., *Emotions in Health and Illness: Theoretical and Research Foundations*, pp. 31–35. New York: Grune and Stratton.

Cohen, S., and S. L. Syme. 1985. Issues in the study and application of social support. In S. Cohen and S. L. Syme, eds., *Social Support and Health*, pp. 3–22. Orlando, Fla.: Academic Press.

Crandall, C. S. 1991. AIDS-related stigma and the lay sense of justice. *Contemporary Social Psychology* 15 (2): 66–67.

Crandall, C. S., and R. Coleman. 1992. AIDS-related stigmatization and the disruption of social relationships. *Journal of Social and Personal Relationships* 9 (2): 163–177.

Cunningham, J. A., L. C. Sobell, M. B. Sobell, S. Agrawal, and T. Toneatto. 1993. Barriers to treatment: Why alcohol and drug abusers delay or never seek treatment. *Addictive Behaviours* 18:347–353.

Denker, A. L. 1990. Stigma and the nursing care of children with AIDS. *International Conference on AIDS* 6 (3): 309.

Draimin, B. 1993. Adolescents in families with AIDS: Growing up with loss. In C. Levine, ed., *Orphans of the HIV Epidemic*, pp. 60–68. New York: United Hospital Fund.

Dubay, W. H. 1987. *Gay Identity: The Self under Ban*. Jefferson, N.C.: McFarland and Company.

Eliason, M. J. 1993. AIDS-related stigma and homophobia: Implications for nursing education. *Nurse Educator* 18 (6): 27–30.

Emlet, C. 1993. Service utilization among older people with AIDS. *Journal of Case Management* 2 (4): 119–124.

Faugier, J., and S. Wright. 1990. Homophobia, stigma and AIDS—an issue for all health care workers. *Nurse Practitioner* 3 (2): 27–28.

Goffman, E. 1959. *The Presentation of Self in Everyday Life.* Englewood Cliffs, N.J.: Prentice-Hall.

———. 1963. *Stigma: Notes on the Management of Spoiled Identity.* Englewood Cliffs, N.J.: Prentice-Hall.

Gottlieb, B. H. 1985. Social networks and social support: An overview of research, practice, and policy implications. *Health Education Quarterly* 12 (1): 5–22.

Green, G. 1993. Editorial review: Social support and HIV. *AIDS Care* 5 (1): 87–104.

———. 1995. Attitudes towards people with HIV: Are they as stigmatizing as people with HIV perceive them to it be? *Social Science and Medicine* 41 (4): 557–568.

Gutheil, I. A., and E. R. Chichin. 1991. AIDS, older people, and social work. *Social Work* 16 (4): 237–244.

Hall, B. A. 1992. Overcoming stigmatization: Social and personal implications of the human immunodeficiency virus diagnosis. *Archives of Psychiatric Nursing* 6 (3): 189–194.

Hays, R. B., H. Turner, and T. J. Coates. 1992. Social support, AIDS-related symptoms, and depression among gay men. *Journal of Consulting and Clinical Psychology* 60 (3): 463–469.

Herek, G. M. 1999. AIDS and stigma. *American Behavioral Scientist* 42 (7): 1106–1116.

Herek, G. M., and J. P. Capitanio. 1992. AIDS-related stigma persists in the United States. *International Conference on AIDS* 8 (2): D524.

———. 1993. Public reactions to AIDS in the United States: A second decade of stigma. *American Journal of Public Health* 83 (4): 574–577.

———. 1998. AIDS stigma and HIV-related beliefs in the United States: Results from a national telephone survey. Conference record of the 12th World AIDS Conference, Geneva, Switzerland.

Herek, G. M., and E. K. Glunt. 1988. An epidemic of stigma: Public reactions to AIDS. *American Psychologist* 43 (11): 886–891.

———. 1993. Public attitudes toward AIDS-related issues in the United States. In J. B. Pryor and G. D. Reeder, eds., *The Social Psychology of HIV Infection,* pp. 229–261. Hillsdale, N.J.: Lawrence Erlbaum Associates.

Herek, G. M., L. Mitnick, S. Burris, M. Chesney, P. Devine, M. T. Fullilove, R. Fullilove, H. C. Gunther, J. Levi, S. Michaels, A. Novick, J. Pryor, M. Snyder, and T. Sweeney. 1998. AIDS and stigma: A conceptual framework and research agenda. *AIDS and Public Policy Journal* 13 (1): 36–47.

Jankowski, S., L. Videka-Sherman, and K. Laquidara-Dickinson. 1996. Social support networks of confidants of people with AIDS. *Social Work* 41 (2): 206–312.

Kelly, J., J. S. St. Lawrence, S. Smith, H. Hood, and D. Cook. 1987. Stigmatization of AIDS patients by physicians. *American Journal of Public Health* 77 (7): 789–791.

———. 1988. Nurses' attitudes toward AIDS. *The Journal of Continuing Education in Nursing* 19 (2): 78–83.

Klingeman, H. K. H. 1991. The motivation for change from problem alcohol and heroin use. *British Journal of Addiction* 86:727–744.

Knox, M., and F. Clark. 1993. Early HIV detection: A community mental health care role. *AIDS Patient Care* 7: 169–172.

Kreibick, T. 1995. Caretakers' support group. In N. Boyd-Franklin, G. L. Steiner, and M. G. Boland, eds., *Children, Families, and HIV/AIDS: Psychosocial and Therapeutic Issues,* pp. 167–178. New York: Guilford.

Lang, N. 1991. Stigma, self-esteem, and depression: Psychosocial responses to risk of AIDS. *Human Organization* 50 (1): 66–72.

Laryea, M., and L. Gien. 1993. The impact of HIV-positive diagnosis on the individual, Part 1: Stigma, rejection, and loneliness. *Clinical Nursing Residency* 2 (3): 245–266.

Lesar, S., M. M. Gerber, and M. I. Semmel. 1995. HIV infection in children: Family stress, social support, and adaptation. *Exceptional Children* 62 (3): 224–236.

Lesserman, J., D. O. Perkins, and D. L. Evans. 1992. Coping with the threat of AIDS: The role of social support. *American Journal of Psychiatry* 149 (11): 1514–1520.

Levine, C. 1990. AIDS and the changing concept of family. *The Milbank Quarterly* 68 (1): 33–58.

Linn, J. G., F. M. Lewis, V. A. Cain, and G. A. Kimbrough. 1993. HIV-illness, social support, sense of coherence, and psychosocial well-being in a sample of help-seeking adults. *AIDS Education and Prevention* 5 (3): 254–262.

Lippmann, S. B., W. A. James, and R. L. Frierson. 1993. AIDS and the family: Implications for counseling. *AIDS Care* 5 (1): 71–78.

Lipson, M. 1994. Disclosure of diagnosis to children with Human Immunodeficiency Virus or Acquired Immunodeficiency Syndrome. *Developmental and Behavioral Pediatrics* 15 (3): S61–S65.

Longo, M. B., J. A. Sposs, and A. M. Locke. 1990. Identifying major concerns of persons with acquired immunodeficiency syndrome: A replication. *Clinical Nurse Specialist* 4 (1): 21–26.

Macks, J. 1993. The psychological needs of people with AIDS. In J. W. Dilley, C. Pies, and M. Helquist, eds., *Face to Face: A Guide to AIDS Counseling,* pp. 2–14. San Francisco: University of California, San Francisco.

Matocha, L. K. 1992. Case study interviews: Caring for persons with AIDS. In J. F. Gilgun, K. Daly, and G. Handel, eds., *Qualitative Methods in Family Research,* pp 66–84. Newbury Park, Calif.: Sage.

McKinlay, J. B., K. Skinner, J. W. Riley, and D. Zablotsky. 1993. On the relevance of social science concepts and perspectives. In M. W. Riley, M. G. Ory, and D. Zablotsky, eds., *AIDS in an Aging Society,* pp. 127–146. New York: Springer.

Mellins, C. A., and A. A. Ehrhardt. 1994. Families affected by pediatric Acquired Immunodeficiency Syndrome: Sources of stress and coping. *Journal of Developmental and Behavioral Pediatrics* 15 (3): S54–60.

Melvin, D., and L. Sherr. 1993. The child in the family—responding to AIDS and HIV. *AIDS Care* 5 (1): 35–42.

Minkler, M. 1985. Social support and health of the elderly. In S. Cohen and S. L. Syme, eds., *Social Support and Health,* pp. 199–216. Orlando, Fla.: Academic Press.

Minkler, M., and K. M. Roe. 1993. *Grandmothers as Caregivers: Raising Children of the Crack Cocaine Epidemic.* Newbury Park, Calif.: Sage.

Moneyham, L., B. Seals, A. Demi, R. Sowell, L. Cohen, and J. Guillory. 1995. Living with HIV: Issues of stigma and disclosure in women infected with HIV. Unpublished paper.

National Association of Social Workers. 1995. Many found daunted by clients with HIV. *NASW News,* September.

Nott, K. H., K. Vedhara, and M. J. Power. 1995. The role of social support in HIV infection. *Psychological Medicine* 25:971–983.

Ogu, C., and L. R. Wolfe. 1994. *Midlife and Older Women and HIV/AIDS.* Washington, D.C.: AARP.

Page, R. 1984. *Stigma.* London: Routledge and Kegan Paul.

Pakenham, K. I., M. R. Dadds, and D. J. Terry. 1994. Relationships between adjustment to HIV and both social support and coping. *Journal of Consulting and Clinical Psychology* 62 (6): 1194–1203.

Pearlin, L. I. 1985. Social structure and processes of social support. In S. Cohen and S. L. Syme, eds., *Social Support and Health,* pp. 43–60. Orlando, Fla.: Academic Press.

Peate, I. 1995. A question of prejudice: Stigma, homosexuality and HIV/AIDS. *Professional Nursing* 10 (6): 380–383.

Perreault, M., M. Reidy, M. E. Taggart, L. Richard, and N. Savard. 1992. Needs assessment of natural caregivers of people with HIV or AIDS. *International Conference on AIDS* 8 (2): B159.

Perryman, S. 1993. Family concerns about confidentiality and disclosure. In C. Levine, ed., *A Death in the Family: Orphans of the HIV Epidemic,* pp. 69–74. New York: United Hospital Fund.

Poindexter, C. 1997. Stigma and support as experienced by HIV-affected older minority caregivers. Ph.D. dissertation, University of Illinois at Chicago.

Poindexter, C., and N. Linsk. 1998. The sources of social support for a sample of HIV-affected older minority caregivers. *Families in Society* (Sept.–Oct.): 491–503.

——. 1999. HIV-related stigma in a sample of HIV-affected older female African-American caregivers. *Social Work* 44 (1): 46–61.

Powell-Cope, G. M., and M. A. Brown. 1992. Going public as an AIDS family caregiver. *Social Science Medicine* 34 (5): 571–580.

Pryor, J. B., and G. D. Reeder. 1993. Collective and individual representations of HIV/AIDS stigma. In J. B. Pryor and G. D. Reeder, eds., *The Social Psychology of HIV Infection,* pp. 263–286. Hillsdale, N.J.: Lawrence Erlbaum Associates.

Rapp, S. R. 1996. Benefits of caregiving: Perceptions of caregivers. Poster presented at Gerontological Society of American, 49th Annual Scientific Meeting, Washington, D.C.

Reidy, M., M. E. Taggart, and L. Asselin. 1991. Psychosocial needs expressed by the natural caregivers of HIV infected children. *AIDS Care* 3 (3): 331–343.

Sauer, W. J., and R. T. Coward. 1985. The role of social support networks in the care of the elderly. In W. J. Sauer and R. T. Coward, *Social Support Networks and the Care of the Elderly,* pp. 3–20. New York: Springer.

Schur, E. M. 1983. *Labeling Women Deviant: Gender, Stigma, and Social Control.* Philadelphia: Temple University Press.

Septimus, A. 1990. Caring for HIV-infected children and their families: Psychosocial ramifications. In G. R. Anderson, ed., *Courage to Care: Responding to the Crisis of Children with AIDS.* Washington, D.C.: Child Welfare League of America.

Sherer, R., and D. Goldberg. 1994. HIV disease and access to care: A crisis within a crisis. In A. Dula and S. Goering, eds., *"It Just Ain't Fair": The Ethics of Health Care for African Americans,* pp. 149–164. New York: Praeger.

Siminoff, L. A., J. A. Erlen, and C. W. Lidz. 1991. Stigma, AIDS and quality of nursing care: State of the science. *Journal of Advanced Nursing* 16 (3): 262–269.

Snyder, M., A. M. Omoto, and A. L. Crain. 1999. Punished for their good deeds: Stigmatization of AIDS volunteers. *American Behavioral Scientist* 42 (7): 1175–1192.

Sobell, L. C., M. B. Sobell, and T. Toneatto. 1992. Recovery from alcohol problems without treatment. In N. Heather, W. R. Miller, and J. Greeley, eds., *Self-Control and the Addictive Behaviours,* pp. 198–242. New York: Maxwell Macmillan.

Solomon, K. 1996. Psychosocial issues. In K. M. Nokes, ed., *HIV/AIDS and the Older Adult,* pp. 33–46. Washington, D.C.: Taylor and Francis.

St. Lawrence, J. S., B. A. Husfeldt, J. A. Kelly, H. V. Hood, and S. Smith Jr. 1990. The stigma of AIDS: Fear of disease and prejudice toward gay men. *Journal of Homosexuality* 19 (3): 85–101.

Turner, R. J. 1983. Direct, indirect, and moderating effects of social support on psychological distress and associated conditions. In H. B. Kaplan, ed., *Psychosocial Stress: Trends in Theory and Research,* pp. 105–155. New York: Academic Press.

Wardlaw, L. A. 1994. Sustaining informal caregivers for persons with AIDS. *Families in Society* 75 (6): 373–384.

Wiener, L. S., H. B. Battles, and N. E. Heilman. 1998. Factors associated with parents' decision to disclose the HIV diagnosis to their children. *Child Welfare* 77 (2): 115–135.

Wiener, L. S., and K. Siegel. 1990. Social worker's comfort in providing services to AIDS patients. *Social Work* (January): 18–25.

4

Death and Bereavement Issues

JOAN LEVINE-PERKELL AND BERT HAYSLIP JR.

The death of a family member, particularly one who is young, brings disorganization to people's lives and shatters the sense of security in believing that there is an orderliness to life and death—that as parents and grandparents, our children and grandchildren will outlive us. To this extent, the death of a child or grandchild is considered nonnormative (Baltes, Reese, and Nesselroade 1988) and idiosyncratic, its likelihood unanticipated. In this respect, the substantial number of AIDS deaths of young children, young adults, and middle-aged persons contradicts the common expectation that it is the old who die in our society (Kastenbaum 2000).

Over and above its nonnormative quality, the outstanding characteristic of an AIDS death of a child is its association with stigmatized behavior. The perception that one acquired HIV disease through male-to-male sexual behavior or by sharing infected needles connected to illicit drug use causes those who are either HIV positive or family caregivers to feel social stigma, shame, guilt, personal failure, or isolation from others (Kastenbaum 2000).

The impact of an HIV-related death of an adult or child and its personal and interpersonal consequences for the surviving child and older adult caregiver must be framed in terms of our culture's death system (Kastenbaum 2000). This system of beliefs and values reflects the manner in which death in general and specific causes of death are conceptualized (e.g., death is to be feared and avoided; dying persons are personally and socially inferior and therefore responsible for their deaths). As a whole, the culture's death system affects our responses to dying persons, their views about themselves, and their access to medical care and support from others. In this context, the stigma associated with AIDS and diminished support from others have important implications for those whose lives must go on after a child's death.

The bereavement adjustment of AIDS survivors is also complicated by the complicated and lengthy death trajectory of HIV disease (Corr, Nabe, and Corr 2000), which makes additional demands on the emotional, economic, spiritual, and interpersonal resources of caregivers. As the overall number of persons living with AIDS who are either African American or Hispanic exceeds that of Caucasians (Centers for Disease Control and Prevention 1999), these issues will have an increasing impact on older AIDS caregivers from these communities. Significantly, T. Rando (1992–1993) predicted that increasing rates of HIV infection would lead to a greater incidence of complicated grief and mourning (e.g., absent, delayed, or inhibited grief; extreme guilt or anger; unanticipated grief; physical or emotional illness). Because of the greater likelihood of persons living into their eighties and beyond, greater numbers of middle-aged and older adults who are experiencing complicated grief will be faced with the task of caregiving and coping with the AIDS death of a young or adult child or grandchild (Rando 1992–1993).

Lund and Caserta (1997–1998) assert that the vast majority of the literature on bereavement has failed to explore the unique impact of AIDS loss of a loved one on individuals of different generations. Because the greatest number of older adults affected by AIDS are the parents of those who are infected or who have died (Riley, Ory, and Zablotsky 1989), it is vitally important to explore the practical and psychological consequences of having adult children predecease their parents (Goodman et al. 1991). Compounding the loss of their adult children, these older caregiving parents often face the task of raising their children's children (Levine-Perkell 1996). This chapter focuses on specifics of loss that influence the bereavement experience of the older adult caregivers of AIDS orphans. To this end, it discusses the interrelated issues of grieving in general, as well as the unique problems in grieving the loss of a parent, a young child, or an adult child who has died of AIDS.

Grief and Bereavement

The experience of bereavement as described by Raphael (1983) is the reaction to the loss of a close relationship. It includes grief, the individual's feelings regarding the loss (e.g., pain and suffering experienced in order to heal and resolve the loss) and mourning, referring to the culturally patterned expressions and rituals that accompany loss and allow others to recognize that a person has become bereaved (e.g., wearing black). Normal grief reactions are somatic (disturbed sleep, loss of strength and energy, diminished appetite, headaches, difficulty in breathing), behavioral (crying, withdrawal, overdependence, inability to perform daily tasks, disinterest in work, restlessness, expression of anger), and intrapsychic/emotional (shock, emotional numbness, sadness, fear, guilt, anger, loneliness, worry, anxiety, hopelessness, helplessness, self-pity) (Cook and Oltjenbruns 1998).

Although there are universal aspects of grief, the process of grief is an individual journey (Humphrey and Zimpfer 1996). Parkes and Weiss (1983) have noted that the work of grieving is a struggle between realization of loss and retention of the lost object. They identify a critical element of healthy grief resolution as the presence of people with whom the individual can share his or her grief. The bereaved person, enriched by warm memories, is then able to forge new relationships and take on a new post bereavement identity, wherein a new relationship to the deceased individual is formed (Parkes and Weiss 1983).

In this context, Worden (1991) identifies four basic tasks of grief: (1) acceptance of the reality of the loss, (2) working through the pain of grief, (3) adaptation to life without the deceased, and (4) engagement in new relationship. Rando (1993) proposed a process of incorporating "six R's":

1. Recognizing the loss (avoidance phase)
2. Reacting to the separation from that which has been lost/experiencing the pain of loss (confrontation phase)
3. Recollecting and re-experiencing the deceased and the relationship
4. Relinquishing the old attachment
5. Readjusting to a new world without forgetting the old (accommodation)
6. Reinvesting in a meaningful life

Factors Influencing Adjustment to Loss

Because grieving is best conceived in terms of an individual in the context of relationships with others' experience, it would not be surprising to learn that one's response to loss is influenced by a number of factors that affect the intensity and course of mourning. These factors include relationship to the deceased, the nature of the attachment, the bereaved individual's history of loss, the availability of social support, the type of death that took the deceased, cultural background, and personal characteristics of the bereaved person. These influences dictate the nature of grief (whether it is complicated or pathological), its intensity, and duration (Cook and Oltjenbruns 1998).

Parkes and Weiss (1983) identified six factors that determine whether the bereavement process will be resolved, be prolonged, or become chronic:

1. MODE OF DEATH   Sudden or unexpected death elicits more intense grief than a death for which the family has had time to prepare emotionally and has experienced anticipatory grief (Sanders 1989). Typically, AIDS deaths are not sudden. However, the experience of watching a person deteriorate physically and mentally is devastating, wherein HIV infection is an emotional roller coaster as patients succumb to opportunistic infections and are left permanently damaged (Walker 1991). In this respect, while it may be said that families caring for AIDS do have the opportunity to grieve beforehand, the impact of having provided care and experienced isolation and loneliness may linger for some time (Sanders 1982). Although some AIDS patients overcome one crisis after the other, it might be argued that, as is the case with families of Alzheimer's disease, AIDS caregivers grieve several times throughout the course of the illness as their children or grandchildren deteriorate progressively.

Regardless of the cause of death, the process of dying disrupts relationships with parents, children, and spouses, interferes with one's future goals and plans, and often undermines one's sense of attractiveness and sexuality. Understandably, a terminal illness or a sudden death leaves family and friends feeling frustrated, angry, and lonely. Because death in childhood or young adulthood is nonnormative, individuals feel angry and cheated that the personal or career goals they have set for themselves are never going to be reached. If middle-aged or elderly persons have experienced the death of adult children or grandchildren, they must experience the sadness of not seeing them grow up, marry, and raise their own children (Rando 1983).

2. SYNCHRONICITY OF DEATH WITH THE EXPECTED LIFE CYCLE As discussed earlier, the death of a child is a nonnormative, "off-time" death. The deaths of children have been termed "high grief" deaths (DeSpelder and Strickland 1999)—few adults expect to bury their children.

3. THE PRESENCE OF MULTIPLE STRESSORS   Burnette (1999) found that most stressful events in the lives of custodial grandparents of color were re-

lated to multiple serious losses. For example, families in which a member has died from AIDS often have been plagued by a history of drug use, the violence of inner city life, poverty, unemployment, poor and overcrowded housing, substandard medical care, and a lack of social support. Multiple losses of loved ones from AIDS, murder, suicide, drug use, and incarceration add an overwhelming component of stress to already taxed families. As persons who have experienced multiple losses tend to respond most poorly, it is quite significant that Fuller-Thomson and Minkler (2000) found custodial grandparents to be more likely to have experienced the death of an adult child in the five years previous to their assuming parental responsibility for their grandchildren.

4. SOCIOECONOMIC CHANGES RESULTING FROM DEATH   Grandparents and other older relative caregivers of "AIDS orphans" often have to stop working or are living on fixed incomes. Families with informal kin-care arrangements function with a much lower level of support and have a higher level of unmet needs such as low financial resources (Minkler and Roe 1993), resulting from current and cumulative economic disadvantage (Burnette 1999).

5. SUPPORT AVAILABLE FROM SOCIAL NETWORKS   A lack of social support predicts a poor response to loss (Cook and Oltjenbruns 1998), and AIDS deaths encourage secrecy and isolation, born of disapproval and rejection by others (Corr, Nabe, and Corr 2000). Elderly parents of adult children who have died of AIDS must therefore deal with shame and social stigma that may cause them to withdraw from others. Fear of contagion causes families to become increasingly isolated, which causes increased stress and impairs communication between family members and friends who try to comfort them and understand their feelings. Family systems are often disrupted by the stigma of AIDS (Levine-Perkell 1996; Maj 1991; Lloyd 1989). Many parents experience the double trauma of learning about their child's homosexuality, promiscuity, or substance abuse at the same time that they learn of his or her AIDS diagnosis (Skeen, Walters, and Robinson 1988). This has been termed the "double death syndrome," where parents must deal with the loss of a "normal" child at the same time that they must deal with their child's illness and impending death because of AIDS (Carl 1986).

6. THE NATURE OF THE RELATIONSHIP TO THE DECEASED   The loss of a dependent or ambivalent relationship can cause intense, prolonged

mourning. In the case of AIDS related deaths, parents are often left with anger at their child's alternate lifestyle, feel guilty that they failed as parents, blame the deceased for becoming ill, and despair that friends and family will reject them (Levine-Perkell 1996).

Adjustment to the loss of a loved one is best expressed as a dual-process model of coping with loss as espoused by Stroebe and Schut (1995). This dual process to grief includes the response to the loss of the relationship to the deceased (a *loss orientation*), involving active grief work (e.g., a preoccupation with the death, heightened emotional responses to the individual's absence), and responses to changes in one's lifestyle and relationships with others (a *restoration orientation*). These two processes often coexist. Over time, individuals alternatively shift from one orientation to another, depending on the individual's life circumstances, needs for social support, health, or requirements to learn new life or work skills. This dual-process model asserts that there are indeed times when denial or avoidance of active grief work would be advantageous, and thus stresses the adaptability and flexibility of individuals' response to loss over time. Moreover, what constitutes a positive bereavement outcome varies along these two dimensions for many individuals. Men may adopt a more problem-focused response to loss, whereas members of various ethnic or racial groups may adopt a more loss-oriented response, where the deceased individual remains a central focus of one's life (for example, through ancestor worship). In such cases, redefining family traditions revolving around the memory of a deceased family member is important (see Stroebe 1992).

In this context, gender and culture often interact to influence bereavement. Strong female ties exist within many extended families, notably African American and Italian. The importance of these female linkage ties cannot be overestimated, especially when considering the significance of the AIDS death of a daughter. The increasing incidence of AIDS-related deaths in young African American women is putting an important family and cultural resource in jeopardy (Nikuradse 1996). According to Troll (1971), the mother-daughter bond is stronger than the mother-son, father-daughter, or father-son bond. Perhaps because of this, mothers often underestimate their daughter's use of destructive behaviors (Pillemer and Suitor 1991); they reported increased distress and more depression and viewed their children's difficulties as signs of their own failures as parents. Minkler and Roe (1993) described the caregiving grandmothers of crack-exposed grandchildren as feeling guilty and full of self-blame related to their child's drug use as well as feeling stigmatized, betrayed, angry, ambivalent, and abandoned by their daughters.

As a rule, one's gender, age, and personality characteristics all interact to influence grief, as well as the availability and acceptability of asking for support from others. Although men are often characterized as grieving less intensely or preferring to share their feelings less so than women (Lund 2001; Staudacher 1991), this is not necessarily the case. To the extent that age predicts one's ability to understand death and be able to reflect on the experience of loss, there is reason to believe that younger and older persons will grieve somewhat differently. Persons who have a history of depression or anxiety, who are intolerant of frustration, who have difficulty communicating with others, or who believe that they have no power to change themselves or events in their lives often respond to loss more poorly (Cook and Oltjenbruns 1998).

Other variables thought to influence the duration and intensity of grief include one's belief that the death was preventable and how central the relationship with the deceased is to the bereaved person (Bugen 1979). Persons who have experienced the loss of a loved one to whom they are emotionally close (psychoanalytically termed an object loss) and who believe that they could have done something to prevent the death have less adaptive responses to loss (Guarnaccia, Hayslip, and Pinkenberg-Landry 1999). In this respect, the death of a child linked to one's failure as a parent or grandparent could easily provoke intense and involved grief reactions among middle-aged and elderly caregivers.

Cultural and Subcultural Responses to AIDS Deaths

Although an in-depth exploration of the culturally diverse response to AIDS deaths is beyond the scope of this chapter, some observations can be made. The United States is a diverse, multicultural society (Burlingame 1999). Bereavement is culturally bound; even in isolation people do not grieve alone, they grieve as part of a community. Each culture has its own views on death and rituals associated with it (Dane 1992). Culturally diverse families draw on culture of origin and current culture for guidelines of family bereavement. As culturally diverse groups within the United States continue to evolve and adopt mainstream values, even families that are highly assimilated seek out the family of origin and funeral rituals that will enhance continuity with ancestral past and balance the discontinuity precipitated by the death of a family member (Shapiro 1996). Acculturation, however, can cause conflicts within a family as levels of assimilation can differ and cause cultural duality.

Families try to balance older cultural values with new ones imposed by experience, school, work, and society in general (Chackes and Jennings 1994).

Because there is little information regarding how older parents interpret the AIDS death of their adult child in ways that allow them to move on with life, cultural values can be a valuable tool in understanding reactions to loss. Beliefs, attitudes, practices, and experiences surrounding death, dying, and bereavement vary among ethnic groups (Kalish and Reynolds 1981). Cultural practices and beliefs, which may vary extensively within ethnic groups, can both facilitate and complicate the grieving process (Doka and Davidson 1998).

Little research has been directed to the historical and cultural relativity of bereavement beliefs and practice (McGoldrick et al. 1999; Shapiro 1996), grief reactions in stigmatized death (Dane and Miller 1992), or the link between mental health, grief, and religious practices among African American and Latino men, women, and children affected by AIDS. In general, research on religion and health has found that older adults who are involved in a religious community consistently demonstrated better mental and physical health (Blasi 1999; Koenig 1998). Religiosity and spirituality are positively associated with health status and coping and protect against mental disorders, depression, suicidal and life-threatening behaviors, anxiety, alienation, loneliness, and substance abuse (Imamoglu 1999). Studies involving religion and ethnicity have shown that 90 percent of African American grandmothers used prayer as a coping strategy as opposed to 60 percent of white grandmothers (Musil 2000), attend church at least once a week (52%) or more (27%) (Brown and Mars 2000), and enjoy an active personal relationship with God, which makes them feel safe, whole, and better able to cope with life's problems (Burke 1999).

In the case of AIDS-related deaths, survivors have no culturally accepted roles for mourning, which makes the successful resolution of grief extremely difficult. Though religion and spirituality play a significant role in both the African American (Brown and Mars 2000; Musil, Schrader, and Mutikani 2000; Johnson-Moore and Phillips 1994) and Latino cultures (Cox, Brooks, and Valcarcel 2000; Chackes and Jennings 1994), in recent years concerns have been raised that African American churches, traditionally the center of the community (Durkin 2000) and a source of social and emotional support for African Americans, especially women (Brown and Mars 2000; Cox, Brooks, and Valcarcel 2000) have not been doing all they could to address the issue of AIDS. As a result, the disenfranchised bereaved keep their grief, guilt, shame, and anger to themselves.

As the number of AIDS cases continues to rise in the inner cities, the African American and Latino communities are becoming doubly disenfranchised, where inner-city families are confronted daily with the negative attitude of society at large, sparse economic resources and health services, crime, drug use, and violence, all of which pose ongoing threats to their lives and create multiple losses that generate increased stress, feelings of vulnerability, guilt, and disengagement. In many inner-city communities 50 percent of the mothers of children being raised by grandmothers were intravenous drug users and/or addicted to alcohol and more likely to be dead than the child's father (Pruchno 1999). Bereavement in the inner city reflects both the strengths and resourcefulness of those who survive, as well as their sense of resignation and defeat (Murphy and Price 1998).

Disenfranchised Grief

Doka (1989) called AIDS the "great disenfranchiser," stating that AIDS has left in its wake hundreds of thousands of bereaved people who are bereft of any recognizable role or opportunity to acknowledge and share their grief publicly. Disenfranchising death can cause intense feelings of anger, guilt, and powerlessness, and such shame and embarrassment that survivors may be reluctant to avail themselves of social support (Doka 1989). It is not uncommon for AIDS deaths to occur in a "cascade effect": parents (especially females and people of color from the inner cities) are plagued by multiple recurring losses, coping with the anticipated deaths of other loved ones, and caring for the children of the deceased. The probability of these multiple losses can cause "psychic numbing." Having grandchildren who need immediate care often means that grandparents do not have time to grieve for their own children. Moreover, the stigma of AIDS often compromises traditional mourning rituals (Richmond and Ross 1995), especially in African American and Latino communities.

Anticipatory Grief

Anticipatory grief is especially relevant to caregivers of young or adult children with AIDS. Lindemann (1944) introduced the concept of anticipatory grief in his study of spousal adaptation to separation and anticipated loss during World War II (see also Sanders 1989). Siegel and Weinstein (1983) have used this term to describe the process that occurs when individuals expect a significant loss and begin their grieving in anticipation of that loss. Anticipatory grief is very different from the work of grief that follows actual loss (Turkoski and Lance 1996). Whereas grief that follows death involves the acceptance of a loss, its resolution, and a moving on with life, anticipatory grief work involves the recognition and acceptance of a future loss and the process of gradual, continued, incremental detachment (Rando 1983). Anticipatory loss is incomplete and there is no moving on until the actual death occurs.

Anticipatory grief can become pathological when it interferes with healthy communication between the dying and their loved ones, decreases the dying person's physiologic comfort, increases stress for the dying person and their loved ones, and makes resolution of grief after the actual death very difficult (Parks 1983). Cues for anticipatory grief include verbal expression of distress, choked feelings, sadness, sorrow, changes in daily habits, libido, activity level, ability to concentrate, and idealization of the anticipated loss (Carpenito 1993). It should be noted that many families deny impending death and continue to hope for recovery (Rando 1993).

For families that witness the progressive mental and physical deterioration of an AIDS patient, the feeling of profound anticipatory loss begins before the final stages of illness and is often painfully prolonged (Boyd-Franklin, Drelich, and Schwolsky-Fitch 1995). AIDS brings with it a myriad of infections and medical complications. Neuropsychological problems as well as gastrointestinal disturbances including unrelenting diarrhea, eye infections that may lead to blindness, peripheral neuropathy that causes pain in the extremities and makes ambulation difficult, chronic fevers, drenching night sweats, profound fatigue, loss of cognitive function, and the loss of muscle and body fat. As Nord (2000) notes, the development of antiviral drug combinations that have the potential to slow the progress of the disease and even to put patients into apparent remission heighten both the AIDS victim's and the caregiver's expectations for success. Yet not all patients respond to such drug combinations, and thus an increased sensitivity to such failures is possible. Such factors lessen the healthy expression of anticipatory grief.

Complicated or Pathological Grief

The frequency of complicated grief is likely to increase, given the increasing incidence of AIDS-related deaths (Rando 1992–1993), the stigmatized and isolated lives of AIDS caregivers, and the "off-time" nature of a child's death. Although "normal" behaviors associated with grief can be identified, it is almost impossible to know what constitutes "normal" behavior in the face of the "unspeakable nature of AIDS related grief" (Oerlemans-Bunn 1988). Persons bereaved by AIDS have few guidelines and resources for grief resolution. Stigma and secrecy restrict traditional grieving practices. For most bereaved individuals, feelings of isolation and alienation from others are major obstacles to asking for and receiving help. These concerns are likely to be exacerbated given the unique nature of AIDS deaths.

Complicated or pathological grief frequently involves a long-term change in the individual's typical behaviors—chronic depression, extended denial of the death, and self-abusive/self-destructive behavior and social isolation (Lindemann 1944) among them. In contrast, normal adaptive grief may or may not last for an extended period depending on a number of factors (personality, health, relationship with the deceased person, support from others). While for many persons grief follows a predictable course, adjustment to the loss of a loved one is nevertheless a complex process, composed of many emotions that necessitate changes in one's relationships with friends, family, and coworkers, others, and views about oneself, as well as impacting one's health as well as one's roles as a citizen in the community and coworker (Schuchter and Zisook 1993).

What further complicates the distinction between normal and pathological grief is the fact that grief is often composed of seemingly contradictory emotions (Stroebe, Stroebe, and Hansson 1993). One can simultaneously experience an intense desire to hold on to the image/memory of the dead loved one and yet also feel guilt, anger, or relief (Cook and Oltjenbruns 1998), and accepting contradictory emotions may predict positive bereavement outcome (Parkes and Weiss 1983). Social isolation further undermines this distinction. Williams-Conway, Hayslip and Tandy (1991) found that professionals attributed more distress and difficulty in older women's adjustment to their husbands' deaths than did widows themselves, while widows yearned more strongly for their husbands and felt more isolated than professionals judged them to feel. Thompson and Range (1990–1991) found that people could not predict the experience of suicidal bereavement regarding the amount and helpfulness of contact with others.

Complicated grief incorporates grief that is either delayed, inhibited, or absent, extreme anger or guilt, or emotional and physical illness (Rando 1992–1993). Perhaps the most distinguishing characteristic of complicated grief is its self-destructive nature; the individual's response to loss works against, rather than for, his/her health and adjustment. Especially with regard to the loss of an adult child, persons may either idealize or mummify (attempt to make things as they once were) their loss or overidentify with the deceased child (e.g., take on the symptoms of the illness from which the child died) (Rando 1986).

Weiss (1991) suggests that ambivalent feelings toward the deceased can result in distress and "obsessive reproaches" that impede emotional acceptance of loss. Inappropriate mourning often reflects negative and highly ambivalent relationships (Bowlby 1980). When an adult child dies of AIDS, many parents have negative thoughts toward the deceased, who might have been a substance abuser or engaged in sexual behaviors of which the parents disapproved. There may have been volatile disagreements that were never resolved, defiance, lies, anger, and guilt. If the deceased left children in the care of elderly parent, ambivalence is heightened even more. Unfortunately, a long illness often leaves the survivor emotionally depleted and subject to intense grief reactions by the time the loss does actually occur.

Older Adults and Grief

Late adulthood is often a period in life often thought of in terms of loss—of good health, relationships with others, and status in the community as independent and productive persons (Kastenbaum 2000). Perhaps the most important losses in later life are deaths of significant others—parents, partners, spouse, siblings, friends—and, ultimately, one's own life. Thus, bereavement becomes an ongoing part of older persons' lives (Rando 1986). Older people are likely to have had more death experiences than younger people, most frequently the loss of a spouse (Parkes 1997). By the age of sixty-five, 50 percent of women have lost their husbands; by the age of seventy-five, two-thirds are widowed (Corr, Nabe, and Corr 2000) This has several consequences: (1) the future seems more definite rather than being infinite, (2) older people may see themselves as less worthy because their future is more limited, (3) desirable roles are closed off to them, and (4) not knowing what to do with one's "bonus time" on earth, one may think that he/she has already used up what years were available. Last, as more friends and relatives die, older persons become more attuned to sadness and loneliness, and to signals from their bodies that say that death is near.

Because of the greater frequency of death in the lives of older adults, bereavement overload is a greater risk. Such persons may appear depressed, apathetic, or suffer from physical problems (Kastenbaum 1978). Because such closely spaced deaths are often sudden, persons who are left behind suffer from acute grief, commonly believed to be more difficult to cope with (Cook and Oltjenbruns 1998).

In general, several factors seem to put bereaved persons at risk for both psychological and health-related difficulties: sudden or especially violent deaths, feelings of ambivalence toward and dependence on the person who has died, poor health before bereavement, other coexisting crises in a person's life, the loss of a parent or child, and a lack of social support from others after the death (Sanders 1993). Elderly persons who coped poorly expressed lower self-esteem before bereavement, had more confusion, a greater desire to die, cried more, and were less able to keep busy shortly after the death (Lund et al. 1986–87).

Loss of An Adult Child

Approximately 10 percent of adults over the age of sixty experience the death of a grown child (Moss, Lesher, and Moss 1986–1987). Not only is the death of an adult child untimely, but a lifelong parent-child bond is also severed forever. Because this loss is comparatively rare, obtaining support from others who have experienced the loss of a grown child can be extremely difficult (Moss, Lesher, and Moss 1986–1987). If a son or a daughter had grandchildren, grandparents may have to raise these children themselves, and yet be faced with caring for themselves (Hayslip et al. 1998).

The single most agreed-on tenet in grief literature is that losing a child eclipses and diminishes other losses (Klass 1988; Pine and Braver 1986). Loss of a child symbolically reflects the loss of one's being and the loss of meaning in life, overwhelming parents with feelings of helplessness and emptiness (Florian 1989), with the death of an adult child being the most traumatic (Levine-Perkell 1996; Gorer 1965). The resulting grief is complicated because of the older parent's social isolation and physical and mental decline, and the fact that the adult child who died is likely to be viewed as irreplaceable by the parent (Brubaker 1985). The older parent may also perceive the death of an adult child as a loss of instrumental support in that this child is typically seen as the person who would have assisted the elderly parent as he or she became more dependent (Brubaker 1985). Older parents may also view their child's death as disappointing in that their expectations for the child were not fulfilled. This disappointment can be expressed as anger and cause the parent to terminate the grieving process prematurely.

Raphael (1983) found that the impact of loss is greater in later life when individuals may also be coping with age-related personal health and social losses as well as confronting their own mortality. Parents who have lost an adult child experience intense and adverse reactions for at least two years; these individuals rated their health as being poorer two to twenty years after the death of an adult child (Raphael 1983). Mothers particularly experienced depression, intense grief, despair, and rumination. They also reported increased levels of anxiety, pervasive feelings of guilt, lack of meaning or purpose in life, and decreased feelings of self-efficacy and control. These negative feelings affected their work, ability to cope, and family relations.

When an adult child dies, the entire family's relationships are affected (White 1999). Consequently, the experience of loss in middle age or late adulthood must be understood in the context of the ongoing family system and its intergenerational relationships (White 1999; Cook and Oltjenbruns 1998). Indeed, the entire family system is altered, as individuals struggle with not only their own feelings in view of the crisis that the loss of a central person in the life of the family creates, but also changes in patterns of communication and in relationships with one another. Moreover, realignments of roles must take place, often in the context of other concurrent stressors (Cook and Oltjenbruns 1998). Guilt, anger, and depression may further cloud family relationships, impede communication, and disrupt family helping patterns and family rituals.

Elderly parents and grandparents experience a profound sense of disbelief and helplessness in their inability to help their children (Reed 2000; White 1999). In general, grandmothers are more likely to discuss the death of a grandchild or adult child than are grandfathers (Ponzetti and Johnson 1991), and grandmothers are more likely to turn to daughters than to sons for comfort and support (Fry 1997; DeFrain, Jakub, and Mendosa 1991–1992).

Available work generally suggests that when a grown child (or grandchild) dies grandparents receive little support from extended family, despite the fact that they may be grieving for themselves, their grandchild, or their adult child, with parents more often providing support and help to the bereaved adult child than vice versa (White 1999). When there exists conflict between grandparents, it is likely that the loss of an adult child or grandchild will be perceived as even more stressful (White 1999). However, when family members agree on the meaning of the loss as it related to the entirety of the family, more positive bereavement outcomes can be expected (Nadeau 1998). In the event of a death due to AIDS, one might predict that these dynamics would be even more stressful. Significantly, in an extensive recent investigation of children's grief (Christ 2000), children who had lost a parent to AIDS were excluded from study.

Children and Grief

The death of a parent is generally recognized as the most stressful event that can happen to a child (Corr, Nabe, and Corr 2000). One's sense of the future and the security associated with having a parent is altered forever. Though children and adolescents vary in their response to the death of a parent as a function of age, gender of child and parent, and cause of death, a parent's death appears to have long-term negative effects on most children (Cook and Oltjenbruns 1998). A parent's death from AIDS further complicates the child's distress because it is a "disenfranchising" loss that often leaves the child overwhelmed. These children have often experienced AIDS deaths of both parents, siblings, aunts, uncles, cousins, and friends. Children who live in a family with HIV/AIDS experience stigma, shame, fear of disclosure, secrecy, multiple losses, and guilt over having survived. Parents with a diagnosis of AIDS are seen by society as undesirable, and their children feel humiliated at school and in the community. As the cause of the parent's death becomes unmentionable, isolation and alienation follow. As the disease progresses and the mental and physical deterioration of the parent becomes more acute, children become very frightened and fear for their own health and those of their siblings. They often have ambivalent feelings about their parents that can lead to excessive fear, guilt, and anger and prolong the resolution of grief. Borus et al. (1998) report that children of parents with AIDS were often anxious and demonstrated behavior problems such as increased fighting at home and at school, using illegal substances and having trouble with the criminal justice system. Children orphaned by AIDS often experience sleep disturbance, night terrors, somnambulism, and decreased self-esteem/due to their self-perception as being defective (Levy and Zelman 1996). Coping mechanisms suffer as the anger, denial, and guilt that the children feel manifest as depression and often find these children exhibiting behavioral problems at home and at school. Children often feel angry about being abandoned or neglected by the deceased parent (Havens, Mellins, and Pilowski 1996).

Children grieve episodically, relying on repression and denial as coping mechanisms to keep their grief under cover, perhaps creating the illusion in the custodial grandparent that the grandchild is over the death of the parent. Indeed, it is not unusual for a very young child to have grief work to do for some time. Many children who are considered "bad" are bereaved, and may be in dire need of professional intervention (Emick and Hayslip 1999; Halter 1996; Kaffman and Elizur 1996). Most AIDS orphans and their grandparents need the help of mental-health practitioners in a variety of settings to enable them to rebuild their lives, start new families, and form new relationships in the face of enormous stress and loss.

Emotionally exhausted and financially insecure grandparents are often ambivalent about their roles as caretakers to their dying child and parent to their grieving grandchild. As their own child becomes sicker, the fear of their death may be replaced by a wish for their death, leading to feelings of enormous guilt and shame that may never be discussed. Niederland (1981) introduced the concept of "survivor guilt" while describing a severe and persevering guilt complex affecting survivors of the holocaust (Dane 1996). Survivors developed symptoms such as anhedonia, anxiety, depression, hyperamnesia, and psychosomatic conditions and often took on personality characteristics of the deceased. For such persons, ambivalent attitudes toward the deceased were important factors in exacerbating guilt and promoting complicated grief. Guilt is experienced in AIDS survivors because of the helplessness they experience in an attempt to assume responsibility for things over which they have no control (Dane and Levine 1994). Significantly, caring for a grandchild may be a means by which the grandmother can replenish or compensate for the loss of her adult child.

The postbereavement relationship of the child and grandparent caretaker is influenced by several issues, among them how the grandmother communicates with the child regarding the death of his or her parent, how the grandmother's own grief and mourning process affects her availability to the child, and the degree to which the grandmother is able to maintain a supportive and developmentally appropriate relationship with the growing child (Borian and Zelman 1996). In this light, the grandparents' own physical condition and mourning may lead to self-absorption and withdrawal from the child. This may cause the child to become excessively fearful, isolated, alienated, angry, and unable to cope in a nontraumatic manner with the loss of the parent

(Levy and Zelman 1996). Importantly, a study by Forehand et al. (1999) indicates that if African American children whose mothers died of AIDS are cared for by maternal grandmothers in a stable home environment, their adjustment difficulties are minimized.

Custodial grandparents face more difficult adjustments when raising a grandchild who is experiencing either behavioral, emotional, or physical illness (Emick and Hayslip 1999; Hayslip et al. 1998). Middle-aged and older persons who are raising a child whose parent has died of AIDS or who is HIV-infected face especially serious challenges. They may either not understand the feelings of the child (who now feels even more vulnerable to loss) about the parent's death, or they may have strong feelings about their adult child's lifestyle. Such grandparents find it difficult to ask for help from others (Emick and Hayslip 1999). For young children who are more severely affected by a parent's death (Ravies, Siegel, and Karus 1999), seeking professional assistance is all the more critical.

Support Groups for AIDS Caregivers

Support groups can facilitate the process of grief, and greater social support is critical in the lives of AIDS caregivers. Operating outside the professional community, the early 1990s saw the birth of self-elevated support groups led by grandparents. Barbara Parkland, the founder of Grandparents United, reported that self-help groups for grandparents serve the purpose of eliminating isolation, gaining perspective, and developing a sense of empowerment (Cohen and Pyle 2000; Kirland 1992). Humphrey and Zimpfer (1996) describe a semistructured adult support group for death-related loss. The expressed goals of the group are to promote a healthy expression of grief, identify coping strategies, facilitate a sense of personal control, and introduce concepts of memorialization and reinvestment in life.

In this light, Weiner (1998) indicates that members of a support group attach a new social meaning to loss through normalization, a process of perceiving that one's thoughts, feelings, and behavior are not aberrant or unusual but are common to those undergoing the same experience. Members struggle to release themselves from guilt or regrets, establish new relationships, and remember the deceased with love in a safe, nonjudgmental environment. Support groups for middle-aged and elderly caregivers of AIDS orphans or HIV-positive adult children and grandchildren that attend to issues of grief as well as to the importance of overcoming stigma have much to offer, consistent with the dual-process model of grief discussed earlier.

In this context, the Multisystem Model of AIDS (Steiner, Boyd-Franklin, and Boland 1995) explores the impact of broader social systems in the lives of HIV/AIDS-infected and -affected children and families, wherein the response to AIDS deaths in African American and Latino communities can be better understood; such persons have been hardest hit by the epidemic and have been especially adversely affected by the stigma and secrecy of the disease. Dalton (1989) points out that the African American community distances itself from AIDS as an outgrowth of its relationship to the dominant society, which threatens people of poverty and color with virtual genocide by neglecting fundamental needs for safety, employment, housing, drug programs, nutrition, education, and adequate health care. Dalton (1989) argues that white America's response to the AIDS epidemic in the inner cities is one of maintaining power and control, treating AIDS as a special concern unrelated to the larger social ecology that nurtures it. These points are of critical importance when conceptualizing social-service programs and support groups for AIDS patients and their caregivers, especially for culturally diverse individuals who may be even less likely to seek help from persons outside their subculture.

An alternative to support groups are approaches that are more explicitly therapeutic in nature. In each case however, being with others establishes a climate of safety and trust and helps destigmatize loss. Anger, fear, sadness, and loneliness can be expressed and shared with one another as well as with the child one is caring for or with a caregiver. For example, Etty (1998) found group psychotherapy over the course of a year to improve relationship skills and school performance and lessen acting-out behavior in adolescent girls whose parent had died of AIDS. Additional goals of therapy with AIDS orphans are to lessen fears of continued abandonment (Mendelsohn 1998), as well as promote honest and open communication with the older caregiver (Ravies, Siegel, and Karus 1999). Communication includes understanding grief responses of other family members, friends, and coworkers, inasmuch as misinterpreting others' behaviors could create perceptions of social isolation and nonsupport. Essential here is the development of tolerance for others' feelings, and both attentive and noncritical listening, especially important when persons of different generations hold different views about AIDS, homosexuality, drug use, the expression of feelings, or the appropriateness of formal funeral rituals (see White 1999). In this respect, Ravies, Siegel, and Karus (1999) found bereaved children to be less depressed and anxious when they perceived their surviving parents to be open in their communication. Longman (1995) found surviving parents of adult children who died of AIDS to benefit from involvement with others through support groups, AIDS-related political causes, and personalized rituals (e.g., going to the cemetery, visiting their child's friends). Such rituals helped them celebrate their children's lives as well as gaining closure about death. For some women, gathering personal mementos or gaining a new identity through career changes were helpful, reflecting the ability to go on with their lives. Schoka and Hayslip (1999) found families that were more cohesive to be more able to discuss and express their feelings in the event of parental loss.

These themes would likely be mirrored in both individual and group psychotherapy as well as in support groups for AIDS caregivers. Additionally, sensitizing the culture at large to the experience of persons living with HIV/AIDS as well as to the stigmatizing, lonely daily existence that many AIDS caregivers face would help to redefine the context in which older AIDS caregivers deal with the emotional, interpersonal, and physical demands of caring for an AIDS orphan, a young grandchild, or an adult child dying of AIDS.

We have much to learn about how such support can be brought to bear on this newly emerging class of AIDS caregivers. Understanding the unique challenges such persons face in the view of issues about loss and grief, aging, grandparenting, and the cultural context in which losses through AIDS are experienced is a first step.

References

Baltes, P. B., H. W. Reese, and J. R. Nesselroade. 1988. *Life Span Developmental Psychology: Introduction to Research Methods.* Belmont, Calif.: Wadsworth.

Blasi, A. J. 1999. *Organized Religion and Seniors' Mental Health.* Lanham, Md.: University Press of America.

Borian, E., and A. B. Zelman. 1996. Strengthening attachment in anticipation of loss: Treatment of a paternally bereaved (due to AIDS) 5 year old girl. In A. Zelman, ed., *Early Intervention with High-Risk Children—Freeing Prisoners of Circumstance,* pp. 189–203. Northvale, N.J.: Jason Aronson.

Borus, M. J., L. Robin, H. M. Reid, and B. H. Draimin. 1998. Parent-adolescent conflict and stress when parents are living with AIDS. *Family Process* 37:83–94.

Bowlby, J. 1980. *Attachment and Loss,* vol. 3, *Loss: Sadness and Depression.* New York: Basic Books.

Boyd-Franklin, N. 1989. *Black Families in Therapy: A Multi-Systems Approach.* New York: Guilford Press.

Boyd-Franklin, N., E. W. Drelich, and E. Schwolsky-Fitch. 1995. Death and dying, bereavement and mourning. In N. Boyd-Franklin, G. Steiner, and M. G. Boland, eds., *Children, Families and HIV/AIDS—Psychosocial and Therapeutic Issues*, pp. 179–195. New York: Guilford Press.

Brown, D. R., and J. Mars. 2000. Profile of contemporary grandparenting in African American families. In C. Cox, ed., *To Grandmother's House We Go and Stay: Perspectives on Custodial Grandparents*, pp. 56–70. New York: Springer.

Brubaker, E. 1985. Older parents' reactions to the death of adult children: Implications for practice. *Journal of Gerontological Social Work* 9:35–41.

Bugen, L. 1979. *Death and Dying: Theory, Research and Practice*. Dubuque: William C. Brown.

Burke, T. C. 1999. Spirituality: A continually evolving component in women's identity development. In C. L. Thomas and S. A. Eisenhandler, eds., *Religion, Belief and Spirituality in Later Life*, pp. 113–136. New York: Springer.

Burlingame, V. S. 1999. *Ethnogerocounseling: Counseling Ethnic Elders and Their Families.* New York: Springer.

Burnette, D. 1999. Custodial grandparents in Latino families: Patterns of service use and predictors of unmet needs. *Social Work* 44:22–34.

Butler, J. 1993. *Bodies That Matter*. New York: Routledge.

Caliandro, G., and C. Hughes. 1998. The experience of being a grandmother who is the primary caregiver for her HIV positive grandchild. *Nursing Research* 47:107–113.

Carl, D. 1986. AIDS: A preliminary examination of the effects on gay couples and coupling. *Journal of Marital and Family Therapy* 12:241–247.

Carpenito, L. J. 1993. *Nursing Diagnosis: Application to Clinical Practice*. Philadelphia: J. B. Lippincott.

Carrier, J. M. 1976. Cultural factors affecting urban Mexican male homosexual behavior. *Archives of Sexual Behavior* 5:103–124.

Casper, J. M., and K. R. Bryson. 1998. *Coresident Grandparents and Their Grandchildren: Grandparent-Maintained Families*. Washington, D.C.: U.S. Bureau of the Census.

Catania, J. A., D. Binson, M. Dolcini, R. Stall, K-H Choi, L. M. Pollack, E. S. Hades, J. Canchola, K. Phillips, J. T. Moskowitz, and T. J. Coates. 1995. Risk factors for HIV and other sexually transmitted diseases and prevention practices among U.S. heterosexual adults: Changes from 1990–1992. *American Journal of Public Health* 85:1492–1499.

Centers for Disease Control and Prevention. 1997. HIV/AIDS and women in the United States. *CDC Update* (July).

Centers for Disease Control and Prevention. 1999. Characteristics of persons living with AIDS at the end of 1997. *HIV/AIDS Surveillance Supplemental Report* (February 28).

Chackes, E., and R. Jennings. 1994. Latino communities: Coping with death. In B. O. Dane and C. Levine, eds., *AIDS and the New Orphans: Coping with Death*, pp. 77–99. Westport, Conn.: Auburn House.

Christ, G. 2000. *Healing Children's Grief.* New York: Oxford University Press.

Cohen, C. S., and R. Pyle. 2000. Support groups in the lives of grandmothers raising grandchildren. In C. B. Cox, ed., *To Grandmother's House We Go and Stay: Perspectives on Custodial Grandparents*, pp. 235–252. New York: Springer.

Cook, A. S., and K. A. Oltjenbruns. 1998. *Dying and Grieving: Life Span and Family Perspectives.* Fort Worth: Harcourt Brace.

Corr, C. 1998–1999. Enhancing the concept of disenfranchised grief. *Omega* 38:1–20.

Corr, C., C. Nabe, and D. Corr. 2000. *Death and Dying, Life and Living.* Belmont, Calif.: Wadsworth.

Cox, C. B., L. R. Brooks, and C. Valcarcel. 2000. Culture and care giving: A study of Latino grandparents. In C. B. Cox, ed., *To Grandmother's House We Go and Stay: Perspectives on Custodial Grandparents,* pp. 218–232. New York: Springer.

Crawford, I., K. W. Allison, L. V. Robinson, D. Hughes, and M. Samaryk. 1992. Attitudes of African American Baptist ministers toward AIDS. *Journal of Community Psychology* 20:304–307.

Dalton, H. 1989. AIDS in black face. *Daedalus* 118:205–227.

Dane, B. O. 1996. Children, HIV infection and AIDS. In C. A. Corr and D. M. Corr, eds., *Handbook of Childhood Death and Bereavement,* pp. 51–70. New York: Springer.

Dane, B. O., and C. Levine. 1994. *AIDS and the New Orphans: Coping with Death.* Westport, Conn.: Auburn House.

Dane, B. O., and S. O. Miller. 1992. Intervening with inner city survivors of AIDS. In *AIDS: Intervening With Hidden Grievers,* pp. 131–152. Westport, Conn.: Auburn House.

DeFrain, J., D. Jakub, and B. Mendosa. 1991–1992. The psychological effects of sudden infant death on grandmothers and grandfathers. *Omega* 24:165–182.

DeSpelder, L., and A. Strickland. 1999. *The Last Dance: Encountering Death and Dying.* Palo Alto, Calif.: Mayfield.

Doka, K. J. 1989. *Disenfranchised Grief.* New York: Lexington.

Doka, K. J., and J. D. Davidson, eds. 1998. *Living with Grief: Who We Are, How We Grieve.* Philadelphia: Brunner Mazel.

Durkin, B. J. 2000. Church gets involved in AIDS education. *Newsday,* March 12, 2000.

Emick, M., and B. Hayslip. 1999. Custodial grandparenting: Stresses, coping skills, and relationships with grandchildren. *International Journal of Aging and Human Development* 48:35–61.

Etty, C. 1998. Traumatized and impoverished minority female adolescents facing parental loss through AIDS: Theoretical and clinical consideration. *Dissertation Abstracts International* 58 (9A): 3722.

Florian, V. 1989. Meaning and purpose in life of bereaved parents whose son fell during active military service. *Omega* 20:91–102.

Forehand, R., J. Pelton, M. Chance, and L. Armistead. 1999. Orphans of the AIDS epidemic in the United States: Transition-related characteristics and psychosocial adjustment at 6 months after mother's death. *AIDS Care* 11:715–722.

Fry, P. S. 1997. Grandparents' reactions to the death of a grandchild: An exploratory factor analytic study. *Omega* 35:119–140.

Fuller-Thomson, E., and M. Minkler. 2000. America's grandparent caregivers: Who are they? In B. Hayslip and R. Goldberg-Glen, eds., *Grandparents Raising Grandchildren: Theoretical, Empirical, and Clinical Perspectives,* pp. 3–22. New York: Springer.

Gilbert, S. 1988. Rising stress of raising a grandchild. *New York Times,* July 28, 1988, F7.

Goodman, M., R. L. Rubenstein, B. B. Alexander, and M. Luborsky. 1991. Cultural differences among elderly women coping with the death of an adult child. *Journal of Gerontology* 46:S321–S329.

Gorer, G. 1965. *Death, Grief and Mourning.* London: Cresset Press.

Guarnaccia, C., B. Hayslip, and L. Pinkenberg-Landry. 1999. Influence of perceived preventability of death and emotional closeness to the deceased on grief: A test of Bugen's model. *Omega* 39:261–276.

Halter, B. S. 1996. Children and the death of a parent or grandparent. In C. A. Corr and D. M. Corr, eds., *Handbook of Childhood Death and Bereavement,* pp. 131–148. New York: Springer.

Hansell, P. S., C. B. Hughes, G. Caliandro, P. Russo, W. C. Budin, B. Hartman, and O. C. Hernandez. 1998. The effect of a social support intervention on stress, coping, and social support of children living with HIV/AIDS. *Nursing Research* 47:79–86.

Havens, J., C. Mellins, and D. Pilowski. 1996. Mental health issues in HIV-affected women and children. *International Review of Psychiatry* 8:217–225.

Hawkins, P. S. 1993. Naming names: The art of memory and the Names Project AIDS quilt. *Critical Inquiry* 19:752–779.

Hayslip, B., R. Shore, C. Henderson, and P. Lambert. 1998. Custodial grandparenting and grandchildren with problems: Their impact on role satisfaction and role meaning. *Journal of Gerontology* 53B:S164–S174.

Hughes, C., and G. Caliandro. 1996. Effects of social support, stress and level of illness in care giving of children with HIV/AIDS. *Journal of Pediatric Nursing* 11:347–358.

Humphrey, G., and D. G. Zimpfer. 1996. *Counseling for Grief and Bereavement.* London: Sage.

Imamoglu, C. O. 1999. Some correlates of religiosity among Turkish adults and elderly within a cross-cultural perspective. In C. L. Thomas and S. A. Eisenhandler, eds., *Religion, Belief and Spirituality in Late Life,* pp. 93–110. New York: Springer.

Imber-Black, E. 1991. Rituals and the healing process. In F. Welsh and M. McGoldrick, eds., *Living Beyond Loss: Death in the Family,* pp. 207–223. New York: W. W. Norton.

Johnson-Moore, P., and L. J. Phillips. 1994. Black American communities coping with death. In B. O. Dane and C. Levine, eds., *AIDS and the New Orphans: Coping With Death,* pp. 100–120. Westport, Conn.: Auburn House.

Joslin, D. 2000. Grandparents raising children orphaned and affected by HIV/AIDS. In C. Cox, ed., *To Grandmother's House We Go and Stay: Perspectives on Custodial Grandparents,* pp. 167–183. New York: Springer.

Joslin, D., and R. Harrison. 1998. The "hidden patient": Older relatives raising children orphaned by AIDS. *Journal of the American Medical Women's Association* 53:65–71.

Kaffman, M., and E. Elizur. 1996. Bereavement as a significant stressor in children. In C. Pfeffer, ed., *Severe Stress and Mental Disturbance in Children,* pp. 203–229. Washington, D.C.: American Psychiatric Press.

Kalish, R. A., and D. K. Reynolds. 1981. *Death and ethnicity: A Psychocultural Study.* Amityville, N.Y.: Baywood.

Kastenbaum, R. 1978. Death, dying, and bereavement in old age. *Aged Care and Services Review* 1:1–10.

———. 2000. *Death, Society, and Human Experience.* Boston: Allyn and Bacon.

Kivett, V. R. 1991. Centrality of the grandfather role among older rural black and white men. *The Journal of Gerontology* 46:S250–S258.

Klass, D. 1988. *Parental Grief: Solace and Resolution.* New York: Springer.

Kirland, B. 1992. Definition of self help group. *Grandparents United Newsletter* (February), p. 1.

Koenig, H. G. 2000. The importance of religious community to older adults: Religion and spirituality in America. *The Gerontologist* 40:112–155.

Levine-Perkell, J. 1996. Care giving issues. In C. Nokes, ed., *HIV/AIDS and the Older Adult*, pp. 115–128. New York: Taylor and Francis.

Levy, A., and A. B. Zelman. 1996. The use of parentally bereaved adolescents as therapeutic assistants in group for parentally bereaved children. In A. Zelman, ed., *Early Intervention with High Risk Children*, pp. 173–188. Northvale, N.J.: Jason Aronson.

Lindemann, E. 1944. Symptomatology and management of acute grief. *American Journal of Psychiatry* 101:141–148.

Lloyd, G. A. 1989. Aids and elders: Advocate, activism and coalitions. *Generations* 32:32–39.

Longman, A. J. 1995. "Connecting and disconnecting: Bereavement experiences of six mothers whose sons died of AIDS. *Health Care for Women International* 16:85–95.

Lund, D. 2001. *Men Coping With Grief.* Amityville, N.Y.: Baywood.

Lund, D., and Caserta, M. 1997–1998. Future directions in adult bereavement research. *Omega* 36:287–304.

Lund, D., M. Caserta, and M. Dimond. 1986. Gender differences through two years of bereavement among the elderly. *The Gerontologist* 26:314–320.

Lund, D., M. Dimond, M. Caserta, R. Johnson, J. Poulton, and J. Connelly. 1986–1987. Identifying elderly with coping difficulties after two years of bereavement. *Omega* 16:213–224.

Macks, J., and D. Abrams. 1992. Burnout among HIV/AIDS health care providers helping the people on the front lines. *AIDS Clinical Review* 9:281–299.

Maj, M. 1991. Psychological problems of families and health workers dealing with people infected with Human Immunodeficiency Virus. *Acta Psychiatrica Scandinavica* 83:161–168.

McGoldrick, M., P. Moore Hines, N. Garcia-Preto, R. Almeida, E. Rosen, and E. Lee. 1999. Mourning in different cultures. In F. Walsh and M. McGoldrick, eds., *Living Beyond Loss: Death in the Family*, pp. 176–206. New York: W. W. Norton.

Mendelsohn, A. 1997. Pervasive traumatic loss from AIDS in the life of a 4-year-old African boy. *Journal of Child Psychotherapy* 23:399–415.

Minkler, M., and K. M. Roe. 1993. *Grandmothers as Caregivers: Raising Children of the Crack Cocaine Epidemic.* Newbury Park, Calif.: Sage.

Moss, M. S., E. L. Lesher, and S. Z. Moss. 1986–1987. Impact of the death of an adult child on elderly parents: Some observations. *Omega* 17:209–218.

Murphy, P. A., and D. M. Price. 1998. Dying and grieving in the inner city. In K. J. Doka and J. D. Davidson, eds., *Living with Grief: Who We Are, How We Grieve*, pp. 113–120. Amityville, N.Y.: Baywood.

Musil, M., S. Schrader, and J. Mutikani. 2000. Social support, stress and special coping tasks of grandmother caregivers. In C. Cox, ed., *To Grandmother's House We Go and Stay: Perspectives on Custodial Grandparents*, pp. 56–70. New York: Springer.

Myerhoff, B. 1978. *Number Our Days.* New York: Simon and Schuster.

Nadeau, J. 1998. *Families Making Sense of Death.* Thousand Oaks, Calif.: Sage.

Niederland, W. G. 1981. The survivor syndrome: Further observations and dimensions. *Journal of the American Psychoanalytic Association* 29:413–426.

Nikuradse, T. 1996. *My Mother Had a Dream: African American Women Share Their Mothers' Words of Wisdom.* New York: Dutton.

Nord, D. 2000. *Multiple AIDS-Related Loss: A Handbook for Surviving a Perpetual Fall.* Washington, D.C.: Taylor and Francis.

Oelermans-Bunn, M. 1988. On being gay, single and bereaved. *American Journal of Nursing* 88:472–477.

Parkes, C. 1997. Bereavement and mental health in the elderly. *Review in Clinical Gerontology* 7:47–53.

Parkes, C. M., and R. S. Weiss. 1983. *Recovery from Bereavement.* New York: Basic Books.

Pillemer, K., and J. J. Suitor. 1991. Relationships with children and distress in the elderly. In K. Pillemer and T. McCartney, eds., *Parent-Child Relations Throughout Life,* pp. 163–178. Hillsdale, N.J.: Lawrence Erlbaum.

Pine, V. R., and C. B. Braver. 1986. Parental grief: A synthesis of theory, research and intervention. In T. Rando, ed., *Parental Loss of a Child,* pp. 257–268. Champaign, Ill.: Research Press.

Poe, L. M. 1992. Black grandparents as parents. Unpublished manuscript.

Poland, J. S. 1991. Helping families with anticipatory loss. In F. Walsh and M. McGoldrick, eds., *Living Beyond Loss Death in the Family,* pp. 144–163. New York: W. W. Norton.

Pollock, S. W., and C. L. Thompson. 1995. The HIV-infected child in therapy. In N. Boyd-Franklin, C. L. Steiner, and M. G. Boland, eds., *Children, Families and HIV/AIDS: Psychosocial and Therapeutic Issues,* pp. 127–141. New York: Guilford.

Ponzetti, J., and M. Johnson. 1991. The forgotten grievers: Grandparents' reactions to the death of a grandchild. *Death Studies* 15:157–167.

Pruchno, R. 1999. Raising grandchildren: The experience of black and white grandmothers. *The Gerontologist* 39:209–222.

Rando, T. A. 1983. An investigation of grief and adaptation in parents whose children have died from cancer. *Journal of Pediatric Psychology* 8:3–20.

——. 1986. Death of the adult child. In T. Rando, ed., *Parental Loss of a Child,* pp. 221–238. Champaign, Ill.: Research Press.

——. 1992–1993. The increasing prevalence of complicated mourning: The onslaught is just beginning. *Omega* 26:43–60.

——. 1993. *Treatment of Complicated Mourning.* Champaign, Ill.: Research Press.

Raphael, B. 1983. *The Anatomy of Bereavement.* New York: Basic Books.

Ravies, V. H., K. Siegel, and D. Karus. 1999. Children's psychological distress following the death of a parent. *Journal of Youth and Adolescence* 28:165–180.

Reed, M. 2000. *Grandparents Cry Twice: Help for Bereaved Parents.* Amityville, N.Y.: Baywood.

Richmond, B., and W. Ross. 1995. Responses to AIDS-related bereavement. In L. Sherr, ed., *Grief and AIDS,* pp. 161–179. Chichester: Wiley.

Riley, M. W., M. G. Ory, and D. Zablotsky. 1989. *AIDS in an Aging Society: What We Need to Know.* New York: Springer.

Sanders, C. 1982. Effects of sudden vs. chronic illness death on bereavement outcome. *Omega* 13:227–241.

——. 1989. *Grief: The Mourning After.* New York: Wiley.

——. 1993. Risk factors in bereavement outcome. In M. Stroebe, W. Stroebe, and R. Hansson, eds., *Handbook of Bereavement: Theory, Research, and Intervention,* pp. 255–267. Cambridge: Cambridge University Press.

Schoka, E., and B. Hayslip. 1999. Grief and the family system: The roles of communication, affect, and cohesion. Paper presented at the Annual Scientific Meeting of the Gerontological Society, San Francisco.

Schuchter, S., and S. Zisook. 1993. The course of normal grief. In M. Stroebe, W. Stroebe, and R. Hansson, eds., *Handbook of Bereavement: Theory, Research and Intervention,* pp. 23–43. Cambridge: Cambridge University Press.

Shapiro, E. R. 1996. Family, bereavement and cultural diversity: A social developmental perspective family process. *Omega* 35:313–332.

Shaw, D. F. 1998. Women and the AIDS memorial quilt. In N. L. Rose and L. K. Fuller, ed., *Women and AIDS: Negotiating Safer Practices, Care, and Representation,* pp. 211–229. New York: Harrington Press.

Siegel, K., and L. Weinstein. 1983. Anticipatory grief reconsidered. *Journal of Psychosocial Oncology* 1:61–73.

Skeen, P., L. Walters, and B. Robinson. 1988. How parents of gays react to their children's homosexuality and to the threat of AIDS. *Journal of Psychosocial Nursing* 26:7–10.

Staudacher, C. 1991. *Men and Grief.* Oakland, Calif.: New Harbinger Publications.

Steiner, G. L., N. Boyd-Franklin, and M. G. Boland. 1995. *Children, Families and HIV/AIDS Psychosocial and Therapeutic Issues.* New York: Guilford Press.

Stroebe, M. 1992. Coping with bereavement: A review of the grief work hypothesis. *Omega* 26:19–42.

Stroebe, M., and H. Schut. 1995. The dual process model of coping with loss. Paper presented at the International Work Group on Death, Dying, and Bereavement, St. Catherine's College, Oxford University.

Stroebe, M., W. Stroebe, and H. Hansson. 1993. *Handbook of Bereavement: Theory, Research, and Intervention.* New York: Cambridge University Press.

Taylor, R. J. 1986. Religious participation among elderly blacks. *The Gerontologist* 26:630–636.

Thompson, K. E., and L. M. Range. 1990–1991. Recent bereavement from suicide and other deaths: Can people really imagine it as it is? *Omega* 28:249–260.

Troll, I. 1971. Family of later life: A decade review. In C. Broderick, ed., *A Decade of Family Research and Action,* pp. 187–214. Washington, D.C.: National Council of Family Relations.

Turkoski, B., and B. Lance. 1996. The use of guided imagery with anticipatory grief. *Home Health Care Nurse* 14:878–888.

Walker, G. 1991. *In the Midst of Winter: Systemic Theory with Families, Couples and Individuals with AIDS Infection.* New York: W. W. Norton.

Weiner, L. S. 1998. Telephone support groups for HIV-positive mothers whose children have died of AIDS. *Social Work* 43:279–285.

Weiss, R. W. 1991. The attachment bond in childhood and adulthood. In C. M. Parkes, J. Stevenson-Hinde and P. Marris, ed., *Attachment Across the Life Cycle,* pp. 66–76. London: Routledge.

White, D. L. 1999. Grandparent participation in times of family bereavement. In B. Dries, ed., *End of Life Issues,* pp. 145–165. New York: Springer.

Williams-Conway, S., B. Hayslip, and R. Tandy. 1991. Similarity of perceptions of bereavement experiences between widows and professionals. *Omega* 23:35–49.

Worden, J. W. 1991. *Grief Counseling and Grief Therapy: A Handbook for the Mental Health Practitioner.* 2d ed. New York: Springer.

5

Physical Health and Emotional Well-Being

DAPHNE JOSLIN AND RUTH HARRISON

Hazel Crooks,[1] a fifty-eight-year-old African American woman, is raising her three grandsons, ages sixteen, fifteen, and ten, in a New Jersey housing project. She also cares for her daughter, the boys' mother, who is dying of AIDS. Now working part-time because of family responsibilities, her daily life is organized by surrogate parenting, maintaining a household for five people on $24,000 a year, and addressing her daughter's need for ongoing personal care. Acknowledging her diminished stamina and strength, her emotional anguish is stark as she explains her helplessness in the face of her daughter's failing health and AIDS-phobic taunts of her grandsons by other children. She has no answers for her grandsons' questions, "Is she dying? Will she die soon?" "I tell them she could. I'm always crying because I can't answer them."

When asked to rate her own health, she answers "fair." It is worse than it was a year ago. Nodding to the living room where her daughter sleeps on the couch, she says tearfully, "I'm dealing with my daughter's poorer health. I look at her and that bothers me, because she was once up and around. This past year has been very hard on me. She was in the hospital, very sick and it was very hard."

Self-reported chronic health problems include high blood pressure, arthritis, and angina (which she describes as being "under control"). Dizziness, shortness of breath, back pain, nervousness, and disabling severe headaches—"sometimes I can't life my head"—are somatic complaints. She is also depressed and is seeking counseling for herself and her grandsons.

Suffering from obesity, she has gained weight over the past year and is getting less exercise. She knows that being overweight may contribute to back and leg pain and shortness of breath, yet is reluctant to say that health problems interfere with caregiving responsibilities. Moreover, she states that she has enough time for her own health, pointing out that when she gets a headache, she tries to sit down and rest. However, instead, of walking with a friend each day before going to work as she used to do, she now uses that time for preparing breakfast for her grandsons and making sure each day that they get off to school. "I want to be sure that everything is just so," she says. "They appreciate what I do for them. . . . But I want to start walking again."

At fifty-eight, she is too young for Medicare and has no health insurance because she is employed only part-time. She says she receives adequate medical attention from a local hospital clinic when she needs care. Her only self-reported unmet health need is mental-health counseling for her depression. Greater concern is expressed about the lack of health insurance for her grandsons, particularly for dental care and for primary care for the thirteen-year-old, who is also asthmatic.

Social class, ethnicity, age, and gender as interwoven hierarchies of privilege and disadvantage (Stoller and Gibson 1997) place Hazel Crooks at increased risk for compromised health. African Americans have a greater prevalence of chronic disease, poorer self-reported health, and greater functional limitations (Clark and Gibson 1997; Markides and Black 1996; Barresi and Stull 1993; Belgrave, Wykle, and Choi 1993), as do women (National Center for Health Statistics 1995), Latinos (U.S. Bureau of the Census 1990; U.S. Department of Health and Human Services 1991) and those with low income (National Center for Health Statistics 1994; U.S. Department of Health and Human Services 1991). Although not yet in her sixties, with three chronic health problems—arthritis, hypertension, and angina—Ms. Crooks reports more health conditions than the average of 1.6 found in a national sample of individuals sixty-five and older (Rice and LaPlante 1988) and the 2.6 chronic problems found in another sample of persons fifty-five years and older (Verbrugge, Lepkowski, and Imanaka 1989). At the same time, self-care for chronic and stress-related conditions is constrained by her responsibility as the sole caregiver to her dying daughter, her own grief, attention to her grandson's anticipatory grief, low household income, and lack of health insurance.

Overall, surrogate parents to HIV-affected children may be healthier than their counterparts who are unable or unwilling to assume this responsibility. In observing grandparents raising children of the crack cocaine epidemic, Minkler and Roe (1993) cite health as a possible "selection factor" in determining parental surrogacy. This heartiness, of course, is both objective and relative; that is, individuals may assume this role despite health problems or disability. One sole parental surrogate for two affected adolescent grandchildren in New Jersey was medically and functionally eligible for adult day care by virtue of her diagnosis of Parkinson's disease. Nonetheless, as relatively "healthy and hearty," HIV affected parental surrogates are potentially "hidden patients" (Joslin and Harrison 1998; Fengler and Goodrich 1979) whose own health needs are likely to be neglected. The implications are serious. Will health problems prevent them from serving as surrogate parents over a number of years, until children are no longer minors? Even if able to continue in this role, will parental surrogacy and HIV care leave these aging adults more vulnerable to health problems and diminished functional capacity? Beyond noting these risks, can we develop policies and programs that will promote their physical and emotional health?

This chapter examines caregivers' physical and emotional well-being, with attention to self-reported health, stress-related conditions, chronic health problems, and depression. Help-seeking, self-care, and access to medical care are discussed, drawing on findings from an exploratory study. Implications for outreach, health promotion, program development, and policy initiatives conclude the chapter.

Physical Health and Well-being

HIV-affected older surrogate parents face compounded health risks, given the multiple roles they assume, as "skipped generation" parents, often to chronically ill children, as caregivers to persons with HIV disease, and as the bereaved.

Whether because of a lifetime of poor health, caregiving stress-exacerbated chronic health problems, or greater likelihood of low income, custodial grandparents report poorer health than noncaregiving grandparents (Marx and Solomon 2000; Minkler and Fuller-Thomson 1999; Fuller-Thomson, Minkler, and Driver 1997; Strawbridge et al. 1997), experience multiple chronic illnesses (Burnette 1999; Grant 1997) fatigue (Minkler and Roe 1993; Burton 1992). Because custodial grandparents are likely to be poor and to have a history of economic disadvantage (Fuller-Thomson, Minkler, and Driver 1997; Strawbridge et al. 1997), many assume the caregiving role with existing health problems. Decreased stamina, lack of respite from the child, and the physical demands of running a household leave many grandparents without adequate time for rest, relaxation, or even time or energy for their own health (Grant, Gordon, and Cohen 1997). Economic pressures, anxiety over grandchildren's physical and emotional health and unsafe neighborhoods, conflict with the children's neglectful or addicted parents, and children's behavioral problems set the stage for persistent somatic symptoms, such as headaches, backaches, gastrointestinal disorders, shortness of breath (Kelley 1993; Kelley and Damato 1995), and exacerbated chronic health conditions such as hypertension, diabetes, asthma, and heart disease (Grant 1997). Not surprisingly, custodial grandparents report lower satisfaction with their own health and significantly more limitations in activities of daily living, such as climbing stairs, doing heavy housework, walking, or even getting around their own home (Minkler and Fuller-Thomson 1999). Women who are alone and raising grandchildren were more likely to report poor health, activity limitations, and health conditions (Marx and Solomon 2000).

Unlike other custodial grandparents and other elder relative caregivers, those raising HIV-affected and orphaned children, like Hazel Crooks, often assume parental surrogacy as they care for an ill or dying adult child. Chapter 7 examines the issues caregivers face in raising infected children and adolescents. The physical, emotional, and financial demands associated with AIDS caregiving can be overwhelming. Caregivers take on a variety of tasks, including personal assistance with bathing, feeding, toileting, transferring, transportation or escort, infection control, medication and pain management, coordinating medical appointments, and interacting with physicians, nurses, social workers, counselors, case managers, and public-benefits staff. While the new antiretroviral therapies extend life and improve its quality, they require precise adherence to drug and food regimens. The caregivers may find themselves stretched between visiting a hospitalized dying or seriously ill adult child or grandchild while worrying about the children at home. As one New York City grandmother stated, "No matter where I was, it wasn't the right place when [my granddaughter] was hospitalized [because her brother and sister were still at home]. I couldn't leave her alone in the hospital but I felt guilty when I had to leave the others alone. I was exhausted from running back and forth, trying to be sure everyone ate and got attention."

Although gerontological research has not established a strong relationship between physical health and caring for a chronically ill family member, greater chronicity and poorer self-reported health are evident in some caregiver populations (Schulz et al. 1995; Wight, Clipp, and George 1993). Among HIV caregivers, myriad somatic symptoms have been identified, including chronic fatigue, physical exhaustion, backaches, headaches, shortness of breath, gastrointestinal complaints, and general malaise (Wight, LeBlanc, and Aneshensel 1998; LeBlanc, London, and Aneshensel 1997; Ravis and Siegel 1989; Turner and Pearlin 1989). In one longitudinal study (LeBlanc, London, and Aneshensel 1997), female AIDS caregivers experienced a greater number of physical health problems than did male caregivers. Fluctuations in the clinical course of HIV disease (Siegel and Krauss 1991; Weitz 1989)—its unpredictable peaks and remission—are reflected in the intensification and easing of stress over the course of HIV caregiving (Pearlin, Aneshensel, and LeBlanc 1997). As earlier diagnosis and more effective therapies extend the disease trajectory (Wight, LeBlanc, and Aneshensel 1998), caregiver health may be compromised because of long-term caregiving (Theis et al. 1997). Physical well-being declined more among female caregivers with lengthy HIV-caregiving careers than among those with relatively short care trajectories (Wight, LeBlanc, and Aneshensel 1998). Moreover, because older surrogate parents, especially in African American and Latino communities, often care for one or more infected adult children and grandchildren, serial or multiple caregiving may exacerbate stress effects (LeBlanc, London, and Aneshensel 1997).

Although death of a close relation is associated in some studies with greater risk of illness through depressed immune function and the inception of chronic disease, data are inconclusive. Bereavement effects on the physical well-being of elder AIDS caregivers are not fully known.

Self-Reported Physical Health, Chronic Conditions and Self-Care

At the end of the pandemic's second decade, the physical well-being of older HIV affected surrogate parents continues to be neglected in research, program and policy. No studies using large, random samples nor longitudinal methods have been conducted. This chapter uses selected findings from an exploratory study of twenty caregivers living in northern New Jersey. Study description appears elsewhere (Joslin and Harrison 1998; Joslin, Mevi-Triano, and Berman 1997). The purpose of the study was to gather descriptive information on self-reported physical and emotional health, chronic health problems, somatic complaints, self-care behaviors, health insurance, and use of medical care. Through semistructured questions participants were asked about the adequacy of time for their own health needs, self-care practices, and the impact of health on daily activities.

Study participants were surrogate parents to affected or orphaned children who were identified through an HIV medical treatment, home care, or social service program in Passaic County, New Jersey. Two-fifths of the caregivers had exclusive responsibility for the affected/orphaned children and 85 percent (N = 17) were the primary caregiver. Where the older adult did not report himself or herself as the primary caregiver, the child's mother, living with HIV disease, was so identified. Six participants had lost an adult child to AIDS within the year and three others were caring for an adult child with AIDS at the time of the interview. Serial and dual caregiving was reflected in several cases. The sample's mean age of 59.6 closely paralleled other studies of grandparents as parents with random (mean age 55: Joslin and Brouard 1995) and convenience sampling (mean age 53: Minkler and Roe 1993; mean age 63: Burnette 1997). Although more than one half reported household income below $19,500 a year, sample data showed some class heterogeneity, with three caregivers being upper-middle income and living in relatively affluent suburban communities.

Fifty-five percent of the sample assessed their physical health as either "fair" or "poor," with 45 percent reporting it as either "excellent" or "good." These global health ratings are slightly worse than those of grandmothers raising crack cocaine-affected children, where one-half reported "fair" to "poor" health (Minkler, Roe, and Price 1992). More dramatic is the comparison with national data, where "excellent" or "good" health was reported by 70 percent of persons age sixty and older (National Center for Health Statistics 1990). A decline in physical well-being over the past year was reported by more than one half of the HIV-affected surrogate parents, compared with less than one-third of the grandmothers affected by the crack cocaine epidemic (Minkler, Roe, and Price 1992); 40 percent reported their health as unchanged. Only one grandmother reported improved health.

Although drawn from a small, nonrandom sample, the health profile of these HIV-affected caregivers marks them as a "high health risk population" with other older surrogate parents (Joslin and Brouard 1995; Minkler and Roe 1993; Burton 1992). Ninety percent reported at least one chronic condition, and 65 percent reported a minimum of two. These prevalence data are comparable to those found among New York City custodial parents using a school-based clinic in East Harlem (Grant 1997). HIV-affected surrogate parents averaged 3.4 chronic conditions (range 0–7), a striking finding when considered against the mean in the two national samples cited earlier. Arthritis (75%), hypertension (45%), and heart disease (30%) were most frequently reported by HIV-affected surrogate parents, followed by diabetes and osteoporosis (15% each). Somatic symptoms included ulcers, stomach problems, headaches, heart palpitations, shortness of breath, chest pains, and dizziness. Ninety percent reported some somatic complaint within the past six months, often requiring immediate rest.

Although poor health and chronic disease may have existed before parental surrogacy, the stressful circumstances of HIV caregiving and surrogate parenting may precipitate onset of or exacerbate chronic conditions. Subgroups of HIV-affected surrogate parents appeared to be more vulnerable. Those with exclusive childrearing responsibility or raising more than one child and/or with lower income households reported poorer global health, physical health decline, and more chronic diseases. Those raising an infected child were more likely to report their health as having deteriorated over the past year. Although caregivers age sixty and older in this sample tended to have more positive global self-reported health and fewer chronic conditions when compared with those age fifty-nine and younger, the physical stamina of the older caregivers may be severely taxed. Forty-five percent gave negative global health ratings, and more than one-half saw their health as worse than in the previous year.

Self-Care Barriers

In recognizing the value of health promotion for older adults, greater attention is being given to *self-care,* as "intentional behavior that a lay person takes on his or her own behalf . . . to promote health or to treat illness" (Levin, Katz, and Holtz 1979), consisting of those activities "to recognize, prevent, treat and manage . . . health problems" (Mettler and Kemper 1993). Because advanced age increases the risk of chronic illness, self-care by older adults is likely to be aimed at not only preventing disease and improving or maintaining health but also at managing chronic illness and its effects (Mockenhaupt 1993). Self-care behaviors include monitoring blood glucose levels if diabetic, engaging in moderate exercise under physician care to manage hypertension, reducing dietary fat to prevent cardiovascular disease, and exercising to reduce the effects of arthritis.

Despite the health problems named earlier, self-care by custodial grandparents is often absent. Instead, custodial grandparents often neglect their own health, diminish its importance, minimize the severity of health conditions, or delay seeking medical attention (Joslin and Harrison 1998; Joslin and Brouard 1995; Minkler and Roe 1993). They may pride themselves on being able to continue as surrogate parents in spite of health problems and chronic pain or inflate their self-assessed health in order to demonstrate their capacity for childrearing, fearful that child welfare authorities might place the child in foster care (Minkler and Roe 1993). All-consuming childrearing and household-management tasks, often on an inadequate income, may overshadow caregivers' attention to their own health needs. As a result, many older surrogate parents lack sufficient time to care for their own health, even to keep medical appointments (Joslin and Brouard 1995; Minkler and Roe 1993). For some, lack of self-care is expressed through unhealthy coping behaviors, such as increased alcohol or tobacco use (Minkler and Roe 1993; Burton 1992).

HIV-affected surrogate parents were asked whether they had sufficient time for their own health and how they coped with their own health problems. Qualitative data from semistructured questions were analyzed through multiple readings of transcribed interviews. Emergent themes were identified which provide a understanding of the complex ways in which individuals perceive their own health needs and define their capacity to respond to them. As Portney and Watkins (1993) observed, a qualitative approach provides a means of understanding "the nature of people's transactions with themselves, others and their surroundings" (p. 239). Although the majority reported having access to medical care (health insurance and regular physician care), less than one-third (N = 6) had sufficient time for exercise, relaxation, medical visits, proper nutrition, and sleep. The remainder either completely lacked adequate time (30%) or only "sometimes" had sufficient time (40%). Nearly all who were raising more than one child reported having insufficient time. Surprisingly, a greater proportion of those without exclusive responsibility reported lacking sufficient time, compared with sole caregivers (75% vs. 63%). It may be that those who are not the sole caregivers also care for an adult child living with HIV disease or another family member, such as a spouse or parent, who also requires assistance.

Both external and internal barriers to self-care were identified (Joslin and Harrison 1998). Internal barriers include beliefs, values, and problem-solving strategies that detract from one's capacity or motivation to engage in health-promoting activities. For example, rather than use the little discretionary time they had to exercise or relax, several caregivers with multiple, stress-related chronic conditions spent this time attending to children's needs (for example, ironing clothes for seven grandchildren). In the face of AIDS stigma and family dissolution, domestic chores may carry more than practical significance.

Imbued with symbolic value, they signify family dignity and self-respect, the value of a stable home and family life, or express love and devotion.

Another internal self-care barrier was a diminished sense of the importance of their own health needs. A sixty-year-old Latina grandmother raising a fifteen-year-old grandson with AIDS in an impoverished household stated, "I must put other's needs ahead of my own" when asked how she attends to her own health problems. Particularly for women, generational and cultural values may cause them to feel selfish when attending to their own needs. Expectations of family responsibility, especially among African American and Latino caregivers, intersect with worldviews that define the needs of the individual within the context of the family, rather than apart from or in opposition to it. Under such circumstances, family caregiving is not perceived as a burden (Pruchno 1999; Young and Kahana 1995; Hinrichsen and Ramirez 1992). Where the basic unit is the family, rather than the individual, caregivers' own health needs are not given expression (Villa et al. 1993).

Identification of health needs may be associated with fear. When asked whether she had any physical health problems, a sixty-three-year-old grandmother caring for her daughter and granddaughter, both with full-blown AIDS, anxiously responded, "Is anyone else going to read this? I'm afraid if something happens [to my daughter] that Amy's father, who has wanted nothing to do with her, will fight me for custody." Fear that authorities would remove the child from their care because of age or health problems was also reported (Minkler and Roe 1993). Grandmothers of the crack epidemic reported physical pain and health problems yet denied any limitation caring for the grandchildren or running a household. Minimization of health problems was found in two other urban, low-income grandparent populations (Grant, Gordon, and Cohen 1997; Joslin and Brouard 1996). HIV-affected surrogate parents were also anxious that calling attention to their own health problems would exacerbate an orphaned child's anxiety that their grandparent would die, as had their mother. A seventy-five-year-old grandmother of Italian descent noted that her twelve-year-old granddaughter expressed great anxiety about her grandmother's health, asking "What would happen to me if you die?" Caregivers themselves worried about being healthy enough to raise the child to maturity. A sixty-eight-year-old grandmother of Greek descent noted her high cholesterol. "The doctor said the values are very bad. I've got to live until she's eighteen, another ten years!"

Does the anxiety about one's health serve as a motivator for self-care? The data are inconclusive. One forty-seven-year-old great-aunt raising an infected ten-year-old girl reported multiple somatic complaints—headaches, ulcers, nausea, vomiting, back pain, menstrual pain, poor appetite, nervousness, and sleep problems. She spoke at length of conscious self-care through rest and slowing down. "I have to keep going for her. I'm all she's got. . . . If they want me to work overtime when I'm tired, I don't. It seems like a hard task but you have to give up other things to take care of your body, to take time out. You need to listen to your body." Reporting her health as excellent, she notes that her cholesterol had been elevated but that she had brought it down through dietary changes. With a family history of breast cancer and diabetes, she is vigilant in screening. Although expressing conscious self-care for the sake of the child, the great-aunt also uses tobacco. "Smoking is my getaway. It calms me down. I am trying to quit."

Denial of health needs may also reflect a caregiver's self-perception as a *survivor*. Because these older adults have outlived or will outlive their infected adult children, their own medical problems seem insignificant. Like other older adults, they also use other age peers as a reference point for self-rated health. "Many people my age are not as active [as I am]."

Caregiver depression has a negative impact on physical health (Vogt et al. 1994; Aneshensel, Frerichs, and Huba 1984), especially among HIV caregivers (LeBlanc, London, and Aneshensel 1998; LeBlanc, Aneshensel, and Wight 1995). Loneliness and social isolation can exacerbate chronic health conditions, even precipitating acute episodes (Grant, Gordon, and Cohen 1997), and may compromise physical health by reducing appetite and water and nutritional food intake (Walker and Beauchene 1991). Decreased immune function (Kiecolt-Glaser et al. 1991; Schultz, Vistainer, and Williamson 1990) may be one of depression's consequences. Motivation to adopt health-enhancing behaviors—to quit smoking, reduce dietary fat, and engage in moderate exercise—is undermined by depressed mood and social isolation. Doubt regarding the efficacy of self-care is magnified by despair and the sense of life being beyond one's control. A complex cycle of hopelessness and negative health behaviors takes hold, "It's like I don't care," said a sixty-two-year-old grandmother, reflecting on having gained ten pounds, which is attributed to eating ice cream when she's feeling blue or lonely. Exhausted from insomnia due to anxiety and interrupted sleep because of the nursing care needs of her infected granddaughter, she turns to cigarettes. She observes that she smokes more when she's tired, and being tired magnifies depressive symptoms. Restricted social contacts due to the intensity of caregiving demands and the stigma of HIV also contribute to depression, which in turn weakens self-care initiative. When asked about the frequency of social contacts, she muses sadly, "I don't have the money to go out and if don't have many people that I trust. I am seeing only doctors and nurses these days."

Internal self-care barriers also include a tendency to explain as "normal aging" a variety of symptoms and complaints (Holtzman, Akiyama, and Maxwell 1986), ranging from gastrointestinal problems to insomnia, shortness of breath, and chronic fatigue. Symptoms viewed as signs of aging rather than disease are likely to be neglected by both medical providers and the older adult, reinforcing the likelihood that the health needs of older surrogate parents will be ignored or neglected.

External barriers to self-care are factors in the individual's environment that limit or interfere with efforts to engage in health enhancing behaviors. Six that confront HIV-affected surrogate parents were identified (Joslin and Harrison 1998): inadequate health insurance, poverty, HIV/AIDS caregiving, child care, transportation, and prior experience with the health-care system.

Lack of access to medical care was an issue for only a small portion of study participants, with 75 percent having health insurance (40% employment-based, 20% Medicaid, and 15% Medicare), 80 percent having visited a physician within the past year, and 85 percent having a regular medical doctor. Caregivers without insurance either used charity care at a local hospital for urgent medical needs or simply went without medical attention. The uninsured ranged in age from fifty-one to sixty-one, below Medicare eligibility; although some were employed, they lacked employer-based coverage.

Poverty's effect on health-care utilization has received several decades of attention, including recent policy initiatives in Medicaid to encourage patient continuity of care through managed care enrollment. Overreliance on emergency rooms, a fatalistic view of health and illness, and lack of patient-initiated preventive care have been ascribed to both the "culture of poverty" (Reissman 1981) and structural conditions in the medical system that create discriminatory and dehumanizing treatment. Sheer economic survival of many HIV-affected families with children reduces the time and attention available for self-care. Notably, grandparents raising grandchildren are likely to be poor, according to recent national data (Fuller-Thomson, Minkler, and Driver 1997). Fifty-five percent of the HIV-affected surrogate parents reported household incomes below $19,500 per year (Joslin, Mevi-Triano, and Berman 1997).

Poverty acts as a grinding force, directing anxious attention to daily survival—to rent, food, and utilities. One grandmother described using her body as warmth to care for her dying son in an unheated apartment in the middle of winter, the heat having been turned off for lack of payment. In such dire circumstances, considering how to exercise, to eat less fat, or even to relax are eclipsed by the enormity of daily survival for oneself and one's family. For low-income families, lack of affordable transportation impedes seeking medical attention for asymptomatic or nonurgent health needs. When asked whether she has enough time to devote to her own health, a Latina grandmother, the sole caregiver to an adolescent grandson with AIDS, stated, "No, I'm careless. I go to a doctor only when I can't go on. I have to think about other people before I think about myself. . . . I have to work to take care of the children. I have no financial help." Grandparents also voiced concern about being unable to get medical attention for uninfected grandchildren who were ineligible for Medicaid and otherwise lacked health insurance. Limited discretionary income was used to seek medical care for the grandchild, often for asthma.

Caring for a family member with AIDS can eclipse all other caregiver concerns, reducing time and energy for self-care. Acute episodes of HIV disease intensify caregiving demands both at home and in the hospital. "Since my daughter was hospitalized with PCP [pneumocystic pneumonia] I have been running between the hospital to visit her, work, and home. Luckily, my sister has helped by caring for Alana [her four-year-old granddaughter] past the usual hours. I'm beat and I know I'm not eating right. . . . I'm smoking more."

Finally, prior experience with the health-care system also interferes with self-care by engendering feelings of alienation and mistrust. These same feelings were expressed by custodial grandparents in an East Harlem school-based program (Grant, Gordon, and Cohen 1997) who described long waits for fifteen-minute medical appointments, delays in scheduling follow-up care, and feeling as if the doctor did not listen and had no time for the patient. A fifty-eight-year-old African American grandmother described "being annoyed with the doctor. He doesn't show any interest in me and I feel that he was disrespectful and doesn't understand anyway. There's no communication or follow-up, I always have to take the initiative, so I have just stopped going."

Interactions with the medical system reinforced feelings of inadequacy and insignificance—poor incentives for self-care. Some HIV-affected surrogate parents expressed feelings of emotional vulnerability, charged with the overwhelming responsibility for the physical well-being of infected grandchildren or adult children and scrutinized or scolded by medical personnel.

Rather than encourage caregivers to attend to their own health, interactions with some HIV and pediatric medical providers reinforced caregiver's beliefs that their own needs were unimportant or that they were failing in yet another area—their own health.

Any discussion of self-care should not overlook the positive ways in which caregivers do attend to their health needs. Prayer, especially as talking with God, was a consistent theme through many interviews. "When things get too rough, I put it in God's hands," said Hazel Crooks. Finding comfort and companionship through prayer and with fellow believers reinforced caregivers' sense of hope. The value of prayer in promoting health has received substantial documentation in recent research (Matthews 1998; Dossey 1993) and should be considered in individual counseling strategies. Reading, gardening, or small craft projects were other pastimes grandmothers mentioned in describing how they coped with the constant demands of caregiving. Assessment of self-care practices and impediments should include discussion of how individuals relax or find enjoyment so that these activities can be encouraged when health enhancing.

Emotional Well-being

The distinguishing features of raising HIV-affected and orphaned children—physical and emotional demands of HIV caregiving, stigma, isolation, death, and bereavement—are significant threats to emotional well-being. Emotional distress is prevalent among AIDS caregivers (Clipp et al. 1995; Irving, Bor, and Catalan 1995; LeBlanc, Aneshensel, and Wight 1995; Ravis and Siegel 1991; Lennon, Martin, and Dean 1990; Pearlin, Semple, and Turner 1988) and grandparents raising grandchildren (Strawbridge et al. 1997; Dowdell 1995; Shor and Hayslip 1994; Kelly 1993; Jendrek 1993; Burton 1992; Minkler and Roe 1992). Because they find themselves in overwhelming circumstances that completely redefine their lives, feelings of role entrapment may increase depressive symptoms among AIDS caregivers (LeBlanc, Aneshensel, and Wight 1995) and grandparents raising grandchildren (Minkler et al. 1997). In several studies, a decline in psychological well-being among custodial grandparents has been associated with increased financial stress, reduced social contacts, family conflict, insufficient social support, fatigue, and role overload (Pruchno 1999; Sands and Goldberg-Glen 1998; Giarrusso et al. 1996; Roe, Minkler, and Barnwell 1994; Shore and Hayslip 1994; Jendrek 1993; Burton 1992).

Depressive symptoms among a sample of predominantly gay white AIDS caregivers were associated with a greater sense of burden as well as financial worry and strain (LeBlanc, Aneshensel, and Wight 1995). Post-traumatic stress disorder symptoms—vivid flashbacks, panic attacks, drug and alcohol use, night terrors, and psychosomatic disorders—were found among the vast majority of mothers caring for adult children who died from AIDS (Trice 1988). Stigma and shame associated with HIV disease in families (Cohen et al. 1995; Sherwin and Boland 1994; Powell-Cope and Brown 1992; see also chapter 3 of this volume), an adult child's incarceration or drug addiction (Minkler et al. 1997) contribute to feelings of humiliation that, in turn, increase the risk of depressive episodes (Brown, Harris, and Hepworth 1995). Caregivers may also experience guilt and powerful feelings of failure and responsibility for their adult children's behaviors that incurred risk of HIV infection (Tiblier, Walker, and Rolland 1989). Those raising HIV-infected children confront unpredictable and complex stressors that contribute to depression and anxiety (Hansell et al. 1998).

"I don't look toward the future," said a grandmother flatly, as she described caring for her daughter and granddaughter, both ill with AIDS. Grandmothers raising infected but healthy grandchildren exhibited a shared anxiety. "There is lots of worry. How will I cope if she gets sick?" Another stated, "One of my worst fears is of her (four year old granddaughter) getting sick." "I am overwhelmed," stated a woman who is caring for a three-year-old granddaughter whose mother and infant brother had died from AIDS the previous year.

More than half of the twenty HIV-affected surrogate parents rated their emotional health as either "fair" or "poor," with 45 percent rating it positively, a similar though slightly poorer profile than crack cocaine-affected grandmothers (Minkler, Roe, and Price 1993). Compared with cocaine-affected caregivers, HIV-affected surrogate parents were more likely to say their emotional health was worse than one year ago (45% vs. 30%). Among HIV-affected surrogate parents, those with poorer emotional well-being, including a sense of deteriorating mental health and greater caregiver burden, were likely to be low-income, raising an infected child, and having lost an adult child to AIDS in the past year (Joslin 2000). Between 45 percent and 50 percent of those studied reported feelings of depression, hopelessness, and loneliness over the past seven days. Patterns of distress were greatest among those with a recent AIDS death. Alternatively agitated and depressed during the interview, Larisse Landers expresses her profound loneliness because of AIDS stigma:

> I never have a break from the kids. No one comes to help. Even going to church, I'm always dragging them with me. What's so hard is seeing the other grandmothers in church with their grandchildren. . . . I've never told anyone at church about my daughter or grandson [who had died]. I lost my best friend—she treated me so cold when she found out about my daughter [having AIDS].

A friend's withdrawal is a wounding experience, adding to the cascade of loss and reinforcing isolation and feelings of shame.

Implications

The epidemiology of HIV infection and mortality among women of child-bearing age in the United States points to disproportionate surrogate responsibility among older African American and Latino women. Greater risk of chronicity at earlier ages marks the health of mid- and late-life parental surrogates from these communities. By age forty-five, Latinos are already coping with chronic diseases such as arthritis, heart disease, and diabetes, conditions that affect white elders in their mid-sixties (Cuellar 1990). Earlier chronicity is also true of African Americans, who are diagnosed with hypertension, stroke, and diabetes at younger ages (Harper 1990). Potential underuse of health and social services by elders of color (Burnette 1999; Angel and Angel 1992; Krause and Goldenhar 1992; Starrett et al. 1990) requires aggressive outreach, case-finding, and development of provider-client rapport in order to encourage older caregivers to seek medical and supportive services for themselves. HIV-affected older surrogate parents can appropriately be considered "hidden patients" (Joslin and Harrison 1998; Fengler and Goodrich 1979) whose health needs are denied, overlooked, or neglected. Efforts to promote their health and well-being must address barriers to health care and self-care.

Given the age, income, and employment profile of the surrogate parents described in this chapter, it is likely that some proportion of HIV-affected caregivers will be ineligible for Medicare or will lack private health insurance, especially if caregiving demands restrict employment to part-time work or otherwise interrupt employer-based health coverage. Extending Medicare benefits to those ages fifty-five to sixty-four through consumer-paid premiums has been proposed in recognition of the greater degree of chronic illnesses occurring in the middle years and the number of mid-life adults in the United States without health insurance (Powell-Griner, Bolen, and Bland 1999). Yet low household income of grandparent-maintained families (Fuller-Thomson, Minkler, and Driver 1997) and the frequent caregiver practice of using limited discretionary income for children's health needs rather than their own make individual cost-sharing and premium payments a burden for the uninsured and underinsured surrogate parent. Because of their fixed incomes, even those with Medicare coverage are likely to be unable to absorb the costs of private supplemental coverage unless they qualify for Medicaid, which assists the elderly poor (Rowland, Feder, and Keenan 1998). Only those poor enough to meet Medicaid eligibility criteria would be able to receive a broad scope of services, including transportation to the physician, prescription drugs, and dental care in addition to primary and specialty care.

Negative experiences with health-care providers deter service use even among those with health insurance and a regular physician (Grant, Gordon, and Cohen 1997). As caregivers, older surrogate parents may be all too familiar with insensitive health-care practitioners within the HIV/AIDS system (Marcenko and Samost 1999) and are wary of medical personnel who may criticize them for their health behaviors. Because public funding for HIV care identifies the infected person as the patient/client, excluding the caregiver from medical or social-work case management, a caregiver's sense that his or her own health care needs are unimportant may be reinforced by interactions with staff during home-care visits or medical or social work appointments at HIV/AIDS treatment centers. Constant caregiving demands without benefit of childcare or respite also restrict health-care utilization to urgent or emergency care. Lack of affordable and accessible transportation is another barrier to low-income elders. Transportation services funded by the Older Americans Act are age-restricted to those above the age of sixty. Funding of supportive transportation services is necessary to promote health-care access.

Despite common usage of the term "hidden patient" (Fengler and Goodrich 1979), there has been no research that has identified factors that contribute to caregivers' neglecting their physical and emotional health. Instead, gerontological research has examined whether physical and emotional health is affected by caregiving stress, but not how caregivers overlook or neglect their own health needs. Although interventions for caregivers of the frail elderly have focused on reducing caregiver strain, they have not considered how to support caregiver self-care practices to manage stress symptoms and manage chronic health problems.

Interview findings related to self-care have implications for outreach and patient counseling. Where self-care was reported, it related to coping with stress and minimizing disabling somatic complaints. Few described efforts to manage diagnosed health problems (e.g., high cholesterol levels, hypertension) actively or to prevent chronic disease. Several noted negative health behaviors—smoking, overeating—as ways they coped with stress or depression. While expressing concern about being healthy enough to continue as the primary caregiver, no surrogate parents considered their own healthy aging an area of concern and thus necessary to promote through self-care. Their primary issue was whether their physical health—or others' perceptions of it—would prevent them from continuing as surrogate parents.

Anxiety about being perceived as too old or too sick to be a surrogate parent may also contribute to caregivers being "hidden patients" (Fengler and Goodrich 1979) and reluctant to identify health needs or seek medical attention. Negative self-assessed health does not necessarily translate into health promotion efforts. Fatalism, social isolation, bereavement, and depression must be addressed in health promotion through individual or group counseling programs. Clergy may also use spiritual guidance as a means of strengthening self-care efforts. In order to encourage self-care, health and human service professionals can affirm caregivers' desire to stay healthy for the children's sake. Legitimizing self-care efforts, professionals can emphasize that health promotion through regular exercise, stress management, adequate nutrition and rest, regular health screenings, primary care, and social support expresses caregivers' devotion to their families and will enhance their capacity to provide a stable home for the children. Where supportive services such as housekeeping, respite, and child care are available so that caregivers can give appropriate time to their health, professionals may need to frame these services as "medical orders" (Joslin and Harrison 1998), especially when surrogate parents view such help-seeking as reflecting their failure as caregivers or their betrayal of family self-sufficiency and independence.

National, state, and local initiatives are needed to address the unmet health needs of HIV-affected and other older surrogate parents. Chapter 13, "Policy Implications for HIV-Affected Older Relative Caregivers," examines key public policies that directly and indirectly relate to caregiver health. Brief mention is given here to three model community programs that address caregiver well-being through comprehensive multidisciplinary services. One is an intergenerational school-based social service and medical care program in East Harlem, New York, that served low-income African American and Latino grandparent caregivers (Grant, Gordon, and Cohen 1997). Central to this program were its family focus and direct recruitment of grandparent caregivers. A multidisciplinary team, including a physician's assistant, social worker, and health educator, was based at the pediatric school-based clinic; where necessary home visits to grandparents were provided. The health-education component of the program demonstrated that program responsiveness to caregiver concerns improved health-care utilization. An Atlanta-based program also provides community-based and in-home services through a multidisciplinary team of social workers, attorneys, nurses, and tutors (Kelley, Yorker, and Whitley 1998). Supportive services including health screening and fitness classes are available in a Boston Grandfamilies House (Roe 2000). These models of health promotion suggest that health promotion can be achieved through comprehensive and well-designed programs. Broader public health and social policies are needed to reduce the conditions of poverty, family disorganization, substance abuse, and community and family violence that erode caregivers' overall well-being and jeopardize their capacity for self-care.

Notes

1. Names have been changed to guard the privacy of respondents.

References

Aneshensel, C. S., R. R. Frerichs, and G. J. Huba. 1984. Depression and physical illness: A multiwave, nonrecursive causal model. *Journal of Health and Social Behavior* 25 (4): 350–371.

Angel, J., and R. J. Angel. 1992. Age at immigration, social connections and well-being among elderly Hispanics *Journal of Aging and Health* 4:480–499.

Barresi, C., and D. Stull. 1993. Ethnicity and long term care: An overview. In C. Barresi and D. Stull, eds., *The Black American Elderly*, pp. 3–21. New York: Springer.

Belgrave, L. I., M. L. Wykle, and J. M. Choi. 1993. Health, double jeopardy and culture: The use of institutionalization by African-Americans. *The Gerontologist* 33:379–385.

Brown, G. W., T. O. Harris, and C. Hepworth. 1995. Loss, humiliation and entrapment among women developing depression: A patient and non-patient comparison. *Psychological Medicine* 25:7–21.

Burnette, D. 1997. Grandparents raising grandchildren in the inner city. *Families in Society* 78:489–499.

——. 1999. Custodial grandparents in Latino families: patterns of service use and predictors of service needs. *Social Work* 44:22–35.

Burton, L. 1992. Black grandparents rearing children of drug-addicted parents: Stressors, outcomes and social service needs. *The Gerontologist* 32:744–751.

Clark, D. O., and R. C. Gibson. 1997. Race, age, chronic disease and disability. In K. S. Markides and M. R. Miranda, eds., *Minorities, Aging and Health,* pp. 107–126. Thousand Oaks, Calif.: Sage.

Clipp, E. C., A. J. Adinolfi, L. Forrest, and C. L. Bennett. 1995. Informal caregivers of persons with AIDS. *Journal of Palliative Care* 11:10–18.

Cohen, F. L., W. M. Nehring, K. C. Malm, and D. M. Harris. 1995. Family experiences when a child is HIV positive: reports of natural and foster parents. *Pediatric Nursing* 21:248–254.

Cuellar, J. 1990. Hispanic American aging: Geriatric education curriculum development for selected health professions. In M. S. Harper, ed., *Minority Aging,* pp. 365–414. Washington, D.C.: U.S. Government Printing Office.

Dossey, L. 1993. *Healing Words: The Power of Prayer and the Practice of Medicine.* New York: HarperCollins.

Dowdell, E. B. 1995. Caregiver burden: grandmothers raising their high risk grandchildren. *Journal of Psychosocial Nursing* 33:27–30.

Fengler, A. P., and N. Goodrich. 1979. Wives of elderly disabled men: the hidden patients. *The Gerontologist* 19 (2): 175–183.

Fuller-Thomson, E., M. Minkler, and D. Driver. 1997. A profile of grandparents raising grandchildren in the United States. *The Gerontologist* 37:406–411.

Giarrusso, R., D. Feng, Q. Wang, and M. Silverstein. 1996. Parenting and co-parenting of grandchildren: Effect on grandparents' well-being. *International Journal of Sociology and Social Policy* 16:124–156.

Grant, R. 1997. The health status of grandparent care givers. Paper presented at the Annual Scientific Meeting of the Gerontological Society of America, Cincinnati.

Grant, R., S. G. Gordon, and S. T. Cohen. 1997. An innovative school-based intergenerational model to serve grandparent caregivers. *Journal of Gerontological Social Work* 28:47–61.

Hansell, P. S., C. B. Hughes, G. Caliandro, P. Russo, W. C. Budin, B. Hartman, and O. Hernandez. 1998. The effect of a social support boosting intervention on stress, coping and social support in caregivers of children with HIV/AIDS. *Nursing Research* 47:79–86.

Harper, M. 1990. *Minority Aging: Essential Curricula for Selected Health and Allied Health Professions.* Washington, D.C.: Department of Health and Human Services, Health Resources and Services Administration.

Hinrichsen, G. A., and M. Ramirez. 1992. Black and white dementia caregivers: A comparison of their adaptation, adjustment and service utilization. *The Gerontologist* 32:373–381.

Holtzman, M, H. Akiyama, and A. J. Maxwell. 1986. Symptoms and self-care in old age. *Journal of Applied Gerontology* 5:183–200.

Irving, G., R. Bor, and J. Catalan. 1995. Psychological distress among gay men supporting a lover or partner with AIDS: A pilot study. *AIDS Care* 7:605–617.

Jendrek, M. P. 1993. Grandparents who parent their grandchildren: Circumstances and decisions. *The Gerontologist* 34:206–216.

Joslin, D. 2000. Emotional well-being among grandparents raising children orphaned and affected by HIV Disease. In R. Goldberg-Glen and B. Hayslip, eds., *Grandparents*

Raising Grandchildren: Theoretical, Empirical and Clinical Perspectives, pp. 87–106. New York: Springer.

Joslin, D., and A. Brouard. 1995. The prevalence of grandmothers as primary caregivers in a poor pediatric population. *Journal of Community Health* 20:383–401.

Joslin, D., C. Mevi-Triano, and J. Berman. 1997. Grandparents raising children orphaned by HIV/AIDS: Health risks and service needs. Paper presented at the Annual Scientific Meeting of the Gerontological Society of America, Cincinnati.

Joslin, D., and R. Harrison. 1998. The "hidden patient": Older relatives raising children orphaned by AIDS. *Journal of the American Women's Medical Association* 53 (2): 65–71.

Kelley, S. J. 1993. Caregiver stress in grandparents raising grandchildren. *IMAGE: Journal of Nursing Scholarship* 25:331–337.

Kelley, S. J., and E. G. Damato. 1995. Grandparents as primary care givers. *Maternal and Child Nursing* 20:326–332.

Kelley, S. J., B.C. Yorker, and D. Whitley. 1998. To grandmother's house we go . . . and stay: Children raised in intergenerational families. *Journal of Gerontological Nursing* 23:12–20.

Kiecolt-Glaser, J. K., J. R. Dura, C. E. Speicher, J. Trask, and R. Glaser. 1991. Spousal caregivers of dementia victims: longitudinal changes in immunity and health. *Psychosomatic Medicine* 53:345–362.

Krause, N., and L. M. Goldenhar. 1992. Acculturation and psychological distress in three groups of elderly Hispanics. *Journal of Gerontology* 47:S279–S288.

LeBlanc, A. J., A. S. London, and C. S. Aneshensel. 1997. The physical costs of AIDS caregiving. *Social Science and Medicine* 45:915–923.

LeBlanc, A. J., C. S. Aneshensel, and R. G. Wight. 1995. Psychotherapy use and depression among AIDS care givers. *Journal of Community Psychology* 23:127–142.

Lennon, M. C., J. L. Martin, and L. Dean. 1990. The influence of social support on AIDS-related grief reaction among gay men. *Social Science and Medicine* 31:447–484.

Marcenko, M. O., and L. Samost. 1999. Living with HIV/AIDS: the voices of HIV-positive mothers. *Social Work* 44:36–45.

Markides, K. S., and S. A. Black. 1996. Ethnicity and aging. In R. H. Binstock and L. K. George, eds., *Handbook of Aging and the Social Sciences,* pp. 153–170. 4th ed. San Diego: Academic Press.

Marx, J., and J. C. Solomon. 2000. Physical health of custodial grandparents. In C. Cox, ed., *To Grandmother's House We Go and Stay: Perspectives on Custodial Grandparents,* pp. 37–55. New York: Springer.

Matthews, D. A. 1998. *The Faith Factor: Proof of the Healing Power of Prayer.* New York: Penguin Putnam.

Mettler, M., and D. Kemper. 1993. Self-care and older adults: making healthcare relevant. *Generations* 17:7–10.

McDonell, J. R., N. Abell, and J. Miller. 1991. Family members' willingness to care for people with AIDS: A psychosocial assessment model. *Social Work* 36:43–53.

Minkler, M., and E. Fuller-Thomson. 1999. The health of grandparents raising grandchildren: Results of a national study. *American Journal of Public Health* 89:1384.

Minkler, M., E. Fuller-Thomson, D. Miller, and D. Driver. 1997. Depression in grandparents raising grandchildren: Results of a national longitudinal study. *Archives of Family Medicine* 6:445–452.

Minkler, M., K. Roe, and M. Price. 1992. The physical and emotional health of grand-mothers raising grandchildren of the crack cocaine epidemic. *The Gerontologist* 32:752–761.

Mockenhaupt, R. 1993. Self-care for older adults: taking care and taking charge. *Generations* 17:5–6.

National Center for Health Statistics. 1994. Current estimates from the National Health Interview Survey: 1994. *Vital and Health Statistics,* Series 10, no. 189.

———. 1995. Current estimates from the National Health Interview Survey: 1994. *Vital and Health Statistics,* Series 10, no. 193.

Pearlin, L. I., C. S. Aneshensel, and A. J. LeBlanc. 1997. The forms and mechanisms of stress proliferation: The case of AIDS caregivers. *Journal of Health and Social Behavior* 38:223–236.

Pearlin, L. I., S. Semple, and H. Turner. 1988. Stress of AIDS caregiving: a preliminary overview of the issues. *Death Studies* 12:501–517.

Portney, L. G., and M. P. Watkins. 1993. *Foundations of Clinical Research: Application to Practice.* Norwalk, Conn.: Appleton and Lange.

Powell-Cope, G., and M. A. Brown. 1992. Going public as an AIDS family caregiver. *Social Science and Medicine* 34:571–580.

Powell-Griner, E., J. Bolen, and S. Bland. 1999. Health care coverage and use of preventive services among the near elderly in the United States. *American Journal of Public Health* 89:882–886.

Pruchno, R. 1999. Raising grandchildren: The experiences of black and white grand-mothers. *The Gerontologist* 39:209–221.

Ravis, V. H., and Siegel, K. (1991) The impact of caregiving on informal and familial care-givers. *AIDS Patient Care* 5:39–43.

Reissman, C. K. 1981. Improving the use of health services by the poor. In P. Conrad and R. Kern, eds., *The Sociology of Health and Illness,* pp. 541–557. New York: St. Martin's.

Rice, D. P., and M. P. La Plante. 1988. Chronic illness, disability and increasing longevi-ty. In S. Sullivan and M. E. Lewin, eds., *The Economics and Ethics of Long-term Care and Disability,* pp. 9–55. Washington, D.C.: American Enterprise Institute for Public Policy Research.

Roe, K. 2000. Community interventions to support grandparent caregivers: Lessons learned from the field. In C. Cox, ed., *To Grandmother's House We Go and Stay: Perspectives on Custodial Grandparents,* pp. 283–303. New York: Springer.

Roe, K., M. Minkler, and R. S. Barnwell. 1994. The assumption of caregiving: Grand-mothers raising the children of the crack cocaine epidemic. *Qualitative Health Research* 4:281–303.

Roth, J. R., S. Siegel, and Black, R. (1994) Identifying the mental health needs of children living in families with AIDS or HIV infection. *Community Mental Health Journal* 30:581–592.

Rowland, D., J. Feder, and P. Keenan. 1998. Managed care for low-income elderly people. *Generations* 22:43–50.

Sands, R. G., and R. Goldberg-Glen. 1998. The impact of employment and serious illness on grandmothers who are raising their grandchildren. *Journal of Women and Aging* 10:41–58.

Schultz, R., P. Vistainer, and G. M. Williamson. 1990. Psychiatric and physical morbidity effects of caregiving. *Journal of Gerontology* 45:181–191.

Sherwin, L. N., and M. Boland. 1994. Overview of psychosocial research concerning pediatric human immunodeficiency virus infection. *Developmental and Behavioral Pediatrics* 15:S5–S11.

Shore, R. J., and B. Hayslip. 1994. Custodial grandparenting: Implications for children's development. In A. E. Gottfried and A. W. Gottfried, eds., *Redefining Families: Implications for Children's Development*, pp. 171–218. New York: Plenum.

Siegel, K., and B. Krauss. 1991. Living with HIV Infection: Adaptive tasks of seropositive gay men. *Journal of Health and Social Behavior* 32:17–32.

Starrett, R. A, C. Bressler, J. T. Decker, G. Walters, and D. Rodgers. 1990. The role of environmental awareness and support networks in Hispanic elderly persons' use of formal social services. *Journal of Community Psychiatry* 18:218–227.

Strawbridge, W. J., M. I. Wallhagen, S. J. Shema, and G. A. Kaplan. 1997. New burdens or more of the same? Comparing grandparent, spouse and adult child caregivers. *The Gerontologist* 37:505–510.

Stoller, E. P., and R. C. Gibson. 1997. *Worlds of Difference*. Thousand Oaks, Calif.: Pine Forge Press.

Theis, S. L., F. L. Cohen, J. Forrest, and M. Zewelsky. 1997. Needs assessment of caregivers of people with HIV/AIDS. *Journal of the Association of Nurses in AIDS Care* 8:76–84.

Tiblier, K. B., G. Walker, and J. Rolland. 1989. Therapeutic issues when working with families of persons with AIDS. In E. D. Macklin, ed., *AIDS and Families*, pp. 81–127. New York: Harrington Park Press.

Trice, A. D. 1988. Post-traumatic stress syndrome-like symptoms among AIDS caregivers. *Psychological Review* 63:656–665.

Turner, H. A., and L. I. Pearlin. 1989. Issues of age, stress and caregiving. *Generations* 13:56–59.

U.S. Bureau of the Census. 1990. *The Need for Personal Assistance with Everyday Activities: Recipients and Caregivers*. Current Population Reports, series P-70, no. 19. Washington, D.C.: U.S. Government Printing Office.

U.S. Department of Health and Human Services. 1991. *Current Estimates from the National Health Interview Survey, 1990*. Washington, D.C.: U.S. Government Printing Office.

Verbrugge, L. M., J. M. Lepkowski, and Y. Imanaka. 1989. Comorbidity and its impact on disability. *Milbank Quarterly* 67:450–484.

Villa, M. L., J. Cuellar, N. Gamel, and G. Yeo. 1993. *Aging and Health: Hispanic American Elders*. 2d ed. Stanford, Calif.: Stanford Geriatric Education Center.

Vogt, T., C. Pope, J. Mullooly, and J. Hollis. 1994. Mental health status as a predictor of morbidity and mortality: A 15 year follow-up of members of a health maintenance organization. *American Journal of Public Health* 84:227–231.

Walker, D., and R. E. Beauchene. 1991. The relationship of loneliness, social isolation and physical health to dietary adequacy of independently living elderly. *Journal of the American Dietetic Association* 91 (3): 300–305.

Weitz, R. 1989. Uncertainty and the lives of people with AIDS. *Journal of Health and Social Behavior* 30:270–281.

Wight, R. G., A. J. LeBlanc, and C. S. Aneshensel. 1998. AIDS caregiving and health among midlife and older women. *Health Psychology* 17:130–137.

Wright, L. K., E. C. Clipp, and L. K. George. 1993. Health consequences of caregiver stress. *Medicine, Exercise, Nutrition and Health* 2:181–195.

Young, R. F., and E. Kahana. 1995. The context of caregiving and well-being outcomes among African and Caucasian Americans. *The Gerontologist* 35:225–232.

6

Stress and Social Support in Older Caregivers of Children with HIV/AIDS: An Intervention Model

PHYLLIS SHANLEY HANSELL, CYNTHIA B. HUGHES, WENDY C. BUDIN,
PHYLLIS RUSSO, GLORIA CALIANDRO, BRUCE HARTMAN,
AND OLGA C. HERNANDEZ

Providing care for an HIV-infected child is a responsibility that often falls to an older adult who may be an extended family member, such as a grandparent or a foster parent. The incidence of orphans resulting from the AIDS epidemic is projected to increase worldwide steadily in the new millennium. Older adults who are extended family members as well as foster parents have assumed a significant caregiving role for children with HIV, providing nurturance, education, and parenting, but it has not been without cost. These older adults, who are the primary caregivers for children infected with HIV, are at increased risk for potential adverse health and psychosocial outcomes. Many factors contribute to these caregivers' risk status. These factors include the normal aging process, which is further compounded by caregiving responsibilities, limited economic resources, and frequently marginalized status as older minority individuals. Often these caregivers are single parents who experience social isolation and responsibility for a child with a stigmatized illness.

Researchers who have investigated the experiences of these elder caregivers of HIV-infected children have consistently documented the negative effects of social isolation and a diminished social support network on these caregivers' coping strategies. Stress also affects the adaptation systems of these caregivers, which are often challenged by the health and behavioral problems of the children as well as of the biological mothers of HIV-infected children.

The purpose of this chapter is to review the impact of caregiver stress on social support and coping among older adult caregivers. We will explore interventions meant to enhance coping strategies relative to social support. Additionally, we will discuss findings from the implementation of a social-support boosting intervention.

Elder Custodial Caregivers of Children

Joslin and Harrison (1998) borrowed the term "hidden patient" from gerontologists to describe the neglected physical and emotional health needs of late-life surrogate parents. In their study of twenty caregivers they found poorer health among single caregivers (aged fifty-nine or younger) of multiple children including an HIV-infected child. They described these caregivers as being reluctant to acknowledge any health-related limitations or needs in spite of existing health problems. Several groups of researchers have also described increased physical health problems and financial, emotional, and social problems such as isolation from peers as a result of custodial grandparenting. Other negative effects reported include restricted freedom, inability to pursue one's own goals, and fears and worries related to the future (Emick and Hayslip 1999; Musil 1998; Kelley, Yorker, and Whitley 1997).

Brabant (1994) highlighted age-related issues that affect kinship caregivers. Financially, elders often live on fixed incomes planned for one or two individuals; they are not prepared to support an expanding family with expanding financial needs. Socially and emotionally, elders experience the loss of significant friends and relatives, reduced social contacts, and loss of status and role in both the family and community.

In January 2000 the New Jersey Assembly Task Force on Grandparenting released an extensive report of findings and recommendations on specific problems relevant to grandparent childrearing. As a state that leads the nation with the highest percentage of women who are infected with HIV and the highest AIDS death rate among women nationally, New Jersey is extremely concerned with the increasing numbers of orphans in the state and the needs of this grandparent caregiving group. Some of the stresses and concerns of grandparent caregivers identified in this report include low annual income; need for public assistance; lack of health insurance for grandchildren; lack of high school education; need for daycare for working grandparents; neglect of their own health; and lack of formal custody arrangements for grandchildren, which affects medical and school decisions. Forty-three recommendations were proposed by this task force, including one to improve the implementation of the new statewide policy, which entitles relatives to receive full foster care rates for child care, improve the dissemination of information about available health insurance supports for this group, and develop and facilitate supportive networks for grandparents with regard to transportation, housing, education, and legal services.

Researchers have reported findings from studies that have compared different groups of caregivers. According to Emick and Hayslip (1999), grandparents caring for a child with a problem (general health or behavioral problem) reported the most distress, the least available social supports, the most disruption of roles, and the most deteriorated grandparent-grandchild relationships. Strawbridge et al. (1997) drew their sample from a large database and compared noncaregivers with a diverse set of grandparent, spouse, and adult-child caregivers. They found that grandparent caregivers experienced poorer physical health and functioning than noncaregivers, while all three caregiver groups had more negative mental health outcomes than noncaregivers. Musil (1999) reported that custodial grandparents (primary caregivers) reported less instrumental and subjective social support and more parenting stresses, distress and parent/child dysfunctional interactions than partial caregivers. Musil found grandmothers in both groups reported high depression and anxiety levels.

From a different perspective, Caliandro and Hughes (1998), using a phenomenological approach, conducted in-depth interviews of grandmothers caring for HIV-infected grandchildren. These authors encouraged the grandmothers to describe their personal experience as caregivers. Relevant themes related to stressful aspects of the caregiving experience include keeping the secret of HIV infection; managing the children's medical care; and living within an environment of diminishing resources and the violence and uncertainty of "the street." Stressful relationships with some of the living biological mothers were also described. These caregivers described ways of coping and managing their caregiving responsibilities by living in the child-centered present, normalizing family life (by, for example, treating the child as much as possible as a "normal" child), finding joy in their special grandchild, maintaining strength as mature women through active decision-making, drawing on their spiritual beliefs, minimizing their own personal illnesses, and, for some, learning to speak out. Grandmothers who were learning to speak out and not hide the HIV infection described solace through seeking social support through groups, the church, or simply talking with a friend. This methodology enabled the researchers to elicit a holistic perspective of their experience. Although stress and diminishing resources were an integral part of their experiences, these grandmothers projected an overall positive outlook. The potential positive effect of caregiving for older adult grandparents is highlighted by Kelley and Damato (1995), who reported that the family often perceived the grandchild as a blessing, offering them another chance at childrearing with a renewed purpose for living.

Two conceptual frameworks provide a perspective on the potential untoward health effects of these late life surrogate parents. Flaskerud and Winslow (1998) propose a model for examining vulnerable populations such as these caregivers. The authors predict that diminished societal and environmental resources (income, jobs, social connections, access to health care) contribute to increased health risk factors such as exposure to violence and abuse, obesity, lack of exercise, and lack of health screenings and, subsequently, increased morbidity and mortality. Flaskerud and Winslow's model is proposed from a community health perspective that views communities as responsible for the collective well-being and health of their citizens.

A second model as proposed by Thoits (1986) focuses more on the impact on the individual and links stress, coping, and social support by drawing on the work of Lazarus and Folkman (1984). According to Thoits, stressors are aspects of one's life viewed as undesirable consequences. Stressors such as negative life events or lack of adequate resources produce stress, which interfere with an individual's performance of role and related activities. The lack of available resources is experienced as a stressor and can contribute to increased risk and adverse health outcomes that compromise the caregiver's ability to actualize the caregiving role.

Lazarus and Folkman (1984) define coping as "the constantly changing cognitive and behavioral efforts to manage specific external and/or internal demands that are appraised as taxing or exceeding the resources of the person" (p. 141). It is a subset of purposeful adaptational activities that includes anything the person does or thinks, the management of stressful conditions, and attempts to master the environment. Two major ways of coping in this paradigm are problem-focused and emotional-focused coping. Problem-focused coping involves taking action on the environment or the self to mitigate stressful situations such as seeking information and turning to others for physical assistance or seeking social support. According to Cohen and Lazarus (1983) successful problem-focused coping depends on the availability and mobilization of resources balanced by constraints. Making use of resources is contingent on a person's appraisal of a stressful situation. Vaux (1988) specifically identified social support as consisting of support network resources, specific supportive behaviors, and subjective appraisal of support. Problem-focused coping includes the appraisal, use, and mobilization of social support. Emotion-focused coping efforts are directed at reducing emotional distress. Strategies used are avoidance, minimization, distancing, selective attention, and positive comparisons, drawing positive value from negative events and self-punishment.

Although investigators have frequently focused on stress and social support in caregiver research, these researchers have relied primarily on convenience samples, variable sample sizes, and descriptive designs. The following research review demonstrates this variability. It is clear in the following research studies that increased stress and decreased social support are linked with adverse health outcomes. Different interventions are described in the literature, which directly or indirectly incorporate aspects of social support. The research reviewed here demonstrates that social support as well as other factors alleviates the effects of some of this stress. Some of the descriptive and intervention studies reviewed here have used direct patient populations but have application for caregiver populations. Furthermore, most models of care proposed by health professionals have not been evaluated through research of outcomes.

Stress and Social Support

Reynolds and Alonzo (1998) studied twenty diverse informal caregivers of AIDS patients. Their results supported previous researchers in that, in addition to providing a range of physical and emotional support, the caregiver also managed multiple sources of loss and uncertainty, stigma and alienation from friends, and the actual or possible risk of becoming HIV-seropositive.

In their descriptive study, LeBlanc, London, and Aneshensel (1997) reported on the impact of caregiving. They studied 642 informal care providers of gay men. More than a third of these caregivers were described as serial caregivers in that they reported previous AIDS caregiving experiences. Many of the caregivers studied reported deterioration in their own health or an exacerbation of their own health problems. Reports of depression among these caregivers were also related to physical health symptoms. LeBlanc, Aneshensel, and Wight (1995) investigated the use of psychotherapy in a caregiver study of 472 AIDS caregivers. Although 31 percent of AIDS caregivers reported high rates of psychotherapy use, caregiver-related stress did not significantly predict this use. Instead, the health status, living arrangements, and relationship between the caregivers and the care recipient predicted psychotherapy use. Caregiver health status and care-related stress did affect reports of depression associated with caregiver psychotherapy use. Frequent use of psychotherapy has not been reported in the grandparent caregiving population.

Caliandro and Hughes (1998) in their qualitative study identified the importance of spiritual connections and the church as sources of support for their grandmothers. To varying degrees, support was also found from family members, mentors, friends, health professionals, and support groups. The grandmothers identified the need for support services aimed at enhancing financial and transportation resources and respite care.

Bennett (1993) reported physical and emotional strains of caregivers in her doctoral study of significant others of gay men who were HIV-positive. These strains included bureaucratic obstacles, maintaining the secrecy of their relationship with the PWA, having to deal with death at an early age, the stigma of organized religion toward AIDS, and social-support issues. The quantitative findings in this study related to caregiver stresses highlighted their financial concerns, their own health problems, and concern regarding the health of their partner. In contrast to those of previous researchers, her sample reported high levels of social support from the gay community and the partner, low levels of threat appraisal, and low levels of emotional distress. These results supported the active problem-solving approach taken by this sample.

Moneyham et al. (1998) investigated the effectiveness of active and passive coping strategies in a sample of 264 women infected with HIV. Active coping was positively related to the presence of physical symptoms and negatively related to emotional distress. Active coping strategies examined included seeking social support, managing the illness, and engaging in spiritual activities. The authors suggest that interventions that support active coping strategies as physical symptoms increase may be effective in promoting adaptation to HIV disease.

In their longitudinal study of 122 caregivers of Alzheimer patients living at home, Goode et al. (1998) found that social support over a one-year period had a protective effect on health symptoms, and conversely, that those caregivers with low levels of social support reported the greatest increases in health symptoms. Lesar and Maldonado (1994) found that social support did not directly influence family well-being among their diverse group of HIV caregivers, although they postulated that social support might indirectly influence child characteristics.

Research-based evidence supporting the effectiveness of social support interventions is sparse. Kalichman, Sikkema, and Somlai (1996) reported on the findings of their study comparing HIV-infected individuals who attended an HIV support group with those who did not. They found social connectedness associated with group attendance and time elapsed since diagnosis. Individuals who did not attend groups experienced greater emotional distress and were more apt to use avoidance coping styles. They suggested that supportive interventions should be focused nearer to the time of diagnosis.

Lutgendorf et al. (1994) reported on the successful effects of a series of ten-week counseling sessions aimed at reducing depression, anxiety, and symptoms of stress in gay men with AIDS at different points in their disease. The ten-week counseling sessions were adapted for different stages of HIV illness but were designed to use cognitive behavioral stress management techniques (CBSM). Sessions included an educational module, CBSM techniques, behavioral change and coping skills training, and assertiveness training. Sessions also included facilitating the use of social support through group interaction and identification of sources of social support and problems with social support systems.

Williams (1995) described using a crisis-intervention model in her work as a social worker with HIV-infected women. Part of the crisis-intervention model included encouraging development of patterns of seeking and using help with actual tasks and feelings by using interpersonal and institutional resources. An example of this is the use of peer support groups so women can share and air their feelings.

Lesar and Maldonado (1994) suggested that interventions should be aimed at the social support network such as education of family members, providing respite care alternatives, and gaining emotional support through joining support groups. A family with HIV infection also needs collaborative case-management services that include the family in problem-solving. Joslin and Harrison (1998) suggested advocating for support programs such as respite care, mental health and counseling services, childcare, and after-school and summer programs to help grandparent caregivers. Littrell (1996) links the use of support groups by HIV-infected people to improved psychological states and better immune function. Schaaf, Sherwen, and Youngblood (1997) described an intervention for the HIV-infected child with an environmental focus aimed at identifying strengths and needs of the environments of the child and caregiver, and emphasized an interdisciplinary, culturally relevant, family-centered approach. The goal of this care is to enhance the competence of the child and increase the caregiver's feelings of efficacy specifically by decreasing stress and increasing coping. The intervention protocol is used by an interdisciplinary team and follows a four-stage protocol that includes an interdisciplinary assessment of the child, planning of intervention by the team, two intervention visits to the home per month, and ongoing evaluation. According to the authors, the home visits are specifically designed to (1) enhance functional ability for children with HIV infection, (2) decrease stress and increase coping of the caregiver combined with identifying environmental barriers and adapting the environment to enhance the child's functional abilities, (3) increase the animate and inanimate characteristics of the environment that promote function, and (4) deliver cost-effective care to children and families (p. 74).

Based on her qualitative study findings of two groups of women caregivers, Rutman (1996) recommended that women find strength through partnership with other caregivers. Family caregiver networks, formal caregiver associations, or support groups may exemplify these partnerships.

As described, frequent themes identified in the literature for enhancing social support include the use of support groups for caregivers and infected individuals and provision of respite care. Other support services suggested include case-management services, mental-health counseling, enhancing linkages with the church, family networks, and involvement in caregiving associations. Research-based evidence to support the effectiveness of these support interventions is sparse.

A Social Support-Boosting Intervention

An intervention model reported elsewhere (Hansell et al. 1999) tested the effects of a social support-boosting intervention on levels of stress, coping, and social support among caregivers of children with HIV/AIDS. This intervention model was derived from a framework in which stressors are conceptualized as aspects of one's life, which are viewed as having undesirable consequences (Thoits 1986). The negative life events that result in stress impede an individual's performance of activities related to role. Therefore, when stressors exceed an individual's resources, behavioral and cognitive efforts are needed to cope with them.

In their work, Hansell et al. (1998, 1999) developed a social support-boosting intervention aimed at enhancing caregiver coping ability by mobilizing the caregiver's social support network. This mobilization of social support would, in turn, help the caregiver change or manage problems that the caregiver identified as stressful.

A two-group experimental design was used to test the effectiveness of social support boosting intervention. Caregivers of children with HIV were recruited from HIV outreach centers and clinics if they met the following inclusion criteria: identified themselves as the biological parent, blood relative, or foster parent of a child with HIV/AIDS; were legally assigned as the primary caregiver; resided in the New Jersey/New York metropolitan area; and could read and write English or Spanish. All biological parents were seropositive and all extended family and foster caregivers were seronegative. Caregivers were stratified and randomly assigned to the experimental or control group. Participants in the control group received standard care without the interventions. Standard care included a multidisciplinary team approach in which the children of the participants received medical treatment and nursing care and the caregiver received caregiver respite and social services. In addition to standard care, the caregivers in the experimental group received the social support-boosting intervention.

The social support-boosting intervention used an individualized case-management approach. According to the intervention protocol, the nurse investigator and caregiver met at monthly intervals for six months. Meetings took place in a private room in the clinic or outreach center for children with AIDS. Each contact for the intervention lasted between thirty minutes and an hour based on individual caregiver needs. The caregiver with the investigator set mutual, objective goals to facilitate caregiver problem-solving. Using this assessment, the investigator and the caregiver identified potential formal and informal social support-network resources for achieving caregiver goals and developed a plan for using them. Social support-boosting strategies included the identification of individuals from the caregiver's social support network who would help to provide resources that meet the individual's support needs. Social support included emotional support, cognitive support, and material support (Cohen and Willis 1985; Thoits 1982). Emotional support consisted of behaviors that generated feelings of respect, comfort, and a sense of worth. Cognitive support refers to knowledge and information. Material or instrumental support refers to services and goods that facilitate problem solutions. The intervention aimed at helping caregivers identify and access network resources that could provide all three types of social support.

Table 6.1 Sample Characteristics According to Caregiver HIV Status

Variable	Sero + (n = 39) n	Sero − (n = 31) n	Total Sample (n = 70) n	%
Ethnic Background				
African-American	26	25	51	73
White	5	4	9	13
Hispanic	7	2	9	13
Marital Status				
Single	18	9	27	39
Separated/divorced	7	11	18	26
Widowed	2	2	4	5
Partnered	8	1	9	13
Married	4	8	12	17
Relationship to Child				
Mother	39	0	39	55
Grandmother/Blood relative	0	12	12	17
Foster Parent	0	19	19	27
Educational Level				
Seventh grade	2	0	2	3
Junior HS	6	2	8	11
Partial HS	14	5	19	27
HS graduate	8	6	14	20
Partial college	8	12	20	29
College graduate	1	6	7	10
Hollingshead Index				
Social Status 1	26	5	31	44
Social Status 2	6	12	18	26
Social Status 3	7	8	15	22
Social Status 4	0	2	2	3
Social Status 5	0	3	3	4
Missing data			1	1

Problems, goals, resources, plans for meeting goals, and the evaluation of the plan were recorded on a structured flowsheet in order to provide continuous monitoring of caregiver progress. The flowsheet incorporated caregiver evaluation (subjective) and investigator evaluation (objective) of intervention outcomes.

The stratified randomized sample included seventy primary caregivers of children with HIV/AIDS. The sample strata were seropositive caregivers (biological parents) and seronegative caregivers (foster parents and extended family members). Of the seronegative caregivers, many were older adults including grandmothers and extended family members with a mean age of fifty-three years (SD = 7.4). Table 6.1 describes sample characteristics.

Results

Outcome measures for the study included the Derogatis Stress Profile (1986) to measure stress; the Tilden Interpersonal Relationship Inventory, a multidimensional measure of interpersonal relationships (1991); and the Family Crisis Oriented Personal Scales (F-COPES) (McCubbin and Thompson 1987), a measure of coping or effective problem-solving.

When initially compared to the control group, the intervention group yielded no significant differences on the outcome variables of stress, coping, and social support. Further analyses were then performed to adjust for the caregivers' HIV status within each study group. A repeated-measure MANOVA was used to test for a group by HIV status interaction. The combined dependent variables were significantly related to the interactions of group by HIV status over time [F $(1,66)$ = 3.47, p = .02]. In order to investigate further the nature of the relationship among the study variables, univariate F values were computed. No statistically significant differences were found for stress [F $(1,66)$ = .197, p = .658] or coping [F$(1,66)$ = 3.27, p = .075]. There were, however, significant differences in measures of social support between the experimental and control group when adjusting for HIV status

Table 6.2   Univariate Analyses of Variance of Three Dependent Variables for Effects of Group by HIV Status Interaction over Time

Variable	F	p
Stress	.197	.658
Coping	3.276	.075
Social Support	10.391	.002

Note: Univariate F-Test with (1,66) D.F.

of caregivers (see table 6. 2). The level of social support for caregivers who were seronegative in the experimental group was significantly different [F (1,66) = 10.39, p = .002] from seronegative caregivers in the control group and seropositive caregivers in both groups (see figure 6.1). Based on these results, seronegative caregivers derived substantial benefit from the social support boosting intervention.

The following cases demonstrate the implementation of the social support boosting intervention.

Case 1.   This case involves a fifty-three-year-old African American, seronegative, biological grandmother who was the primary caregiver for her six-year-old granddaughter. The child acquired HIV through perinatal transmission from her mother, who is the biological daughter of the grandmother caregiver. Although infected with HIV, the child appeared to be clinically well and attended school while receiving treatment at a children's HIV/AIDS clinic for an occasional ear infection. This grandmother was a widow living with a male partner in a single-family home along with her granddaughter. Problems identified by this caregiver included dealing with the shock and stigma of her granddaughter's diagnosis of HIV and not feeling able to disclose

Social Support

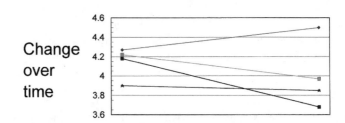

	Data Collection 1	Data Collection 2
✱ Exp. (sero+)	4.18	3.68
✦ Exp. (sero-)	4.27	4.50
✶ Control (sero+)	3.90	3.85
▪ Control (sero-)	4.22	3.97

F (1,66) = 10.39, p = .002

Figure 6.1 Changes in mean social support levels over time.

the diagnosis to others. Another problem was the hostility that the grandmother had toward her daughter for the havoc she had created within the family. The biological mother of this child had a history of intravenous drug abuse and expired from AIDS shortly after this participant was entered into the study. The grandmother, attempting to grieve for her lost daughter, was concerned that she hadn't cried enough for her daughter following her death. Issues related to what can be expected as part of the normal grief process were discussed.

This caregiver identified her live-in male partner as a most important member of her social support network. She was able to discuss most of her concerns with him openly but felt that there were some concerns she could not discuss even with him. She did identify other individuals in her support network that were available to provide additional support. However, these sources of support were not used until the caregiver dealt with issues of disclosure of the HIV status. She was afraid to disclose the diagnosis of HIV in fear that people would distance themselves from her and her granddaughter. She also mentioned that she did not want her granddaughter to be treated differently. This caregiver was helped to identify issues related to fear of rejection and isolation. Through talking first with a few close family members and friends, she discovered how emotional support, companionship, and help with errands could be beneficial. Gradually she was able to open up to others and offered that she was relieved of the burden the diagnostic nondisclosure of the child's HIV/AIDS status. This case demonstrates how the fear of AIDS stigma prevented this caregiver from reaching out for social support. This in turn exacerbated the stress she experienced. Through implementation of the social support-boosting intervention this caregiver was able to access members of her network and acquire the necessary support to deal with the many stressor associated with caring for a child with HIV/AIDS.

Case 2. Case 2 involves a fifty-six-year-old married African American grandmother who is the primary caregiver of two HIV-infected grandchildren aged six and eight years. Her only daughter who had AIDS, committed suicide at the age of twenty-one, before the grandmother became involved in the intervention. Subsequently, the grandmother and her husband obtained custody of the daughter's two HIV-infected children. Unfortunately, the husband had colon cancer of two years' duration and was in the terminal phase of this disease. They all lived together in a cramped four-room apartment in an urban setting in the New York metropolitan area.

Problems associated with caring for the children included frequent illnesses requiring medical attention, behavioral-developmental problems, and sibling rivalry. The six-year-old was described as "mentally slow" and required special education consideration. The eight-year-old was suspended from school for three weeks. She and a classmate were caught commingling blood from self-inflicted cuts—the objective having been to become "blood sisters."

Personal problems of this older caregiver are related to strained financial resources, unresolved grief and anger toward her daughter, resentment of her confinement to the house because of the increased demands of caring for her dying husband, and the potential role of being a single parent at the age of fifty-six.

Members of the caregiver's social support network were identified, using the social support-boosting intervention protocol, and were used to help solve problems associated with the caregiving needs of the children. Her unmarred forty-five-year-old sister was identified as her confidant and helped out on weekends. The local association for retarded children and school guidance counselor, hospice and grief and bereavement counseling, and home health services enabled her to have some free time from her steadily increasing responsibilities. Outcomes for this caregiver included successful resolution of some of her problems related to the caregiving needs of her two grandchildren.

These cases demonstrate how two older seronegative caregivers were able to access and use a variety of social support resources to deal with caregiving problems over time following six monthly interventions. The social support-boosting intervention's effectiveness for these caregivers holds significance from both a research and practice perspective. For many older individuals responsibilities associated with caring for a child with HIV/AIDS is a new experience requiring substantial role redefinition and adjustment. Issues related to disclosure of the HIV status of the child often create situations whereby the caregiver becomes isolated from members of his or her support network due to stigma of HIV/AIDS, and the accumulation of stress becomes immobilizing. Findings from this study suggest that older seronegative caregivers in the experimental group were able more effectively to solve problems with the use of the social support-boosting intervention, which ultimately increased levels of perceived social support and reduced stress.

Clinical Implications Relative to Health Care for
Older HIV/AIDS Caregivers

A critical component of holistic care for the HIV-affected family is provision of social support. Caregiver problems need to be identified and validated in tandem by the health care practitioner and the caregiver in order to solve problems effectively. Evaluation of the achieved outcomes of the plan of care implemented also occurs in tandem with subjective evaluation by the caregiver and objective evaluation by the health care provider.

Caregiver social support-network density seems to be related to the caregiver's HIV status, with HIV-positive caregivers having more limited social support networks than HIV-negative caregivers who are either foster parents or extended family members (Hansell et al. 1993). Boosting the social support network of the older seronegative caregiver is a realistic goal that will facilitate the building of their social support network as well as enable more effective use of their social support network to enable the effective resolution of caregiver problems.

Social support boosting for the seropositive caregiver is extremely difficult. For these caregivers with multiple complex needs overlying progressive HIV/AIDS, more is needed than simply boosting social support. These caregivers need numerous active interventions with referrals to various social service agencies in order to begin to solve problems that entangle their lives. In the experience of the HIV-positive caregiver recurrent illnesses often complicated with frequent hospitalization are quite commonplace. In order to augment effectively the social support network of these caregivers, health-care providers need to be sensitive to the intense needs of the HIV-infected caregiver.

The health professional who provides care for HIV-infected children and their families is confronted with a most challenging situation. Using the social support-boosting protocol has been demonstrated to be effective for older seronegative caregivers.

Acknowledgments

The authors gratefully acknowledge the participation of the AIDS Resource Foundation for Children, Newark, New Jersey; Jersey City Medical Center, Jersey City, New Jersey; and Newark Beth Israel Medical Center, Newark, New Jersey. The study was supported by a grant received from the National Institute of Nursing Research, National Institutes of Health, Grant number 5R01 NRO 2903–03.

References

Bennett, C. 1993. Factors which impact coping and health outcomes of significant others of persons with AIDS. Ph.D. dissertation, University of California at Los Angeles.

Brabant, S. 1994. An overlooked AIDS affected population: The elderly parent as caregiver. *Journal of Gerontological Social Work* 22 (1/2): 131–144.

Caliandro, G., and C. Hughes. 1998. The experience of being a grandmother who is the primary caregiver for her HIV-positive child. *Nursing Research* 47 (2): 107–113.

Cohen, F., and R. S. Lazarus. 1983. Coping and adaptation in health and illness. In D. Mechanic, ed., *Handbook of Health, Health Care and the Health Professions,* pp. 608–635. New York: Free Press.

Cohen, S., and T. Willis. 1985. Stress, social support, and the buffering hypothesis. *Psychological Bulletin* 98:310–357.

Derogatis, L. 1986. *The Derogatis Stress Profile (DSP): A Summary Report.* Baltimore: Clinical Psychometric Research.

Emick, M., and B. Hayslip. 1999. Custodial grandparenting: Stresses, coping skills and relationships with grandchildren. *International Journal of Aging and Human Development* 48 (1): 35–61.

Flaskerud, J., and B. Winslow. 1998. Conceptualizing vulnerable population's health-related research. *Nursing Research* 47 (2): 69–78.

Goode, K., W. Haley, D. Roth, and G. Ford. 1998. Predicting longitudinal changes in caregiver physical and mental health: A stress process model. *Health Psychology* 17 (2): 190–198.

Hansell, P., C. Hughes, G. Caliandro, P. Russo, W. Budin, and B. Hartman. 1993. Stress, coping, social support and problems experienced by caregivers of HIV infected children: A comparison of HIV infected caregivers to non HIV infected caregivers. Paper presented at the Ninth International Conference on AIDS, Berlin.

Hansell, P., C. Hughes, G. Caliandro, P. Russo, W. Budin, B. Hartman, and O. Hernandez. 1998. The effect of a social support boosting intervention on stress, coping and social support in caregivers of children with HIV/AIDS. *Nursing Research* 47 (2): 79–86.

———. 1999. Boosting social support in caregivers of children with HIV/AIDS. *AIDS Patient Care and STDS* 13 (5): 297–302.

Joslin, D., and R. Harrison. 1998. The hidden patient: Older relatives raising children orphaned by AIDS. *Journal of the American Women's Medical Association* 53 (2): 65–71.

Kalichman, S. C., K. J. Sikkema, and A. Somlai. 1996. People living with HIV infection that attend and do not attend support groups: A pilot study of needs, characteristics and experience. *AIDS Care: Psychological and Socio-Medical Aspects of AIDS/HIV* 8 (5): 589–599.

Kelley, S. J., and E. G. Damato. 1995. Grandparents as primary caregivers. *Maternal Child Nursing* 20:326–332.

Kelley, S., B. Yorker, and D. Whitley. 1997. To grandmother's house we go . . . and stay:

Children raised in intergenerational families. *Journal of Gerontological Nursing* 23 (9): 12–20.

Lazarus, R. S., and S. Folkman. 1984. *Stress, Appraisal and Coping*. New York: Springer.

LeBlanc, A., C. Aneshensel, and R. Wight. 1995. Psychotherapy use and depression among AIDS caregivers. *Journal of Counseling Psychology* 23:127–142.

LeBlanc, A., A. London, and C. Aneshensel. 1997. The physical costs of AIDS caregiving. *Social Science Medicine* 45 (6): 915–923.

Lesar, S., and Y. Maldonado. 1994. Infants and young children with HIV infection: Service delivery considerations for family support. *Young Children* 6 (4): 70–81.

Littrell, J. 1996. How psychological states affect the immune system: Implications for interventions in the context of HIV. *Health and Social Work* 21 (4): 287–295.

Lutgendorf, S., M. Antoni, N. Schneiderman, and M. Fletcher. 1994. Psychosocial counseling to improve quality of life in HIV infection. *Patient Education and Counseling* 24:217–235.

McCubbin, H., and A. Thompson. 1987. *F-COPES: Family Assessment Inventories for Research and Practice*. Madison: University of Wisconsin Press.

Moneyham, L., M. Hennessey, R. Sowell, A. Demi, B. Seals, and Y. Mizuno. 1998. The effectiveness of coping strategies used by HIV-seropositive women. *Research in Nursing and Health* 21: 351–362.

Musil, C. 1998. Health, stress, coping and social support in grandmother caregivers. *Health Care for Women International* 19:441–455.

New Jersey Assembly Task Force on Grandparenting Report of Findings and Recommendations. January 2000. http://www.census.gov/population/socdemo/grandparents/gp-2.txt.

Reynolds, N., and A. Alonzo. 1998. HIV informal caregiving: emergent conflict and growth. *Research in Nursing and Health* 21:251–260.

Rutman, D. 1996. Caregiving as women's work: Women's experiences of powerfulness and powerlessness as caregivers. *Qualitative Health Research* 6 (1): 90–111.

Schaaf, R., L. Sherwen, and N. Youngblood. 1997. An interdisciplinary, environmentally-based model of care for children with HIV infection and their caregivers. *Physical and Occupational Therapy in Pediatrics* 17 (3): 63–85.

Strawbridge, W., M. Wallhagen, S. Shema, and G. Kaplan. 1997. New burdens or more of the same? Comparing grandparent, spouse, and adult child caregivers. *The Gerontologist* 17 (4): 505–510.

Thoits, P. A. 1982. Conceptual, methodological, and theoretical problems in studying social support as a buffer against life stress. *Journal of Health and Social Behavior* 23:145–159.

——. 1986. Social support as coping assistance. *Journal of Consulting and Clinical Psychology* 54 (4): 416–423.

Tilden, V. P. 1991. The interpersonal relationship inventory (IPRI): Instrument development summary. Paper, Oregon Health Science University School of Nursing.

Vaux, A. 1988. *Social Support: Theory, Research and Intervention*. New York: Praeger.

Williams, J. 1995. Afro-American women living with HIV infection: Special therapeutic interventions for a growing population. *Social Work in Health Care* 21 (2): 41–53.

7

Caring for the HIV-Infected Child

JENNY GROSZ

Identification of the first pediatric AIDS cases occurred in the early 1980s, reported by Dr. Arye Rubenstein in the Bronx, New York, and by Dr. James Oleske in Newark, New Jersey. Babies born to women who were intravenous drug users presented with recurring bacterial infections, interstitial pneumonitis, and failure to thrive (Oleske et al. 1983; Rubenstein et al. 1983). Sickly babies were being abandoned in city hospitals and were developing devastating infections, often resulting in death. By 1987 AIDS had become the third leading cause of death among African American children between the ages of one and four years in New York and New Jersey. Although the majority are concentrated in large urban areas such as Miami, Washington, New York, Newark, Los Angeles, and San Juan, pediatric AIDS cases have been reported in forty-nine states (Centers for Disease Control and Prevention 1999).

Although it shares characteristics with other chronic illnesses, such as the need for long-term medical care, slow deterioration of health, and a foreshortened sense of future, HIV disease continues to present unique issues. The diagnosis of HIV in a young child or infant often results in the identification of HIV in the mother and possibly other family members. Families may experience the loss of several children, one or both parents, and extended family members who may also be infected. Fear of stigma leads to further withdrawal from community supports, isolating families. Unlike other chronic diseases of childhood, HIV/AIDS can lead to the breakdown of the family. This devastating diagnosis can result in the deterioration of fragile, marginal families that are already struggling with the effects of poverty, stigma and social isolation, drug addiction, and poor health care.

In the United States growing numbers of children are being cared for by older caregivers (Hackworth 1998). HIV/AIDS, with its associated medical, psychosocial, and emotional complexities, presents an overwhelming dilemma to older caregivers who must set aside their own lives to care for ill children with uncertain futures. This chapter provides an overview of issues confronting older caregivers who are raising infected children and adolescents. It draws on the shared experiences of a group of caregivers who have met on a biweekly basis for the last six years at the Children's Evaluation and Rehabilitation Center (CERC). Part of the Albert Einstein College of Medicine, the center provides the neurodevelopmental and mental health component of the Bronx Pediatric and Adolescent AIDS Consortia (BPAAC), a Ryan White Title IV–funded program. The women range in age from the mid-forties to the early eighties. They are grandmothers and adoptive mothers who have raised at least one generation of children in the past and who are now caring for chronically ill children whose own biological mothers were unable or too sick to care for them. They come together for support, to celebrate birthdays and holidays, to share each other's joys, and to comfort each other in times of mourning. They have established their own community, replacing the one they gave up when they became caregivers of a child with HIV/AIDS (Edell 1998).

Epidemiology and Demographics

The third decade of the HIV/AIDS epidemic is marked by the development of new treatments that have brought a renewed sense of hope to those living with the disease. AIDS is becoming a manageable, chronic illness, no longer the universally fatal disease that it once was. Death rates among persons with AIDS have dropped significantly over the past few years (Centers for Disease Control and Prevention 1998). However, death rates among women, especially women of color, have dropped less dramatically, and HIV/AIDS continues to disproportionately affect poor, minority, and traditionally underserved populations from the inner cities. Rates of transmission are increasing at an alarming rate in women, especially young women of color, most notably in the African American and Hispanic communities. Many women of childbearing years are infected in adolescence, with progression to AIDS taking anywhere from eight to ten years. In 1992 women accounted for 13.8 percent of persons living with AIDS compared with 19.1 percent in 1997. More than thirteen thousand new cases of AIDS in women were reported in 1997.

Twenty percent of those cases were in women between the ages of thirteen and twenty-nine. Sixty percent of the women reported with AIDS in 1997 were African American, and the rate of AIDS cases was seven times higher in Hispanic women than in white women (HRSA Care Action 1999).

As of December 1998 a cumulative total of 8,461 pediatric AIDS cases had been reported in the United States since the beginning of the epidemic (Centers for Disease Control and Prevention 1999). It is important to note that although some states report all cases of HIV infection, the majority of states with large populations of persons infected with HIV only report cases of full-blown AIDS. As a result, the CDC statistics underreport the actual number of cases of HIV infection in adults and children. The total number of children infected with HIV is estimated at two to three times the number of known AIDS cases. By adding the number of HIV-infected children reported by those states that have HIV reporting with the numbers of children reported to have full-blown AIDS, the CDC concluded that 5,237 children under the age of thirteen were living with HIV infection and with AIDS in the United States in 1998. The New York State AIDS Institute's Bureau of HIV/AIDS Epidemiology estimated that 121 perinatally infected adolescent AIDS cases were presumed alive in New York in 1997, reflecting the growing population of long-term surviving children reported around the country. By 1996 the number of children who were diagnosed with AIDS declined 43 percent, primarily due to the continued success of efforts to reduce perinatal transmission through voluntary HIV testing and AZT treatment for pregnant HIV infected women and their infants (Institute of Medicine 1998).

Transmission in Children

Maternal transmission is the most frequent cause of Pediatric Human Immunodeficiency Virus (HIV) in the United States, representing 91 percent of the total cases according to the CDC (Centers for Disease Control and Prevention 1998). In more than half of such cases the infected child's father or the mother's domestic partner is also HIV-positive. Mothers with HIV infection, in the vast majority of cases, have acquired HIV either by direct intravenous drug use or heterosexual contact with an intravenous drug-using partner.

Transmission from mother to child is known as vertical transmission. A very small number of children have acquired the disease from blood products or sexual abuse. All children born to HIV-infected women are "sero-exposed" and will test positive for maternal HIV antibodies. However, this does not mean that all babies born to infected women will develop HIV. Transmission rates vary. In the United States, they range at about 25 percent to 30 percent. New technology such as the use of polymerase chain reaction (PCR) and actual culturing of the HIV virus can determine the HIV status of newborns within the first few weeks of birth (American Academy of Pediatrics 1998). When babies no longer test positive for maternal antibodies, they are said to serorevert. These babies were never actually infected with HIV, and within twelve to eighteen months will no longer test HIV-positive when given an antibody test. Infants and children who are infected are considered seropositive and will have positive PCR test results and positive viral cultures for the rest of their lives. Although the incidence of HIV in women has increased, a dramatic decrease in the incidence of new pediatric AIDS cases has been noted over the past few years. The treatment of pregnant, HIV-positive women with AZT during pregnancy and delivery and treatment of the newborn in the first six weeks of life have resulted in transmission rates' dropping from 30 percent to 8 percent. Transmission rates have been further reduced to less than 2 percent when the babies are delivered by cesarean section (U.S. Public Health Service Task Force 1998). The trend toward mandatory HIV counseling and voluntary testing of pregnant women has further resulted in early identification of HIV infection in women who can then receive appropriate reproductive-health counseling. Infected women will be able to make educated decisions about whether to have children and whether to participate in drug regimens and delivery procedures that could potentially eliminate pediatric HIV/AIDS.

Testing and Diagnosis

Some states, including New York, mandate HIV testing of all newborns as part of the routine Newborn Screening Test. Though not optimal because of the lost opportunity to provide intervention in utero, the results of these tests yield information about the mother's HIV status. The diagnosis of HIV in a young child or infant often results in the identification of HIV in the mother and possibly other family members. Positive identification of maternal antibodies can lead to referral for medical care including early intervention with antiretroviral treatments and PCP prophylaxis to delay and possibly prevent the progression from HIV infection to AIDS.

However, HIV testing of newborns presents a serious ethical dilemma. By testing the newborn, the mother's status is automatically revealed, regardless of her consent to be tested. This violates the principle of the confidentiality of the mother who is being tested through her newborn. Controversy has developed between advocates for women's rights who feel that women continue to receive second-class HIV-related treatment and advocates whose goal is the reduction of perinatal transmission.

Mandatory counseling and voluntary testing of all pregnant women provide important information and the opportunity for the women to accept testing. The right of the mother to consent to be tested preserves her confidentiality while encouraging early diagnosis of maternal HIV and the benefits of early treatment for the newborn.

Although technology exists to definitively diagnose HIV infection in children at a very early age, children born before the implementation of universal newborn testing were not routinely tested for HIV and may be undiagnosed until the onset of symptoms. In some cases children are tested because of the birth of a younger sibling who has been identified as HIV-positive through newborn screening or due to illness in that infant. Testing of all family members is strongly recommended at that time, and many mothers report that they learned of their own HIV diagnosis and that of other family members after the birth of an infected child. Children who have been completely asymptomatic in early to middle childhood test positive for the virus.

Diagnosis of HIV in older children can also occur as a result of sudden onset of a serious illness such as neurological deterioration unrelated to injury or intractable opportunistic infection such as recurring shingles. The following cases highlight the diagnosis of perinatally acquired HIV in two preadolescents who had not been previously tested.

At age eleven Jimmy was hospitalized with a serious case of shingles, a painful and potentially scarring rash caused by the same organism that causes chickenpox. Aggressive treatment did not prevent repeat recurrences over a four-month period. His mother had died of AIDS when Jimmy was three years old. His father had been diagnosed with HIV in 1995. Although the family had received consistent, comprehensive medical care from a family physician, Jimmy had not been tested for HIV before this episode. At the time of his diagnosis he had an alarmingly high viral load and low T-cell count despite no prior symptomatology.

• • •

Hannah is a thirteen-year-old girl who had been in the care of her paternal grandmother since infancy. The mother, a drug user, had abandoned the child at birth and had had intermittent contact with the family through the years. The grandmother was not aware of any health problems in the mother, who had moved to New Jersey.

The grandmother noticed that Hannah was losing her hair when she was thirteen. She took Hannah to her pediatrician at New York City Municipal Hospital, located in an area of the Bronx with an especially high prevalence of HIV infection. The child was referred to dermatology clinic and given medication to treat the hair loss. The grandmother was not satisfied with the results and took the child to a medical clinic in the neighborhood. The physician at the clinic examined the child and suggested that she have an HIV test. The grandmother did not believe there was any possible risk but consented. The child tested HIV-positive. Ultimately, the grandmother learned from Hannah's mother that she was also infected but well.

These two cases underscore the continued reluctance to test children for HIV. In the first case, there was sufficient cause for testing following the mother's death and later on, the father's diagnosis. In the second case, while the risk factors were less evident, the child's mother had a history of drug use, lived in an area of very high seroprevalence, and had abandoned the child. The child had received all of her wellness care from a municipal hospital with a large HIV patient population. Yet in both cases the children remained untested until they developed symptoms. Opportunity to provide early intervention was lost for these children, who had severely compromised immune systems by the time they were diagnosed. Diagnosis of perinatally infected adolescents has been increasingly reported by pediatric HIV/AIDS clinics in New York and Miami.

HIV Disease Progression and Symptomatology

The spectrum of pediatric HIV disease ranges from asymptomatic infection to a child severely ill with AIDS. The latency period between infection with HIV and the first symptoms of AIDS in children varies widely (Wolters, Brouwers, and Moss 1995). Some children have such mild symptoms that they may be undiagnosed for years until they develop a serious AIDS-defining illness. Children diagnosed with HIV-related symptoms, such as lymphadenopathy, hepatomegaly, splenomegaly, recurrent or multiple opportunistic infections such as septicemia or PCP pneumonia, or encephalopathy before one to two years of age are considered "rapid progressors" and have a significant decrease in survival rates (Blanche et al. 1990). Other children may not develop HIV-related symptoms until after two years of age but may then develop AIDS-defining illnesses such as encephalopathy with loss or regression of motor milestones. This group may have multiple hospitalizations and a difficult medical course characterized by failure to thrive, anemia, hair loss, and recurrent or chronic diarrhea. With the use of new antiretroviral drugs, protease inhibitors, and powerful antibiotics, survival into the mid-childhood years is likely. A third group of children, considered "long-term survivors," consists of youngsters who were infected at birth but who have remained free or only mildly symptomatic of HIV-related symptoms and are living into their teen years (Grubman et al. 1995).

The clinical manifestations of HIV infection in children are extremely varied. The virus can affect many organ systems, such as the cardiovascular (heart), hepatic (liver), central nervous system (brain and neuromuscular), or pulmonary (lungs). Multiorgan dysfunction leads to an array of health problems that can range from mild, recurring ear and upper respiratory infections to severe neurological deterioration due to encephalopathy and central nervous system involvement. Problems seen most often in children are failure to thrive and short stature, reactive airway disease, recurrent serious bacterial infections, and developmental delays. Children with early onset of opportunistic infections, infections that affect persons with weak immune systems, such as PCP- or HIV-related developmental delays within the first year of life, tend to have a poorer prognosis and earlier death (Blanche et al. 1990). Early diagnosis of HIV infection can lead to simple intervention with antibiotic treatment to prevent the development of PCP in young children that can result in a healthier course for many infected babies.

Neurodevelopmental and Behavioral Difficulties

In addition to severe immune deficiency, leading to opportunistic infections, and possible dysfunction of multiorgan systems, impairment of the central nervous system (CNS) is a major consequence of HIV infection (American Academy of Pediatrics 1998). Early studies of infected children reported that between 78 percent and 90 percent had neurodevelopmental abnormalities (Ultmann et al. 1987; Epstein et al. 1986). These included mental retardation, cerebral palsy-like symptoms, varying degrees of developmental delay and HIV associated progressive encephalopathy (PE).

PE is most often seen in children who are rapidly deteriorating. The predominant features of PE are impaired brain growth, progressive motor dysfunction and loss, plateauing, or inadequate rate of achieving neurodevelopmental milestones (American Academy of Pediatrics 1998). Children with PE require neurodevelopmental follow-up and rehabilitation including physical, and occupational therapy to improve fine and gross motor impairment and speech and language therapy to address feeding difficulties and language deficits. More recent data indicate that children with a slow progression of HIV infection can have a wide range of deficits, many with less severe cognitive and motor dysfunction (Fundaro et al. 1998; Moss et al. 1998; Wolters, Brouwers, and Moss 1995; Cohen, Papola, and Alvarez 1994). Mild neurodevelopmental symptoms in less impaired children, such as mild cognitive deficits, attentional problems, memory loss, perceptual and organizational difficulties, and language-processing problems might not be identified by caregivers who are more focused on the acute symptoms of HIV disease. This can lead to an array of school difficulties that include learning disabilities, issues of self-esteem, behavioral problems, and difficulties with peers. Academic difficulties may also be the result of genetic, familial issues, or prenatal drug exposure. Hyperactivity and attentional problems may be due to CNS involvement or medication side effects such as asthma treatments or be symptomatic manifestation of childhood depression or anxiety, which can reduce concentration. Distractibility, inactivity, and irritability can also be markers of childhood depression. Behavioral difficulties may be expressions of children's distress over illness in other family members, maternal depression, multiple family losses, or bereavement (Wolters, Brouwers, and Moss 1995). HIV-positive children who have no other symptoms can exhibit memory loss, organizational problems, and attentional difficulties. Fatigue, inconsistent school attendance due to illness and a general feeling of malaise, and medication side effects also affect school performance. Early interventions, including differential diagnosis, can diffuse behavioral and emotional difficulties that affect social function, school performance, and self-esteem.

Antiretroviral Treatments

Antiretroviral therapies have significantly improved the quality of life of persons living with HIV/AIDS. As the life cycle of the virus is better understood, new drugs are being developed and used in combination therapy to combat the virus more effectively.

Standard-of-care guidelines assist clinicians in determining the most effective treatments. AZT, one of the most widely used drugs in HIV care, and other antiretroviral drugs have been effective in reversing the effects of PE to some extent (American Academy of Pediatrics 1998). New drugs known as protease inhibitors (Norvir, Crixivan, Viracept, and Sequanavir), when used in conjunction with AZT or ddI, another commonly used antiretroviral drug, seem to inhibit the growth of the virus more effectively than with AZT or ddI alone. These drug combinations are considered highly active antiretroviral treatments (HAART). Generally, protease inhibitors increase CD-4 counts, one marker of how the immune system is functioning. Blood tests to determine the amount of virus in the blood, known as viral load testing, are used to monitor the effectiveness of the drugs in keeping viral loads below undetectable levels.

As is true for many drugs, clinical trials for pediatric HIV drug use are limited. Prior to approval for pediatric use, physicians, sometimes at the urging of parents who understood the drug benefits in adult HIV symptomatic patients, started "compassionate use" of these new drugs on children with some dramatic benefits, in some cases even reversing serious deterioration. Recent legislation providing incentives to pharmaceutical companies to conduct clinical trials for efficacy in children has led to a greater number of available pediatric HIV clinical trials. Despite the benefits, HAART can have serious drawbacks. Complicated medication regimens with as many as thirty to forty-five pills daily and at specified times with relation to meals (with food or after fasting) can lead to poor adherence. Physician's reluctance to put older children and adolescents on HAART is due to the high rate of drug resistance if the drugs are not taken as prescribed.

Many drugs have many unpleasant side effects. Children and adults alike complain of nausea, light-headedness, nightmares, abdominal cramps, and bad aftertaste. Caregivers report major difficulties in managing the complicated schedules required for compliance with these medications. Children who may otherwise be asymptomatic feel sick and can experience weight loss and diarrhea. One grandmother was forced to confront quality-of-life issues and the major dilemma of either insisting that her teenage grandson take medication that made him too sick to attend school or choosing not give the medication despite the implications for a very poor prognosis. Medical providers did not know how to deal with these issues and resorted to reporting the grandmother to protective services to try to force her to administer the medications. Ultimately, therapeutic work with the adolescent led to a brief hospitalization to help get him onto the regimen and past the side effects so that he could return home. The difficulty with medication adherence is not unique to HIV infection, as documented in the pediatric literature relating to other chronic diseases such as juvenile diabetes (Anderson and Ho 1997). Working closely with medical providers and social workers can help the child and family deal with the complex decisions surrounding HAART.

Dealing With Debilitating Illness

Coping with HIV illness takes a dramatic toll on caregivers, infected and affected children, and other family members. Caregivers and patients alike must cope with the prospect of an uncertain future. Onset of an acute episode of HIV-related illness could leave a medically stable child in a critical state with significant loss of functioning. The following case illustrates this.

Ten-year-old Samantha was a healthy, well-functioning child who had been diagnosed as HIV-positive at age five following the birth of her brother. She had been doing well in school and had not experienced any medical problems. One morning she awoke with mild memory loss, and had difficulty walking, with motor problems that included poor balance and weakness on the left side of her body. The episode was not accompanied by any other symptoms (e.g., fever or apparent infection). Samantha's condition was stabilized by a change in medication, but she required months of intensive occupational, physical and speech therapy to help her regain the lost skills.

In advanced stages of disease, the child may experience physical pain and deterioration of motor function. Families experience a roller coaster ride of highs when new medications halt or even reverse deterioration and improve prognosis, and lows when the treatments no longer prevent a downward decline. Many caregivers have held vigil over their children in intensive care and made funeral arrangements at the suggestion of providers, only to have the child make such dramatic improvement that they are able to return to relatively normal functioning. Caregivers who maintained the belief that their love and care would reverse the inevitable outcome of HIV disease are devastated by their inability to change the situation (Lieberman 1989). Confusion and mixed emotions around whether they can emotionally cope with another death frequently plague family members who may be reliving painful memories of other loved ones that rebounded from pseudo health and eventually died.

During a caregivers' support group session at CERC Cherry tearfully spoke of the deterioration of her little niece, Janie, seven, who had suffered a stroke. She had become incontinent, dependent for feeding and all self-care needs. The caregiver, who had no outside help, described her state of exhaustion at trying to keep the child comfortable. She spoke of her sister, the child's mother, who had died several years before after lingering between life and death for several weeks. The child's illness had brought back unresolved feelings of guilt and regret that she had not done enough for her sister.

• • •

Sarah, an eighty-three-year-old grandmother, tearfully described her ambivalence around her twelve-year-old granddaughter's slowly improving health, stating that she didn't know what to wish for—that the child get better or that the child die.

Caregivers are also confronted by unresolved grief over the physical and/or psychological deaths of their own children. Many question whether they have the strength to weather a child's debilitating illness as they age and become debilitated themselves (Poe 1999).

One grandmother in the caregiver's group, Maddie, age seventy-four, poignantly spoke of her granddaughter Dolly as the fourth set of children she had raised. She shared feelings of failure in raising Dolly's mother, who had become an intravenous drug user. She talked about her other grandchildren, now adults, whom she had raised when her daughter was unable to care for them. She wearily added that before Dolly had come to live with her, she had finally been looking forward to a life of decreased stress with her husband and friends. However, instead of going to the theater with her peers, she was running to hospitals and clinic appointments with her granddaughter. Dolly, thirteen, had lived with her mother and father in a suburb of New York City. Family visits were infrequent. When Dolly's mother Annie became desperately ill, the father brought Dolly to Maddie for care. Maddie was unaware of Dolly and Annie's diagnosis of AIDS. While Annie lay dying in the hospital, Dolly developed severe neurological symptoms, described by Maddie as strokelike. Struggling to understand what was happening to her daughter and granddaughter, Maddie confronted a wall of silence on the father's part; he refused to disclose any information about the nature of the disease. It was only after he relinquished guardianship of Dolly that Maddie was able to learn that the cause of the illness was HIV infection. Against the wishes of the father, but on the strong advice from medical professionals that Dolly would die without aggressive treatment, Maddie gave permission for Dolly to receive combination therapy. Looking back on that time in her life, Maddie reflects on whether her daughter might still be alive had she had treatment. More importantly, she is convinced that without her intercession Dolly would probably have died for lack of treatment. Totally devoted to Dolly's needs, Maddie is struggling with feelings of guilt that she is not attentive to her husband who has recently developed prostate cancer. Loyalties are torn between her responsibilities as a wife, and those of a caregiver of a child, making the golden years more difficult than she could ever imagine.

Care of a chronically ill child places exceptional demands on any caregiver. Because the spectrum of HIV disease can be extremely broad, day-to-day management of the illness can be very taxing. Caring for a youngster who is in an acute stage of disease can entail running between the hospital and home during lengthy hospitalizations, learning to perform lifesaving procedures such as suctioning tracheotomy tubes, or adjusting to the presence of visiting nurses and home attendants who may be perceived as intrusive. Caregivers have little regard for their own needs, and rest, health care, and emotional needs are commonly ignored. Caregivers try to juggle the routine demands of caring for a family with the extraordinary pressures of dealing with their child's discomfort and their own fear regarding the child's prognosis. Often, they try to do this without any additional support to handle the daily tasks of managing a household or caring for other children or family members in the home.

The mildly symptomatic HIV-infected child presents an equally exigent burden on the family caregiver. Medical management requires regularly scheduled doctor visits, lab work, and routine monitoring. Ancillary interventions such as psychoeducational support, occupational, physical, and/or speech therapy, and mental-health services place extra demands to participate in weekly clinic visits. It is not uncommon for a youngster to have two or three weekly therapy sessions in addition to medical visits. Some kids spend so much time in clinic that they jokingly refer to clinic as a second home. Helping the caregiver prioritize what interventions are most beneficial is an important task of medical providers to avoid overloading the child and the caregivers and causing additional distress. A balance between supportive interventions and quality of life must be stressed to give caregivers who feel that they are obligated to accept all recommendations regardless of the difficulties these may create.

Stigma and Disclosure of HIV Diagnosis

Fear of stigma and ostracism associated with HIV cause caregivers to remain secretive about the child's and the family's diagnosis. Although disclosure may lead to additional sources of support, it can also lead to rejection and persecution resulting from ignorance and fears surrounding transmission (Weiner and Septimus 1991). Though progress has been made in educating the public about HIV, societal attitudes persist to maintain the need for secrecy (Lewis, Haiken, and Hoyt 1994).

Infected children live with grandparents and other surrogate caregivers when their parents are unable to care for them due to HIV-related illness, substance abuse, mental illness, or death. In many instances, the caregivers have not been informed of their adult child's HIV-positive diagnosis and learn of it only at a time of crisis, such as the parent's hospitalization or death, when they are called on to assume care of the children. It is not uncommon for caregivers to report that they have not been given direct information and only surmise that their loved one has died of AIDS. Consequently, caregivers are often ill prepared to discuss the situation with anyone. Feelings of embarrassment and guilt prevent them from discussing the reasons of their loved one's death or inability to care for the children. Often they withdraw from traditional sources of support such as their religious congregation for fear of what others might think.

Antonia, age sixty-eight, a grandmother in the CERC Caregivers Group, looks back on the time that she got custody of her young granddaughter Terri. Antonia, who feared that her daughter Karen's drug addiction compromised her ability to care for Terri, reported Karen to Child Protective Services. Terri was placed in the grandmother's care.

The child was suffering from recurrent and painful ear infections that did not respond to treatment. After some discussion with the family doctor, Antonia gave consent for the child to be tested for HIV. Much to her surprise, the test was positive. When Antonia told her daughter about the results of the test, Karen immediately accused the grandmother of exposing Terri to sexual abuse that had led to the HIV diagnosis. Mortified at this possibility, Antonia sought help to understand how her grandchild could be infected. It was not until several years later, after the birth of another infected baby that Karen admitted to being positive herself. Antonia had lived with the guilt of thinking that she had caused her granddaughter's infection. She did not know anyone else in her situation and had no where to turn for support.

Caregivers need support and guidance as they deal with feelings around disclosure. Making a distinction between the family's right to privacy and "keeping a secret" can remove negative connotations. Knowing when, how and to whom to disclose information can free families from fear of stigma and its associated isolation. Once released from the burden of secrecy the family can enjoy many social benefits including attendance in school and church, and support from friends and family.

Not all families choose to disclose the diagnosis. Learning to understand the purpose of the disclosure and to identify the benefit to the child and family helps to minimize the sense of isolation and stigma. For example, disclosure to the Child Study Team in school can help caregivers to gain access to educational placement and services that would otherwise be difficult to arrange. Disclosure can be limited to the review team and need not be shared with the actual teachers or personnel in the school. Helping caregivers to explore the "HIV savvy" of different providers can lead to identifying important resources in the community. Families should be encouraged to ask questions about the makeup of the student population (such as "How do you handle children with chronic medical problems like sickle cell, seizures, or HIV?") that would provide insight into the level of comfort among staff in dealing with HIV-positive children.

Disclosure to Children

Caregivers often express concern about disclosing the diagnosis to the infected child, worried about causing undue distress in the child. Some worry that the child will discuss the family secret and create problems in the neighborhood when intolerant people learn of the diagnosis. However, caregivers overlook the stress that the children experience when they know something is wrong and have no one to talk to. All too often children try to protect their parents from the knowledge that they, the children, suspect about their illness. A seven-year-old child told his therapist that he had AIDS and asked the therapist not to tell his mother because he did not think the mother could handle the information. Another child shared his relief with his therapist when he found out that he was the one with the illness, while all along he had feared that his caregiver aunt was dying because she was always crying.

When disclosure is handled sensitively, children who participate in a support group report little distress over the information. Disclosure at an early age and at a time of relative good health can lead to acceptance of the diagnosis as a matter of fact. Often the child will want to share the information with a friend or significant adult as a way of testing out the reactions of others. It is important for parents and caregivers to help the child understand that the diagnosis is private and personal information. Children need guidance in developing good judgment about whom to share the information with, just as they would with any other private family issue.

The American Academy of Pediatrics published recommendations on disclosure of diagnosis to children and adolescents living with HIV infection (American Academy of Pediatrics 1999a). Citing the more than eight thousand cases of AIDS in children under age thirteen and three thousand cases in teens, the Academy recommends that "disclosure of the diagnosis to an HIV-infected child should be individualized to include the child's age, psychosocial maturity, the complexity of the family dynamics and the clinical context." It suggests that parents and caregivers of an HIV-infected child should receive counseling from knowledgeable health professionals about disclosure to the child about their infection status.

Confounding Family Factors

Caregivers deal with many issues aside from childcare responsibilities. One common dilemma can occur when called on to care for their ill adult child and an ill grandchild and other grandchildren living in the home. As helpers in the home, they try to allow the child's mother to maintain a role over the children, yet feel the responsibility to ensure the child's well-being. Ill parents can "parentify" children by placing too many adult responsibilities on them. The intervention of a grandmother can be perceived as meddling or usurping of the mother's parental role causing conflict between the mother and well-meaning caregiver. At the same time, caregivers struggle to deal with their feelings around the declining health of their loved ones and fear of the future. The friction can cause difficulties in the relationship between the adults, leading to added distress.

Nina, age thirty-four, was extremely ill and had become wheelchair-bound and emaciated. She and her three sons—Charlie, ten; Arnie, four; and Tim, two and HIV-positive—lived in a two family house that they shared with Shelley, her fifty-six-year-old mother. During the day the grandmother helped with childcare and prepared meals. She made sure that the children got to school, did homework and monitored Tim's medical appointments. The grandmother worked as a night home attendant in a local nursing home. The children were left alone with Nina, who often had pain and difficulty sleeping. Charlie was responsible for the younger boys and for helping his mother to get to the bathroom during the night. Shelley knew that the arrangement was a poor plan, and attempted to have a homemaker come into the home at night. Nina refused, saying that she could not understand why the mother could not quit her job to care for her. Charlie started doing very poorly in school, was extremely preoccupied that his mother was going to die while he was in charge and developed serious behavioral problems. The grandmother was at a loss for what to do because Nina perceived every attempt she made at getting help as a lack of confidence. Ultimately, with the help of the clinic providers, Nina was helped to understand the impact on Charlie and the other children. She eventually accepted help in the home. However, as her health improved with the use of HAART, she regained charge of her family and became estranged from her mother.

The presence of mentally ill or drug-using parents further complicates the responsibility of caring for children, making the task overwhelming. Emotional and physical absence of the parents and the abandonment of young children may lead to foster-care placement. In some cases, the Child Protective Services Agency has removed the children from the care of the natural parents and prohibits contact. Allowing the parent to visit the caregiver's home, whether it is for a hot meal or to spend time with the children, puts the children at risk of being removed from the home for violation of the non-visitation order. Caregivers are confronted with painful choices between the needs of their adult child vs. the needs of the children for whom they care.

Perinatally Infected Children Becoming Adolescents

At the onset of the pediatric HIV epidemic, when the long-term prognosis was very bleak, caregivers took on the task of caring for terminally ill children. Many expressed the hope that their loving care would reverse the devastating outcome of the disease. They accepted this task with grace and love, hoping to make the short lives of these children as enriched and fulfilled as possible. Many hoped but very few believed that they would still be caring for these kids into adolescence. Yet this is becoming the reality for many caregivers of the first generation of perinatally infected teenagers.

Members of the Caregivers Support Group meet to gain strength from each other, to provide each other support, and to commiserate on the difficulties of raising children in the new millennium. Many have said that although they fully expected to nurse sick children, none of them ever thought that they would have to confront issues of schooling and homework, sleepovers and overnight camp, adolescence and emerging sexuality. Though thrilled at the prospect of seeing the children live well beyond anyone's expectations, caregivers and professionals alike cope with the challenges this poses. One adoptive mother shared her dilemma about her desire to give her teenage daughter an opportunity to date and to have a romantic experience while fully aware of the need to safeguard the well being of others. Another caregiver discussed her concern that the infant born to her perinatally infected granddaughter might also be infected despite adherence to guidelines to reduce perinatal transmission.

Adolescence is a time of tremendous physical and emotional growth, of experimentation, and separation. For youngsters living with HIV disease, adolescence is complicated by fears of disclosure, stigma and isolation, and concern about the future. Coping with delayed sexual maturation, short stature and a fragile, sickly appearance can be devastating to a teenager who just wants to be like everyone else. The need for peer acceptance is never stronger than in adolescence. This can lead to risk-taking behaviors such as experimentation with drugs and alcohol, sexual relationships, and a lack of discipline with regard to medication adherence. For young people living with HIV, their sense of a foreshortened future means there is no time to lose.

Young people ages fourteen to seventeen who participate in a support group for perinatally infected youth speak openly about their feelings. Issues related to taking medication set the tone for the discussions. Most say, "Why take medicine? I'm going to die anyway." Feelings of uncertainty about the future highlight an underlying sense of depression that the teenagers express.

Caregivers in the group sit around the large conference table and share their concern that they are not sure how to help the situation. Daisy, seventy-one, speaks for everyone when she says, "I didn't know that I was going to have to face the challenge of raising a teenager." Separated from the children by a large generational gap, these caregivers talk about how the rules have changed with regard to childrearing since the last time they had teenagers in the home. Issues such as reproductive health and sexuality, preparation for entry into adulthood, and the challenges of adolescence are now integral in the daily lives of these families. They are frightened by the prospect of getting it wrong again, inasmuch as many of them harbor guilt over having failed their own children. Some have said that they are not sure whether they would have taken on the task of raising these children if they had known they were going to survive into adolescence. They reach out for help from clinicians who are equally stumped.

Conclusion

Pediatric HIV disease has a major impact on the lives of older caregivers who have assumed responsibility for the care of ill and orphaned children. Selfless and determined to provide an optimal life for these youngsters, they have set aside their own needs and lives to devote themselves to their task.

Caring for any chronically ill child is stressful and demanding. HIV/AIDS brings with it additional burdens of social stigma and isolation, issues of disclosure, and often bereavement and anticipated loss. The transition from "dying of AIDS" to "living with HIV" has had a major impact on the lives of these families as caregivers have been learning how to deal with the new challenges of HAART and perinatally infected adolescents. Working to help the youngsters overcome their foreshortened sense of future and helping them learn to integrate management of chronic disease within the context of self evolution are two major tasks that caregivers and clinicians must tackle together to ensure positive outcomes for the kids.

Supportive interventions are needed to assist older caregivers to cope with evolving and increasing demands placed on them. Support groups are effective tools by which caregivers can be encouraged to care for themselves and to articulate their needs and those of their families to service providers. In addition, service providers must work collaboratively to provide interventions for the caregivers—who, too, are long-term survivors.

References

American Academy of Pediatrics. 1991. Policy statement: Education of children with HIV infection, Task Force on Pediatric AIDS. *AAP News,* June.

———. 1998. Anti-retroviral therapy and medical management of pediatric HIV infection. Supplement, *Pediatrics* 102:1052–1054.

———. 1999a. Disclosure of illness status to children and adolescents with HIV infection. *Pediatrics* 103:164–166.

———. 1999b. Planning for children whose parents are dying of HIV/AIDS. *Pediatrics* 103: 509–511.

Anderson, B., and J. Ho. 1997. Parental involvement in diabetes management tasks: Relationships to blood glucose monitoring adherence and metabolic control in young adolescents with insulin-dependent diabetes mellitus. *Journal of Pediatrics* 130 (2): 257–265.

Belman, A. L, G. Diamond, D. Dickson, D. Houroupian, J. L. Llena, G. Lantos, and A. Rubenstein. 1988. Pediatric acquired immunodeficiency syndrome: Neurological syndromes. *American Journal of Diseases in Children* 142:29–35.

Blanche, S., M. Tardieu, A. Duliege, C. Rouzioux, F. Le Deist, K. Fukunaga, M. Caniglis, C. Jacomet, A. Messiah, and C. Giscelli. 1990. Longitudinal study of 94 symptomatic infants with perinatally acquired human immunodeficiency virus infection. *American Journal of Diseases of Children* 144 (11): 1210–1215.

Centers for Disease Control and Prevention. 1998. *HIV/AIDS Surveillance Report, December 1998.* Washington, D.C.: U.S. Department of Health and Human Services.

———. 1999. *HIV/AIDS Surveillance Report, June 1999.* Washington, D.C.: U.S. Department of Health and Human Services.

Cohen, H. J., J. Grosz, K. Ayoob, and S. Schoen. 1997. Early intervention for children with HIV infection. In M. J. Guralnick, ed., *The Effectiveness of Early Intervention,* pp. 429–454. Baltimore: Paul H. Brookes.

Cohen, H. J., P. Papola, and M. Alvarez. 1994. Neurodevelopmental abnormalities in school age children with HIV infection. *Journal of School Health* 64 (1): 11–13.

Diabetes Control and Complications Trial Research Group. 1993. The effect of intensive treatment of diabetes in children and progression of long-term complications in insulin-dependent diabetes mellitus. *New England Journal of Medicine* 329:977–986.

Draimin, B. 1993. Adolescents in families with AIDS: Growing up with loss in death. In C. Levine, ed., *The Family: Orphans of the HIV Epidemic,* pp. 13–23. New York: United Hospital Fund.

Edell, M. 1998. Replacing community: Establishing linkages for women living with HIV/AIDS—a group work approach. *Social Work with Groups* 21:49–62.

Epstein, L. G., L. R. Sharer, J. M. Oleske, E. M. Connor, J. Goudsmit, L. Bagdon, M. Robert-Guroff, and M. R. Koenigsberger. 1986. Neurological manifestations of HIV infection in children. *Pediatrics* 78 (4): 678–687.

Fundaro, C., N. Miccinesi, N. Figliola Baldieri, O. Genovese, C. Rendeli, and G. Segni. 1998. Cognitive impairment in school age children with asymptomatic HIV infection. *AIDS Patient Care and STDs* 12 (2): 135–140.

Grosz, J., and K. Hopkins. 1992. Family circumstances affecting caregivers and brothers and sisters. In A. C. Crocker, H. J. Cohen, and T. A. Kastner, eds., *HIV Infection and Developmental Disabilities,* pp. 43–51. Baltimore: Paul H. Brookes.

Grubman, S., E. Gross, N. Lerner-Weiss, M. Hernandez, G. D. McSherry, L. Hoyt, M. Boland, and J. M. Oleske. 1995. Older children and adolescents living with perinatally acquired human immunodeficiency virus infection. *Pediatrics* 95:657–663.

Hackworth, S. 1998. Grandparents raising grandchildren. *Contemporary Pediatrics* 9:75–83.

HRSA Care Action. 1999. *HIV Disease in Women of Color.* Rockville, Md.: HRSA HIV AIDS Bureau.

Institute of Medicine. 1998. *Reducing the Odds: Preventing Perinatal Transmission of HIV in the United States.* Washington, D.C.: National Academy Press.

Lieberman, A. 1989. Characteristics of foster families caring for HIV positive children. Abstract, Proceedings of the Fifth National Pediatric AIDS Conference, Los Angeles.

Lewis, S., H. Haiken, and L. Hoyt. 1994. Living beyond the odds: Long-term survivors of pediatric HIV infection. *Developmental and Behavioral Pediatrics* 15:S12–S17.

Lipson, M. 1993. What do you say to a child with AIDS? *Hastings Center Report* 23:6–12.

——. 1994. Disclosure of diagnosis to children with HIV or AIDS. *Journal of Developmental Behavioral Pediatrics* 15:S61–S65.

Michaels, D., and C. Levine. 1992. Estimates of the number of motherless youth orphaned by HIV in the U.S. *Journal of the American Medical Association* 268:3456–3461.

Moss, H., S. Bose, P. Wolters, and P. Brouwers. 1998. A preliminary study of factors associated with psychological adjustment and disease course in school-age children infected with HIV. *Developmental and Behavioral Pediatrics* 19:18–25.

National Center for Health Statistics. 1994. *Underlying Cause Mortality Files, U.S.* Hyattsville, Md.: National Center for Health Statistics.

Oleske, J., A. Minnefor, R. Cooper, et al. 1983. Immune deficiency in children. *Journal of the American Medical Association* 249:2345–2349.

Poe, L. M. 1999. The changing family: Psychosocial needs of grandparents parenting a second shift. *The Source* 9:7–8.

Popola, P., M. Alvarez, and H. J. Cohen. 1994. Developmental and service needs of school-age children with human immunodeficiency virus infection: A descriptive study. *Pediatrics* 94:914–918.

Richardson, L. 1998. Born with HIV: Struggling with teen-age lives. *New York Times,* April 18, 1998.

Rubenstein, A., M. Sicklick, A. Gupta, et al. 1983. Acquired immunodeficiency with reversed T4/T8 ratio in infants born to promiscuous and drug addicted mothers. *Journal of the American Medical Association* 249:2350–2356.

Tasker, M. 1992. *How Can I Tell You?* Bethesda, Md.: Association for the Care of Children's Health.

Ultmann, M. H., G. Diamond, H. A. Ruff, A. Belman, B. E. Novick, A. Rubinstein, and H. J. Cohen. 1987. Developmental abnormalities in children with AIDS: A follow-up study. *International Journal of Neuroscience* 32:661–667.

U.S. Public Health Service Task Force. 1998. Recommendations for the use of antiretroviral drugs in pregnant women infected with HIV-1 for maternal health and for reducing perinatal HIV-1 transmission in the United States. *Morbidity and Mortality Weekly Reports* 47 (RR-2): 1–30.

Weiner, L., H. Battles, et al. 1996. Factors associated with disclosure of diagnosis to children with HIV/AIDS. *Pediatric AIDS and HIV Infection: Fetus to Adolescent* 7 (5): 310–324.

Weiner, L., and A. Septimus. 1991. Psychosocial considerations and support for the child and family. In P. A. Pizzo and C. M. Wilfert, eds., *Pediatric AIDS, The Challenge of HIV Infection in Infants, Children and Adolescents,* pp. 577–594. Baltimore: William and Wilkins.

Wolters, P. L., P. Brouwers, and H. A. Moss. 1995. Pediatric HIV disease: Effect on cognition, learning and behavior. *School Psychology Quarterly* 10:305–328.

Zayas, L. H., and K. Romano. 1994. Adolescents and parental death from AIDS. In B. O. Dane and C. Levine, eds., *AIDS and the New Orphans,* pp. 59–64. Westport, Conn.: Auburn House.

8

Their Second Chance:
Grandparents Caring for Their Grandchildren

LOCKHART McKELVY AND BARBARA DRAIMIN

Grandparents are being a called on in record numbers to care for their grandchildren. In 1997, 3.7 million grandparents were caring for approximately 4 million grandchildren. These grandparent-headed families represent 13.5 percent of African Americans, 4.1 percent of whites, and 6.5 percent of Hispanics (Lugaila 1997). The inner city marks the convergence of multiple factors that contribute to mothers' losing their role as primary caregivers. Teenage births, the frequency of single-parent households, the increased numbers of women in prison, drug abuse, random violence, and the assault on this population by the AIDS epidemic are all part of the toxic mix that displaces and kills parents. From the AIDS epidemic alone, homes had to be found for 82,000–120,000 children and adolescents by the year 2000 (Michaels and Levine 1992). Although the advent of combination therapies has slowed the death rate, people of color living in disenfranchised neighborhoods with poor access to health care remain the hardest hit by the epidemic.

Caregiving grandparents and family members have been the subject of many books and articles. Much of this work is cited in other chapters of this book. However, there is much less information on the relationship between caregivers and their children. Solomon and Marx (1995) have looked at how the overall health and school performance of children are influenced by the caregiving relationship, but in general very little is known about what goes on inside the homes of these families. Through a combination of case experiences from our practice and data from several studies, this chapter will bring the reader closer to the struggles, successes, and strengths of "skip-generation" families. The chapter's particular focus will be on how a parent's death from

AIDS affects both children and elderly caregivers. We will examine financial, cultural, emotional, and social challenges. Ultimately, the data will show that although these families are stressed, elderly family members derive pleasure from heading skip-generation households. However, in contrast to the positive report in our interview sample, a fair number of grandparents ask for our help with the children placed in their custody. We will discuss the difficulties presented by these families and finally recommend implications for practice and service delivery.

Program Data on Elderly Caregivers and Their Families

Although this chapter is not a research publication, data available from three different projects illustrate important points that both corroborate and differ from our field observations. The first data set is drawn from the Family Center's Project Share, whose interviewers gathered data on eighty-seven caregivers and the children in their care. The purpose of Project Share was to gather data to create a description of caregivers and their children, with particular emphasis on physical and mental health, permanency planning, and disclosure. Seventeen of these caregivers were over fifty-five. The second project, the Family Center's Project Care, helps parents with a chronic, terminal illness such as AIDS or cancer to create a legal, permanency plan for their children (see chapter 9).

The third set of data used in this chapter comprises the results from the work of Project Talk of the Family Studies Unit of the University of California at Los Angeles. Project Talk was a long-term study that followed three hundred parents with AIDS and their adolescent children. Group interventions were used to help families through the crisis of having a parent with an AIDS diagnosis. The Caregiver branch of the study was a sample of about seventy families who were followed after the death of the parent. Of that sample, approximately thirty were elderly. These families were given a variety of interviews and norms tests to improve our understanding of the stress and strengths of skip-generation families. The data's most striking conclusion, which is fairly consistent across the three studies, is that although the financial, social, and health difficulties seem overwhelming, grandparent caregivers feel a sense of pride and accomplishment in caring for their grandchildren. However, Project Care caseworkers and mental health-team social workers often observe a less positive picture, especially when adolescents are a part of these "off-time" families. Problems in these families include school truancy, angry outbursts, gang involvement, and complicated bereavement. Although some difficulties can be overcome with time, counseling, and lots of patience, the first year is often especially challenging for both generations. This is illustrated in the following case.

Maria is a sixty-one-year-old Puerto Rican grandmother who is separated from her third husband. She has already raised five daughters and is currently caring for five of her grandchildren, four girls—Casey, eleven; Sophia, nine; Jasmine, eight; and Monique, seven—and a boy, José, eight. Three of the girls are from her daughter Irma. José and Monique are from another of Maria's daughter's, Luz. Maria lives in a two-bedroom apartment in section 8 housing.

Maria became the caregiver for Irma's children from a neglect case founded against Irma three years ago. The three girls were found steps away from the scene of a drug transaction that involved Irma and her partner Roberto. On short notice, Maria was called from Puerto Rico to come to a Long Island police precinct to pick up her grandchildren who were in the custody of Administration for Children's Services (ACS). After establishing herself in an apartment and on the recommendation of the ACS worker, Maria was granted kinship care of her grandchildren. After three years, Irma died of AIDS-related causes. Maria was told by her ACS caseworker that she had to petition the family court to obtain guardianship of the children or the children might eventually be removed from her care. When she went to court, the girl's father, who had been brought from jail and never signed the children's birth certificates, requested visitation rights. Maria's lawyer objected stating that he had neither established paternity nor had he ever expressed interest in the children before being in court. Maria was also very upset by the possibility of Roberto's being in her life because she believed that this man had infected her daughter with HIV. Ideally, Maria wanted to adopt the girls but she was told that she would lose the subsidies she needed from the foster care agency.

Maria came to care for Luz's children José and Monique in a somewhat different fashion. A neglect petition was founded against her daughter, and the children were removed from her care. When Maria learned of this, she went to court and petitioned to have the children placed with her. Maria wanted to keep the children in the family, even though accepting guardianship meant that she would only be able to receive public assistance for the children, not the generally higher foster-care subsidies.

During the process of obtaining guardianship for José and Monique, Maria was told she might have lung cancer. Obviously, this put additional stress on a family that was already under enormous pressure. To Maria's great relief, the medical tests were negative. However, when the family specialist visited, Maria frequently complained of pains and medical problems that were clinically unfounded. She also was having difficulty talking about the death of her daughter Irma with her children. All three of Irma's girls attend special education programs and counseling with a local mental-health clinic. She has not been able to talk to the children about the cause of their mother's death, and, although she has attended several grief workshops in the community, she does not see the value of "remembering such a bad time with children who already have problems."

Maria's case is typical in a number of ways, including her conviction that even though she could barely afford their care, her grandchildren were better off with her than with strangers. She was also caring for two sets of children with different visitation and guardianship requirements. Finally, all members of the family were affected by multiple losses, losses made more complicated by Maria's reluctance to talk about her daughter. Her reasons were not uncommon. She felt that it would make life harder for the children, and because the family had suffered enough already, there was no sense talking about pain from the past.

The Family Center was able to intervene with Maria in several important ways. First, she was assigned a family specialist, an experienced, bilingual worker, who helped Maria sort through custody options and informed her of their financial and legal implications. Maria was assigned a Family Center lawyer who began with helping her sort through the available childcare options in the state of New York. For Maria, it was very important to have a lawyer assigned to her case as soon as possible because she had already arranged for court dates and needed representation. As Maria's case progressed, the family specialist provided counseling sessions to address a variety of stressors. In particular, Maria spoke about the loss of her daughter; her anger at Roberto; her fears concerning her health; and whether or not to talk to the children about the death of their mother. Maria felt that it was her duty to protect her grandchildren from painful feelings. However, the family specialist felt that she was so guarded that the children had no opportunity to discuss their sadness. Mental-health services are an option at the Family Center, but the children were already seeing a mental-health professional at a clinic, so they were not referred to the Family Center clinical team. The legal team's work with Maria concluded after she received legal documentation for all the children in her care. However, Maria has not yet been able to speak freely to the children about the losses in their lives, especially the death of their mother. Because feeling sad about losses at home is not an option, it is hoped that the children are able to express themselves more openly in their psychotherapy sessions.

There are also caregivers who are not elderly. Melva's case, for example, is typical of caregivers who are still parenting their own children. This case illustrates some of the common problems that we see in the field with overwhelmed caregivers of any age and frustrating children.

Melva is a thirty-five-year-old African American who has six children with her live-in companion Andrew. Both her parents are deceased and her extended family provides her with little or no extra help. Andrew is an active drug user and does not see himself as a primary caregiver for his family. Two years ago Melva's best friend and sister Jackie died of throat cancer, leaving Melva to care for two more children, Jerome, eleven, and Tanya, one. This brought the total number of children in Melva's care to eight. Two of Melva and Andrew's children have severe developmental delays. When they all moved in together, the children, ranging in ages from one month to eleven years, shared just two bedrooms. There were four high chairs in the living room. Melva desperately needed additional space, money, and an extra hand.

While Melva's sister was alive, a case manager from the Family Center helped her and Jackie work out the details of caring for Jackie's children. The case manager also provided supportive counseling to Jackie and encouraged the two sisters to meet frequently and discuss plans for the children. Unfortunately, the problem of space could not be addressed until after Jackie died. As with many poor caregivers, Melva lived in public housing that does not allow tenants to move until they can prove that they have custody of additional children. After establishing guardianship, she requested a transfer and waited for two years for a larger apartment. After the move, some of the stress caused by little or no privacy abated, but the true stress in Melva's life was and remains feeling exhausted and unhappy that she will never be able to meet the needs of all of the children in her care.

The case manager and Melva agreed that she and her family would benefit from counseling on an ongoing basis, and Melva was referred to the mental-health team. When the social worker met with Melva he was impressed with her strength and resolve to take care of all eight children, and they contracted to meet every two weeks in her home. Because there were such diverse counseling needs in the family, they decided to refer the older boy, Jerome, to counseling at a community agency. Melva requested that his younger sister, her niece, be evaluated by the state for an early intervention program. Unfortunately, any agency or medical appointment meant that Melva had to arrange to either have some of the children with her or find someone to care for the children at home. When Melva first began caring for this family, she felt guilty when she missed an appointment, especially when agency workers scolded her, but after time and talking with the social worker about what was truly possible, she began to relax and not chastise herself so severely. She finally began to feel that "sometimes I can only do what I can do."

Because the Family Center social worker was able to visit Melva in her home, they decided that the best use of his time was to provide an hour of counseling and support for her alone. She spoke about several issues, including her concern about Andrew's on-and-off drug use and his lack of support, her guilt when setting limits with the children, and her depression and sadness from the multiple losses in her life. The social worker has been meeting every other week with Melva for almost two years. She is still exhausted most of the time, but she also knows that because she has made the decision to care for them, she has to live with feeling that she cannot do enough. To complicate matters further, her oldest grandchild, Jerome, is generally angry and unappreciative, and Melva has a difficult time with his poor attitude. Tanya, his much younger sister, has been more receptive to Melva's care. She now calls her "mom," and although in the beginning she cried frequently, she is now much happier and adjusting well in school. For Melva, being called "mom" is complicated. On one hand, she is glad that Tanya is bonding with her. On the other hand, it also makes her feel sad and alone because she knows that her sister will never return.

The Toxic Environment of the Inner City

The combined effect of deaths from AIDS-related causes, violence, incarceration, and drug use has created an inner city environment that is traumatic for families (Draimin, Levine, and McKelvy 1998). In particular, young people whose grandmothers were interviewed for Project Talk and Project Share live with multiple stressors including overcrowded schools, gangs, fights, drugs, poverty, and families with multiple losses. The elderly especially talk about their fear of raising grandchildren in dangerous neighborhoods; they feel powerless against the young people and gangs who are in the streets. One grandparent in Brooklyn put it this way: "When I was coming up it wasn't so bad. Sure there was bad stuff, but you could avoid it and people didn't bother me or the children. Now I don't know anyone in the neighborhood and if I talk to other children they are rude. I tell the kids to stay right in front of the building where I can see them." Moving out of the inner city is not an option for most elderly caregivers. It may even move them from supports and family that are crucial for their ability to care for grandchildren.

Social workers can best help elderly caregivers by referring the young people in their care to community youth programs. In addition, workers can educate grandparents about the real risks that kids are facing in the community from drugs, gangs, and violence. In one example, a neighborhood gang believed that twelve-year-old José, who lives with his elderly aunt, was "disrespecting their colors" and threatened to kill him. Because he was so afraid, José stopped going to school. His aunt became very upset and threatened to throw him out of the house. A social worker from the Family Center was referred to the family and explained to the aunt that José could be in real danger and that they should consider requesting a school transfer. After the aunt heard from the social worker about the seriousness of the danger, she understood why José was so afraid and helped him with his transfer.

The Effect of Multiple Losses

Often older caregivers are assuming parental surrogacy for children who are coping with severe loss. From our sample of seventeen elderly caregivers, 70 percent of the mothers and 29 percent of the fathers of these children were deceased. Seventeen percent of the children have also experienced the death of another family member in addition to their parents. Twenty-nine percent of the children never knew their mothers, and 47 percent never knew their fathers. Many of the children who did know their parents, had relationships impaired by drug use and incarceration. Forty-one percent of their fathers and 47 percent of their mothers had or currently have problems with drug use, 17 percent of the mothers have been in prison, and 29 percent of their fathers are currently in prison. For young people these statistics represent staggering losses, and for elderly caregivers these losses are not only painful, but they also represent a source of guilt. Many caregivers feel that when their adult children die from drug use, HIV/AIDS, or even street violence they have failed as parents. New caregivers must struggle to overcome both the sadness and guilt they feel concerning their children in order to "refocus" their parenting efforts on the next generation. Counseling, mentoring programs, and family interventions combined can help children and grandparents find some relief from these burdens, but for both generations these deficits will always remain a part their identity.

Childhood Bereavement

Symptoms of "normal bereavement" for children include difficulties in school, sleep disorders, and withdrawn behavior (Silverman and Worden 1992; Wolkind and Rutter 1985; Van Eerdewegh et al. 1982), but in families where loss is pervasive young people's reactions can be more severe. Their responses can range from the "numbing" associated with post-traumatic stress disorder to intense feelings of sadness and anger. To an uninformed caregiver, grieving children can appear distant, angry, and ungrateful; they seem uninvolved in the life of their new family. During the transition from parent to grandparent, many adolescents are referred to the clinical social workers, but few engage in ongoing treatment. Adolescence is generally a time of separation from adults, and this separation is further complicated by the fact that a young person's who has lost a parent believes that adults are not going to be there for him or her. If adolescents are not willing to attend counseling sessions, the Family Center tries to keep young people involved in programs such as computer and activity groups, with the hope that relationship can develop slowly in a more nonthreatening way. Often, after meeting clinical staff through activity groups, teenagers are more willing to meet for more formalized counseling sessions.

Children with Special Needs

Children with special developmental or mental health needs require a higher level of energy from their elderly caregivers. According to Project Share's sample of seventeen grandparent caregivers, 41 percent of the young people in their care have some kind of ongoing health problem such as obesity, hyper-activity, or a learning disability. An equal percentage were perceived by the caregiver to be sad or depressed, and of the seventeen children who were scored by their caregivers on the Child Behavior Check List, or CBCL (Achenbach 1991), 18 percent of the children scored in the clinical range, meaning that almost one in five has a DSM-4 diagnosis. Results from one study of caregivers (Minkler et al. 1997) indicate an increased amount of stress for the grandparent when the skip-generation family included a child with special needs. Children who demand more attention, who do not fit into a norm, and who need more help from professionals will increase the level of stress in any family; but when these children are also grieving and changing homes, the challenge for an elderly caregiver is significantly increased. In families where there are children with special needs, caseworkers can help ensure that children are referred to clinics where their counseling and healthcare needs can be met, ideally in the same setting. Linkages such as these will reduce stress for elderly caregivers.

Adjustment from Ill Parent to Caregiver

When a child moves from a home where a single parent has AIDS or any terminal illness, to a new home with an elderly caregiver, he or she must make adjustments. For example, some children who have lived with an ill parent have been in situations where limits are few and often not reinforced. Parents are often too ill to follow through. Some teenagers either abuse this freedom or learn to care for themselves. In either case, they no longer expect adults to be concerned about their behavior. Parents who are ill also become dependent on their older children, and when "parentified" adolescents are forced by their new caregivers to give up their positions of responsibility a struggle frequently ensues. These young people are reluctant to allow caregivers, even with a strong previous connection, to tell them what to do. On occasion, the transition can be made even more difficult by a teenager's belief that asserting their independence shows loyalty to their deceased parent. The combination of these factors often leads to problems with the caregiving relationship when it involves adolescents. One of the ways this can be overcome is for agencies to follow these families after the death of a parent and begin working with the elderly caregiver and the older children before problems occur.

Who Are the Elderly Caregivers?

At this writing, in Project Care there are twenty-three new caregivers ranging in age from twenty-two to eighty-one. Of these, eleven are elderly; three are grand-mothers, five are aunts, two are uncles, and one is a grandfather. The remain-ing caregivers are siblings or non-blood relatives. Results from Project Share's interviews of seventeen caregiving grandparents, including demographics, health, stress, and relationship indexes, tell us that skip-generation families are generally headed by disenfranchised and undereducated elderly. Specifically, half of our fifty-five-and-older group live in New York City public housing; half did not complete high school; almost all receive some kind of public assistance such as monthly checks, food stamps, or Medicaid; most do not have their child (the parent of their grandchild) or any other adult living in their home. Fully half see themselves as poor and struggling to survive. The facts seem bleak, but, interestingly enough, some of these grandparents view themselves in a some-what different light.

Sixty percent of the Project Share sample of seventeen grandparents said they were happy with their housing, and 40 percent said they were comfortable financially. Fifty-seven percent said there had been no change in their financial status, and 10 percent said it had slightly improved. Because all of the elderly caregivers are on public assistance, it seems hard to believe that 40 percent could feel that they are comfortable financially. Perhaps their mood or general life ex-perience accounts for a more positive view of their circumstances. Another way to explain their satisfaction might be that although we cannot imagine how these caregivers survive, they cannot imagine having more, or they may receive help from outside resources that they do not report to us during interviews. However, if this is the case, based on field observations, the lifestyles of these elderly caregivers are not substantially altered by these contributions. Elderly caregivers also bring a lifetime of skills to stretching their money, consistently placing their needs second to those of the young people in their care. As one caregiving grandparent said, "I haven't had a new pair of shoes in years. Every-thing extra I have goes to the children." Whatever the reason, it is surprising that these caregivers are not more vocal to caseworkers and interviewers about their housing and financial challenges. Perhaps there is a perceived threat from social workers who, with many of these families, were the ones who "removed" their grandchildren from their children's substandard housing and economic conditions. In this light it is easier to understand that minimizing the hardships associated with caring for grandchildren is, in some way, protecting them from possible removal. Sometimes a careful explanation of the worker's role and building a trusting relationship with the family will help the elderly caregiver be more forthcoming with their needs for practical assistance.

Elderly Caregivers' Responses to Loss

Elderly caregivers experience the same multiple losses as the children in their care. Perhaps even more difficult, however, is the fact that these grandparents are grieving for their children, an experience no parent anticipates, and many caregivers are grieving for more than one child. Grandparents have described their losses in these words:

"I don't think I could handle any more bad news. I've had as much as anyone should have in a lifetime."

"I just go on no matter what happens. I don't have the time to feel sad."

"I gave up feeling anything at all."

"Giving up feeling" is a strategy commonly used by people who feel they cannot manage another painful experience. This approach, though necessary at times, implies that one should not discuss painful feelings if one is to cope. Unfortunately, this can result in a grandparent who is unwilling to talk about the loss of the child (or children) with their grandchildren. Another factor contributing to their silence is that the natural progression for talking about painful losses is to begin with your husband or wife, and many elderly caregivers are without adult partners. All of these circumstances, as well as young people's natural propensity to take cues about "taboo" topics from adults, can result in new caregiving families where there is little mention of the lost parent.

Data from Project Share also show that the stigma associated with AIDS contributes to a caregiver's wish for silence. Ninety-eight percent of grandparents, as compared to 32 percent of the children, knew that their child/parent had died from AIDS-related causes. Whether to protect the grandchildren or to keep additional stigma out of an already painful situation, or from fear that a young person cannot keep a secret, new caregivers are often unwilling to talk about the true cause of parental death. As a result, a parent's death can become shrouded in a layer of shame and secrecy. Sadness and loss become a private, individual experience, limiting one family member's ability to care for another. Ideally, agency or clinic interventions will focus on a caregiver's grieving and feelings about stigma before talking with the children in their care. The elderly thus have the experience of beginning to integrate their own grief, so they are better prepared for the difficult questions and sadness of the children in their care.

Another common response to multiple losses is an elderly caregiver's temptation to overindulge or spoil a grieving child. Many caregivers feel that their grandchildren have been through enough, and they are therefore reluctant to contribute to a child's suffering by setting a limit or punishing them. Unfortunately, this belief runs contrary to what children need to feel safe and reassured in a new home. Social workers assigned to these caregivers can educate them about the needs of children in new homes. Support groups can be particularly effective with elderly caregivers. For example, Carol Cox's program at Fordham University brings caregivers together to talk about relevant issues such as grief, loss, and effective parenting strategies in a training and discussion forum (Cox 2000).

Loss of Confidence in Parenting Ability

Caregivers who have lost their adult children to AIDS, drugs, incarceration, and/or violence sometimes lose confidence in their ability to raise children. They second-guess their attitudes about a child's demand for freedom and their ability to set limits in general. If they were strict with their children, they may be more permissive with their grandchildren. If they were lenient, they may feel that this time being strict will make the difference. Most children feel misunderstood in the face of strict and rigid limits. They want the same opportunities to explore as their peers, and ultimately, they will be forced to make the same decisions their parents had to make concerning drugs and sex. For grandparents who are more confident, however, the caregiving experience provides a valuable second chance to be a parent. For them, caregiving is an opportunity to change the painful legacy of a lost generation.

The Generation Gap

Elderly grandparents who are first-generation immigrants with young people in their care often see their grandchildren as more "American." The differences in this culture gap can include attitudes about food, language, drugs, sex, dress, and dating. Adolescents do not often accept warnings from grandparents about heated topics like drugs and sex. They do not see the older person as able to relate to their challenges. Grandparents also feel this distance, making statements to caseworkers such as, "I don't understand these kids and their music," "That girl thinks she's twenty and she's only thirteen," or "I didn't dare fool around like my grandson does." Other more confident grandparents are amused by their grandchildren's assertion that they have no understanding of the problems they face. As one grandparent said, "They think I don't know anything, but I am not stupid. They have a crazier world, but I dealt with lots of the same things they have to." Caseworkers can work with the elderly to ensure that whatever the beliefs of the different generations, communication between child and caregiver remains a priority.

The Stress of Isolation

Isolation from his or her peer group significantly affects the level of stress in an elderly person's life. In Jendrek's (1993) sample of 114 caregivers, 58.6 percent felt they had less privacy, 58 percent had less time to themselves, and 53.6 percent had less time to get things done. Many report not having time to "generate and maintain a network of friends" (Burton 1992). When caregivers meet at the Family Center they are enthusiastic about the opportunity to share ideas, strategies, and, like most parents, they complain and boast about the children in their care. As one grandparent said, "I have never been around other grandparents who are doing what I do. I can learn from these people." This departure from the appropriate life stage clearly has its costs, yet increasing numbers of skip-generation families in the inner city are changing the norm. Another grandmother who lives in a large city housing project said, "I think that all the children in my building are being cared for by their grandparents." Furthermore, 43 percent of the grandparents studied by Sands and Goldberg-Glen (1998) reported that during their childhood they had spent at least ten years in the same household as a grandparent. Therefore, although the occurrence of skip-generation families is on the rise, it is not without precedent. The community's response to these families should be to provide opportunities for supportive, educational groups so that caregivers can share knowledge and combat their isolation. The more successful caregiver programs schedule groups or activities simultaneously with programs for the young people in their care.

Time with Bureaucracies

Time spent negotiating large and cumbersome bureaucracies further reduces recreational opportunities for elderly caregivers and their families. At a minimum, caregivers must interact with the Board of Education and a pediatric clinic or hospital. Because 45 percent of the children in the Project Share's sample have a chronic health condition, health-care appointments are not infrequent. In addition, fully half of the children in the same sample have received counseling during the past six months. Because many of these children are identified by the Board of Education as having special needs, there is always a demand for advocacy in order to be sure that grandchildren receive appropriate services and school placements. In short, caregiving means getting out of the house in all weathers and being persistent with overwhelmed and stressed agencies. Social work with elderly caregivers should include helping them to advocate for children and adolescents in their care so that they receive the best possible education, psychotherapy, and health services. When children are engaged in the community, a caregiver is more relaxed and able to focus her energy life at home.

Poor Health

When grandparents become caregivers, their often poor health can be further taxed by the stress, responsibility, and physical activity of childcare (see chapter 5). According to Burton (1992), 35 percent of the caregivers in her sample reported heightened medical problems. In Sands and Goldberg-Glen's (1998) sample of 123 caregiving grandparents, 65 percent said they had a particular health problem. Twenty-five percent of this sample stated that their health had gotten worse since caring for their grandchildren, but, conversely, 18 percent said it had improved from the additional responsibility. Perhaps this can be explained as either a shift in priorities or that caregiving brings these grandparents "back in life," which many of the elderly feel is essential for good health. In Project Share's sample, fifteen of seventeen caregivers report at least one health condition such as high blood pressure, arthritis, or heart disease.

On occasion, caregivers report that physical limitations have prevented them from accomplishing tasks that they feel are important to childrearing; but for the most part, grandparents will push themselves to fulfill required childrearing tasks.

A caregiver's health also effects the children who are living in the home. A young person who has lived at length with an ill parent and then lost him/her to AIDS can be especially anxious and even obsessive about the health of their elderly caregiver. For example, after the death of his mother, a six-year-old boy began living with his grandmother. He became very anxious when she took a nap and would try to waken her by pulling her eyelids open. This child's response to his caregiver's sleep illustrates how his fears after the death of his mother have entered into his relationship with his grandmother. After the caregiver spoke to her caseworker, she felt relieved to discover that her grandson's behavior was not unusual for a grieving child. Although this child's reaction was probably temporary, for others fear about the death of a caregiver can become more complicated when a caregiver's poor health is evident.

Caregiver Mental Health

In order to understand the general mental heath of the elderly caregiving population, thirty caregivers in Project Talk were given the Brief Symptom Inventory Index (Derogatis 1993). Four areas were found to be significant. Thirty-three percent of the grandparents felt their feelings were hurt easily, and 40 percent felt more than moderately annoyed. Finally, 33 percent of the grandparent caregivers had trouble falling asleep. Thirty percent of caregivers experienced nervousness or shaking. One possibility for this high incidence of nervousness may be cultural. For example, many Latinas describe *ataques de nervios* when they feel stressed or overwhelmed. Whatever the culture, all four symptoms are indicative of the effects of stress, yet there were many choices in the BSII that the caregivers did not feel were significant. Difficulty trusting people, feeling lonely or blue, suffering from an upset stomach, or experiencing temper outbursts were all responses that caregivers felt did not describe their current circumstances. Caregivers in the Project Share sample took the Psychiatric Symptoms Index (Ilfeld 1976). Their mean score was 13.5; the community norm is 10.5, with a score above 20 indicating "high symptoms of distress." Because our sample of caregivers scored only slightly above the mean we can assume that our caregivers are doing fairly well. However, four grandparents scored above 20 and two above 30, suggesting that there are elderly caregivers who are having a very difficult time.

Other researchers found their samples to be more distressed. Eighty-six percent of the African American grandparents studied by Burton (1992) reported that they were depressed or anxious most of the time. Ninety-three percent reported concerns of robbery, drive-by shootings, and drug trafficking, but the majority of this sample also stated that "they deeply loved and were committed to their grandchildren and that at times their role was very gratifying" (Burton 1992:748). Minkler et al. (1997) found that 158 elderly primary caregivers were twice as likely as the norm to have depressive symptoms with health, time spent caregiving, and age being the most significant factors. The data from these studies indicate that it may not be the children, financial strain or even the adolescents who are causing stress for their caregivers as much as health concerns, feelings of incompetence as caregivers, and the violent, urban environments in which they live. However, social workers with Project Care often find that caregivers identify the rebellious behavior of adolescents as a major stress in their family lives. Many of the referrals to the clinical department are requests from caregivers for help with their adolescent charges. Whatever the source of stress, caregivers who are isolated and without social or family support are more at risk themselves for physical and mental-health problems (see chapter 6).

Spiritual Strength

The most common and significant strength of the caregivers in both the Family Center's Project Share and Project Talk of the Family Studies Unit is that caregivers see themselves as very religious or somewhat religious/spiritual. The importance of spirituality is corroborated by Burnette's work with Latinas who are caregiving. In her sample of seventy-four Latinas raising grandchildren, 90 percent state that religion is extremely important in their lives. This is not unusual for minority communities or the elderly. Spiritual and religious beliefs are clearly a factor in how people manage hardship and loss. Because these caregivers already view the church as significant to their survival, these organizations represent a gathering point for off-time families. Religious leaders have an opportunity to serve caregivers by designing programs where their spiritual and socialization needs can be addressed.

The Positive Relationships Between Caregiver and Child

The data that describe the relationship between elderly caregivers and their children create a picture of families that are doing well despite the many challenges. The Family Relationship cohesion subscale (Moos and Moos 1981) was given to the thirty elderly caregivers working with the New York City site of the Family Studies Unit of the University of California at Los Angeles. Using true-or-false questions such as "Family members really help one another," the scale measures togetherness, conflict, and expressiveness. The community norm for families is a mean score of 6.61 on a scale from 1 to 9, with 9 being the highest level of cohesion. The mean score for the skip-generation families was 7.32, suggesting that they are getting on rather well. Time together is not taken into account in this scoring, which may be a factor, but generally even in families where there has been significant loss there is cohesion. Perhaps this can be explained by some of the maturing that can take place in an adolescent's life when he loses a parent (Tyson-Rawson 1996; Oltjenbruns 1991), or these families may bond as a result of facing multiple tragedies together. In the Family Center's Project Share sample 100 percent of the caregivers felt proud of their grandchildren, felt loved by their grandchildren, loved their grandchildren like their own children, liked spending time with their grandchildren, and had fun with them. Ninety-four percent of the caregivers feel that raising grandchildren has increased their purpose in life. Certainly these statements are striking in the face of the adversity described in this chapter, but the data confirm a positive experience for both the elderly caregivers and the children in their care. Considering the difficulties these families experience, their successes with or without professional help, is a tribute to their resilience and perseverance.

Issues for Social Workers

In summary, there are areas where agency professionals need to interface in order to identify and work with skip-generation families. Perhaps the most challenging area is engaging a skip-generation family. Given the time constraints of caregivers, there is much to be gained by visiting them in their homes, churches, and health-care clinics. In terms of training, workers should have a good understanding of AIDS services, the bereavement process, the needs of the elderly, and family therapy. Agencies that focus on the elderly, mental health clinics, legal clinics, and AIDS-service and cancer programs can all play a role with skip-generation families. The goals of each agency will vary, but in our experience an elderly caregiver needs to understand the legal-custody and entitlements options that are available as well as the community services such as schools, clinics, and mental-health centers. Caseworkers should be aware that although these caregivers may be elderly, they are generally up to the job, and for both generations, an off-time relationship can be very satisfying. Professionals involved in these families should keep in mind that a caregiver's mental health affects both the mood in the home and the stability of the caregiving relationship; consequently, they should be ready to refer to community mental-health programs when appropriate. These families have shown us that even under difficult circumstances they can take care of their own, and although they may not need us, professionals and a variety of community supports can help to be sure that children will not be "passed around" and that the caregiving experience is gratifying for both generations.

References

Achenbach, T. M. 1991. *Child Behavior Checklist/4–18 and 1991*. Burlington: University of Vermont Department of Psychiatry.

Burnette, D. 1999a. Custodial grandparents in Latino families: Patterns of service use and predictors of unmet needs. *Social Work* 44 (1): 22–34.

———. 1999b. Social relationships of Latino grandparent caregivers: A role theory perspective. *The Gerontologist* 39 (1): 49–58.

Burton, L. M. 1992. Black grandparents rearing children of drug-addicted parents: Stressors, outcomes and social service needs. *The Gerontologist* 32 (6): 744–751.

Cox, C. 2000. Empowering grandparents raising grandchildren. In C. Cox, ed., *To Grandmother's House We Go and Stay: Perspectives on Custodial Grandparents*, pp. 253–267. New York: Springer.

Derogatis, L. R. 1993. *Brief Symptom Inventory*. Minnetonka, Minn.: NCS Pearson.

Draimin, B. H., C. Levine, and L. McKelvy. 1998. AIDS and its traumatic effects on families. In Y. Danieli, ed., *International Handbook of Multigenerational Legacies of Trauma*, pp. 587–601. New York: Plenum.

Ilfeld, F. 1976. Further validation of a psychiatric symptom index in a normal population. *Psychological Reports* 39:1215–1228.

Jendrek, M. P. 1993. Grandparents who parent their grandchildren: Effects on lifestyle. *Journal of Marriage and the Family* 55:609–621.

Lugaila, T. 1997. *Marital Status and Living Arrangements: March 1997*. Washington, D.C.: U.S. Bureau of the Census.

Michaels, D., and C. Levine. 1992. Estimates of the number of motherless youth orphaned by AIDS in the United States. *Journal of the American Medical Association* 268 (24): 3456–3461.

Minkler, M., E. Fuller-Thomson, D. Miller, and D. Driver. 1997. Depression in grandparents raising grandchildren. *Archives of Family Medicine* 6:445–452.

Moos, R. H., and B. S. Moos. 1981. *Family Environment Scale.* Palo Alto, Calif.: Consulting Psychologist Press.

Oltjenbruns, K. A. 1991. Positive outcomes of adolescents' experience with grief. *Journal of Adolescent Research* 6 (1): 43–53.

Sands, R. G., and R. S. Goldberg-Glen. 1998. The impact of employment and serious illness on grandmothers who are raising their grandchildren. *Journal of Women and Aging* 10 (3): 41–58.

Silverman, P. R., and W. J. Worden. 1992. Children's reactions in the early months after the death of a parent. *American Journal of Orthopsychiatry* 62 (1): 93–104.

Solomon, J. C., and J. Marx. 1995. To grandmother's house we go: Health and school adjustment of children raised solely by grandparents. *The Gerontologist* 35 (3): 386–394.

Tyson-Rawson, K. J. 1996. Adolescent responses to the death of a parent. In C. A. Coor and D. E. Balk, eds., *Handbook of Adolescent Death and Bereavement,* pp. 155–172. New York: Springer.

Van Eerdewegh, M. M., M. D. Bieri, R. H. Parrilla, and P. J. Clayton. 1982. The bereaved child. *British Journal of Psychiatry* 140:23–29.

Wolkind, S., and M. Rutter. 1985. Separation, loss and family relationships. In M. Rutter and L. Hersov, eds., *Child and Adolescent Psychiatry: Modern Approaches,* pp. 34–57. London: Blackwell Scientific.

9

Custody and Permanency Planning

JAN HUDIS AND JEROME BROWN

Planning for the future care and custody of children is a complex process for all families. For parents, the thought of not being present for the milestones of a child's life is extremely sobering and painful, more so when the parent is facing a life-threatening illness. For caregivers, the decision to care for the child after a parent's death takes place against a backdrop of many interwoven and often competing interests and needs. These include the caregivers' love and commitment to the children, their feeling of obligation to the dying or deceased parent, their own grief about the anticipated loss of a loved one, the expectations of other family members that they will or should take on the caregiver role, their own health needs, and many other logistical, personal, and economic concerns.

Ideally, mothers and fathers with AIDS make plans for their children's futures well before they become terminally ill. This gives them time to weigh carefully the various custody options available, to speak with the proposed caregiver, and to gain the proposed caregiver's commitment to care for the child. It also allows them to document their wishes and inform others who have an interest or stake in the children's lives. By planning early, parents with AIDS can get expert professional assistance to help them in putting into place the paperwork that documents their wishes and to assist them in gaining everyone's agreement to the plan well before it is implemented. It is also best for the parent to include in the planning those who might object to their choices for the child's future care, such as a noncustodial parent, in order to resolve any challenges to the plan early and with certainty.

Many mothers and fathers with AIDS rely on their own parents or other older family members to take responsibility for their children when they are no longer able to care for them. These older adults caring for young children form what are known as "skip-generation" families, where those providing the care and those receiving the care are separated by more years than is traditional in parent/child relationships. Although skip-generation families are not a new phenomenon in American society, older caregivers in the past often took on the parenting role on a temporary basis. For example, grandparents, aunts, or uncles were often solicited to care for a child while the child's biological parent was away working, going to school, or taking care of other business. The skip-generation family might be in place for an extended period, but rarely was the arrangement seen as permanent and often the child's mother and or father remained at least peripherally involved in the rearing and nurturing of the child.

Today's skip-generation families, formed as a result of AIDS-related illness and death, are permanent by necessity, and often neither parent is alive to participate in the guidance and oversight of the child's development. Hence, the AIDS epidemic in the United States has spawned a growing group of aging Americans with primary responsibility for the parenting of bereaved children, many of whom have complex educational and emotional needs. These older caregivers have a unique constellation of service needs. Although some have raised their own children in the past, their current knowledge of health, education, and social institutions may be limited and their ability or willingness to negotiate these institutions may be hampered by their own health needs or those of others in the newly formed family (Burton et al. 1995).

This chapter explores the benefits and challenges of planning for the future care and custody of children before parental death, with emphasis on the importance of involving the proposed caregiver in that planning. Case examples are presented to illustrate the difficulties experienced by caregivers when plans are not made in advance and the benefits to both caregivers and children when parents have created clear plans for their children's futures.

Background on the Family Center

The authors have more than ten years' combined experience serving and researching New York City families affected by AIDS at the Family Center, a community-based agency founded in 1993 to strengthen children, families, and new caregivers as they move through the transitions caused by the loss of a parent. All services are free. The Center has an active caseload of two hundred families and has served more than two thousand families with AIDS in New York City since its opening. The Family Center is a unique model of service, weaving together legal and social services. The Family Center provides mental-health counseling, substance-abuse counseling, and entitlement services as appropriate to the client's needs through a coordinated system of case management. The Family Center provides linkage, support, and follow-up to clients needing services not directly provided by the Center. Because each family's needs are unique and often complicated, the multifaceted aspect of the Family Center's services is instrumental in developing long-term plans for the care of children following parental death (Draimin and Hudis 2000).

Almost all families served by the Family Center are Medicaid-eligible and live in economically disadvantaged communities. More than 90 percent are of African or Latino descent, and 89 percent of families are headed by single mothers. Eleven percent of the families served are headed by fathers with AIDS who are caring for their children. Family Center clients live in communities burdened by violence, poverty, drug abuse, homelessness, discrimination, illness, and inadequate health care. They are in the lowest income bracket; 99 percent live below the poverty level. Many are past or current drug users. Some are mentally ill. Others are victims of domestic abuse. Generally, their education levels are low and their communication and self-advocacy skills poor. Additionally, because HIV/AIDS continues to be a stigmatized illness, many experience social and familial isolation.

Although families served by the Family Center are among the most needy, their experiences in dealing with the anticipated death of one or both parents from HIV are instructive for anyone facing a terminal illness and seeking to secure the children's futures. Issues facing the parents, as well as concerns and needs of the intended caregivers, are similar regardless of the socioeconomic status, medical diagnosis, or other personal situations. One reality that the HIV epidemic has brought to light is that all parents should anticipate the potential that another caregiver might have to assume responsibility for their children's growth and development. This chapter examines a strategic and supportive approach to helping parents and caregivers make this important decision and secure its enactment. This process is referred to as permanency planning.

Permanency Planning

The first step in assisting parents to plan for the future care of their children is to help them to recognize the importance of this issue and to examine all their options. Many parents feel considerable stress at the prospect of securing a future caregiver for their children, and their anxiety frequently results in hesitation to engage a potential caregiver in the process and to confirm their choice in a legally sanctioned way.

Counseling focused on the selection of the most ideal future caregiver begins with assisting parents in setting out goals for the children's future and determining which potential caregiver is realistically situated to support those goals. For example, desires about the future education and religious upbringing of the children may guide the selection to a specific family member or friend. An assessment about the likelihood that the caregiver is prepared and willing to accept the responsibility must then be made. Essential to this selection is the participation of the potential caregiver in serious discussion about the implications of the proposed new family structure on their lives and others in the new family unit.

Because each family is unique, it is impossible to anticipate the course of the permanency planning process. Often, as a plan develops, a spectrum of issues—such as family communication problems or implications of disclosure about a health condition—may surface and redirect the selection process or affect the final decision. Additionally, entitlements and financial supports are extremely important to most clients and may affect the viability of the initial plan. Professionals providing permanency-planning services need to be well versed in the ramifications of current and future entitlement or social benefits on the various options being discussed with the family.

Legal Options

Once a caregiver has been selected and accepts that role, uncertainty about the available legal options and the complex requirements of the law may further deter the parent from completing a plan for the future. Permanency-planning legal options vary by state, and all families are best served by expert legal assistance in the state of residence before decisions are finalized. It is best for them to know and assess all the options available and to select the mechanism that best reflects their personal situation and has the greatest likelihood of supporting their wishes for their children's future.

The Family Center's mission, which is to assure a secure future for children of parents with life-threatening illnesses, directs the focus to identifying and confirming the best plan for the children and to stabilize that plan through the most protective legal means. The following description of legal options is provided as background for better understanding of the case material that follows. Those interested in legal options available in specific states should contact their state Bar Association. More information about the Family Center can be found at www.thefamilycenter.org.

A WILL   In many states, terminally ill parents planning for their children's future custody have several options to chose from when putting a plan in place. All parents may document their wishes for the future care and custody of their children in a will. However, a will has no legal standing in the eyes of the court and, if contested by a party who has a legitimate interest in the welfare of the child, a custody proceeding of uncertain outcome may take place. This has the potential of resulting in a custody arrangement different from that envisioned by the deceased parent. For example, a noncustodial parent who has had little or no involvement in a child's upbringing might contest the deceased parent's designation of a grandparent as caregiver and, with limited understanding of the implications on the child, the court system may assign custody to the living parent. Because the courts do not generally recognize the will, it provides the least assurance that the person chosen by the parent will actually become the caregiver.

The advantages of doing a will over other options are primarily that it can be done quickly if needed, and does not require going to court.

COURT APPOINTED STANDBY GUARDIANSHIP   Recognizing the unique needs of parents with terminal illnesses, many states now have legal mechanisms in place to provide parents with better ways to ensure that their wishes for the child are put in place at the time of their death by designating a future guardian for the child prior to the parent's death. This is known as a standby guardianship. The standby guardian is someone who cares for the child only when the parent dies or becomes too incapacitated to continuing caring for the child. At all other times the parent maintains legal custody of the child without the actual transfer of legal guardianship to the caregiver until the occurrence of a triggering event, such as death or incapacity, that prevents the parent from fulfilling his or her parental duties. At that time the standby guardian must petition the court for full guardianship, and his or her caregiver duties are activated.

The court application process for securing a standby guardianship can be quite lengthy and usually includes background checks and a home study of the intended guardian or guardians. Parents must consult the intended caregiver regarding this designation and obtain consent for these investigations. Some potential caregivers are reluctant to participate in this application.

Another significant barrier for many families is that the designation of a standby legal guardianship may limit the financial benefits available for the family more than those available to kinship foster families. For example, in New York, a court-appointed standby guardian is ineligible to serve as a foster parent for those same children. Foster care is generally viewed as an alternative for families who have no other options. Therefore, neither the parent nor the standby guardian can later request that the guardian be designated as the child's foster parent, even if the financial supports and benefits available through foster care would be greater.

GUARDIANSHIP AND ADOPTION   Guardianship and adoption are court processes that involve the transfer of parental rights from the parent to the nominated caregiver. In the case of adoption, the transfer of parental rights is permanent and immediate, thereby terminating all parental rights and responsibilities. In the case of guardianship, transfer of parental rights may be revoked under petition. Although the guardianship option is available in a number of states, parents rarely execute it because they do not desire the immediate termination or suspension of parental rights and decision-making authority. The standby option, if available, is generally better suited to the situation in most families.

Following the death of a parent, a caregiver must petition the court for guardianship or adoption in order to be recognized officially as the person vested with the legal authority and right to make decisions for and on behalf of the child. Caregivers whom the courts have not legally recognized run the risk of being denied the ability to make important decisions for those children in matters related to education, health, and access to other needed services and benefits. This is an insecure and undesirable situation for the family.

FOSTER CARE   Some states have kinship foster-care programs that allow children to be placed with a suitable relative who then becomes the certified foster parent of the child. The primary advantage of the kinship foster-care arrangement as a permanency planning option is the increased payments for the support of each child as compared with public assistance. A large network of foster-care social services also becomes available to the family and can be accessed free of charge once the designation of foster parent has been made. However, this option has disadvantages that both the parent and caregiver need to consider. Generally, the commissioner of social services in the locale where the family resides retains the legal guardianship of the child and, as such, the commissioner must provide consent for all major decisions regarding the care of the child. These might include authorization for invasive surgery or the transfer of a child to a different school. Additionally, the foster care agency that oversees the certification of the foster parents continues its involvement with the family by making regular visits to the foster home.

Do Parents Plan?

From research conducted by the Family Center with parents who have AIDS, we know that most mothers and fathers have someone in mind whom they would like to care for their children, but many have never spoken with the proposed caregiver about the plan in terms concrete enough to gain his or her commitment to care for the child. In interviews with ninety-five mothers with AIDS in New York City conducted by the Family Center in collaboration with the Albert Einstein College of Medicine, 28 percent of mothers reported not having identified a future caregiver for their children, and 17 percent reported having identified someone as a potential caregiver, but not having spoken with them about the plan. The remaining 55 percent had spoken with the proposed caregiver about the plan and had obtained his or her commitment to care for the child. Of these 55 percent, fewer than 10 percent had documented their wishes in writing. As we continue to follow and serve these ninety-five women over time, we expect that some of those with no plan or without committed caregivers will make plans and speak with the proposed caregiver about the plan. We also expect that more mothers will document their wishes in writing. Nevertheless, there will be families in which the parent does little or no planning before death, leaving surviving family members to put together the best possible plan, at one of the worst times in the family's life.

Additional research at the Family Center that examines the planning process from the caregivers' perspective confirms that many parents do not involve the proposed caregiver in making a plan before they die. Of seventy-nine caregivers of children orphaned as a result of AIDS in New York City,

34 percent reported that the parent of the child they were caring for had not made a custody plan before death, and 23 percent of the caregivers had not realized that taking care of the child would be their responsibility. Not surprisingly, caregivers reported a complexity of feelings and circumstances associated with deciding to care for the child. Although all of the caregivers interviewed said that "they really wanted to care for the child," they also reported a number of pressures and assumptions related to the decision. Almost one-quarter (24%), reported that they would not have agreed to care for the child if someone else had offered to take responsibility, and 11 percent reported that they felt pressured to care for the child. More than one-half (62%) reported that it was assumed they would care for the child, and 43 percent said it was expected of them to care for the child. Added pressures included there being no one else to care for the child (42%), the caregiver's involvement being the only way for the child and his or her siblings to remain together in one household (47%), and the fear that the child would be put in foster care with an unfamiliar family (57%). This research confirms the complexity and difficulty that parents and potential caregivers face in planning for the future. Many questions need to be addressed, including:

How many children need plans?

What are the ages of the children?

Do any of the children have special needs?

Is the family willing to go to court to legalize a plan?

Who is available and interested in caring for the children?

Can they care for all of the children in the family?

Will they be able to care for the children until they reach majority?

What backup supports are available to the proposed caregiver, particularly those caregivers who are elderly, ill or are caring for other children and/or adults?

If the children are separated, will they be in contact regularly?

As evidenced by successful Family Center cases, the process of permanency planning, though complex, is achievable and can result in the effective transition of children into new family environments. Careful planning is key to this success.

The Planning Process

Family Center services are designed to accomplish a number of specific goals, including (1) enhancing disclosure and communication between ill parent and child, ill parent and future caregiver and future caregiver and child; (2) developing an appropriate and feasible custody plan before the parent's death; (3) working with the caregiver and child after parental death to facilitate the transition to the new family; and (4) enhancing access to concrete resources and social support. The model is based on the belief that appropriate disclosure to the child and caregiver, combined with a viable custody plan, will increase the likelihood that children will have a stable future, with the necessary resources available to make it happen (Armistead et al. 1999; Burton et al. 1995).

Family Center services provide parents with support to acknowledge the need for a plan, educate clients about all planning options, and provide in-home legal services and court representation when needed. Services are provided in the home by a team of a case manager called a family specialist, a clinical social worker, and lawyer. The expertise of a substance use counselor is also available when needed. Continuity of services is stressed. The family specialist works with the family throughout the planning process, accessing clinical and legal services when appropriate. Family communication is emphasized and, whenever possible, families are encouraged to use mediation and other methods to resolve family communication problems and to avoid court battles over child custody. Caregivers are encouraged to go to court for guardianship of the children in their care, and parents are presented with the option of going to court under New York's standby guardianship law to gain the court's approval of their plan prior to incapacitating illness or death. Continuity is maintained following the death of the parent, with services provided to the new caregiver and children. Services provided after the death of the parent focus on helping the family deal with grief and loss issues, assisting with benefits and entitlements problems, and supporting all family members' adjustment to the new household.

Unfortunately, even with a package of services designed to be flexible enough to meet the varied and complex needs of families with AIDS, the ideal frequently is not met. The worst-case scenario occurs when the parent did no planning and told no one that he or she was ill, and when the death came as a complete surprise to family members and friends. A more common situation is that the family did know that the parent was ill but may not have known how serious the illness was or, despite knowledge of the seriousness of the illness, may not have had the resources to create a workable plan. In some families, the parent may not have been able to acknowledge that a plan was needed until it was too late. In others, the parent may not have had someone she trusted to name as a caregiver or avoided naming any one person caregiver out of fear of alienating other family members or friends who might have an interest in raising the child.

Parents working with the Family Center are encouraged to involve proposed caregivers early in the planning process and one of the goals of service is to have a meeting that brings together the parent, the proposed caregiver, and the family specialist to assess the strengths and weaknesses of the plan. This meeting is a kind of "reality check" and is an important test of the viability of the plan. Planning with the parent often proceeds smoothly until the family specialist suggests involving the proposed caregiver, at which point the work slows down, meetings are missed, and phone calls are not returned. There are a number of reasons the parent may be unwilling to involve the caregiver, including reluctance to disclose an HIV infection to the caregiver and the feeling on the part of the parent that the discussion cannot take place without full disclosure. Other reasons for avoiding a discussion with the intended caregiver include fear that the caregiver will say no, cultural prohibitions around planning for death, and, in some communities, the feeling that discussing the plan in any way will insult the family member whose intention or expectations would always be to care for the child, if needed.

The following case illustrates what may happen when a parent with AIDS postpones speaking concretely with the proposed caregiver about the plan, and then dies suddenly. It also demonstrates the difficulty service providers experience when a parent keeps important information from the caregiver. In this case, the caregiver did accept services from the Family Center after her daughter's death but has had a great deal of difficulty following through on obtaining guardianship for her two grandchildren. She is always pleasant and courteous, but staff believe that her ability to work with them has been compromised by her feeling of having been betrayed by the very service that was supposed to help her be in a better position to care for the children. Services designed to work with both HIV-infected parents and the proposed caregivers of their children must be prepared for difficult discussions about who is the client, and for developing guidelines and support for staff who find themselves working with families with many complex secrets, including HIV disclosure.

Frances is a forty-four-year-old mother of six and grandmother of four. She is a client of the Family Center, working on guardianship for two of her grandchildren, Terry and Shawnee. Terry and Shawnee came to live with Frances after their mother, Elizabeth, died of AIDS, eighteen months earlier. At the time of her death Elizabeth had been working with the Family Center for four months on a permanency plan for her children. During the planning process, Elizabeth was open to having her mother involved but was adamant that she did not want her to know her HIV status or the fact that nine-year-old Terry was also HIV-positive. She believed that her mother would care for the children regardless of Terry's HIV status but was reluctant to talk to her about HIV. Elizabeth did inform her mother that she and Terry were sick, choosing to tell her that they had sickle cell anemia rather than AIDS. Elizabeth began discussing the various planning options available in New York state when she died suddenly, without any written documentation of her wishes for her children's future care.

As Elizabeth assumed, Frances did take her grandchildren into her home. With no other option for the children, she decided to care for them as long as she could despite her bad health. At the time of her daughter's death, Frances was informed by the hospital about her grandson's HIV status, and given information necessary for his continued medical care. The family was shocked by the suddenness of Elizabeth's death and surprised to learn of her and Terry's HIV status. Frances appeared overwhelmed by all of the decisions she had to make following her daughter's death and by the obstacles she was encountering in obtaining the children's entitlements and in enrolling them in school.

The Family Center lawyer and family specialist assisted Frances with letters to the Board of Education and Department of Social Services, and the children began receiving benefits and were enrolled in school in time for the new academic year. Frances met with the lawyer to review the guardianship process, and decided to pursue this avenue for legalizing her caregiving role with Shawnee and Terry. The guardianship process generally takes about four months to complete. In this case, the process met with a number of obstacles, including Shawnee's father, who saw his daughter regularly and whose consent to the plan was needed. Shawnee's father finally consented to the plan, and eighteen months after Elizabeth's death the paperwork was ready for submission to the court.

In the meantime, Frances was increasingly ambivalent about pursuing the guardianship because she feared the court-ordered home study would find her apartment too crowded. In addition to Frances, Shawnee, and Terry, her three-bedroom apartment housed four of Frances's daughters and four of their young children.

Although Frances has not directly conveyed her ambivalence about pursuing the guardianship further, she has made it clear that it is not her first priority. With the children in school and in receipt of benefits, there is no immediate need for the legal paperwork. Frances clearly has reservations about subjecting herself and her family to the scrutiny of the court. She is still overwhelmed by her added responsibilities, and she frequently expresses resentment that Elizabeth did not do more to secure the plan before she died. If Elizabeth had planned in a way that realistically informed Frances that she would be taking care of Shawnee and Terry, it is possible that better housing arrangements could have been obtained earlier. It is also possible that had Elizabeth included her mother in the planning process, Frances would now be more motivated to complete the guardianship and might be more open to receiving additional assistance from The Family Center and other services.

Even when parents make a plan, there can be significant vulnerabilities to the arrangement that the caregiver may have to deal with after the parent's death. One of the most common vulnerabilities is failure to obtain the noncustodial parent's consent to the plan. Eighty percent of parents planning for the future care and custody of their children are mothers, many of whom are estranged from the fathers of the children. The average mother has three children, not all fathered by the same man. Many mothers are reluctant to involve one or more father in the planning process, leaving their plans vulnerable to future interference. Mothers with AIDS resist involving fathers for many reasons, including a history of abuse with the former partner, possible current drug use activity by the father, a lack of disclosure of HIV and bitterness over his noninvolvement and lack of financial support of the child. A mother with AIDS will commonly resist involving the father because she fears he will seek immediate custody of the child when he learns that she is planning, regardless of his current involvement in the child's upbringing. Even when the father knows her HIV status and may himself have HIV, a mother with AIDS will often avoid involving him because she fears that his antagonism toward her and his anger at not being named caregiver will set in motion an immediate custody battle, even if he has no real interest in caring for the child. Animosity between the parents frequently is played out in the court system and can have negative repercussions for the child's future. Many mothers in this situation believe that the father will not contest the plan after their death because they believe that the primary motivating factor is the fight with them and not who cares for the child.

The problem with this kind of a plan is that it is more of a wish than a plan. If the mother's assumptions about the father are incorrect, it may result in the father's contesting the plan put in place by the mother and agreed to by the caregiver. If the father has maintained contact with the child and has no other attributes that would call into question his ability to parent the child, it is quite likely that a judge will award him custody. If this happens, the caregiver is then left with the choice of going to court to battle the father for custody or allowing the father to exercise his parental rights without the involvement of the court. Very frequently, the proposed caregiver in a case like this is the mother's mother or mother's sister, women without the financial, emotional, or physical resources to engage in a protracted and costly custody battle.

Regardless of the outcome, no one really "wins" in a contested custody case. If the father is awarded custody, the proposed caregiver loses custody and perhaps even contact with her grandchild or niece, the child loses an important part of his or her support network, and the father loses a potential ally in the raising of the child. For the caregiver, the emotional toll is often great as she deals with a complex array of feelings, which may include anger toward the child's mother for having misjudged the father's intentions, sadness and guilt over her perceived failure to implement the plan, and feelings of grief over the loss of contact with the children, an important living link to her dead daughter. If the caregiver is awarded custody, she too loses a potential ally in the raising of the child and may still struggle with feelings of anger toward her daughter for not completely "taking care of business" before she died and with feelings of sadness and guilt over involving the child in a court battle.

Ideally, planning involves all interested parties in the process as early as possible. This approach may lengthen the time it takes to put a plan in place, but the increased strength of the plan makes its smooth implementation more likely. The following case illustrates how the Family Center's approach to planning, including involving the father whenever possible, increases the viability of the plan. It also illustrates the complexities of planning for children with different fathers.

Susan, fifty-four years old, is the mother of Mary Alice, a thirty-year-old woman with AIDS. Susan had five children, three of whom are living. In the last six years she has lost two sons to AIDS. She has a son who lives in Massachusetts with his wife and two young children, and another son who lives in Florida. Susan is close to all of her children and the children are in close contact with one another.

Susan is aware of Mary Alice's HIV status and is a frequent visitor in her daughter's home, helping with childcare and other tasks when needed. Mary Alice is the mother of four children. Her daughters are thirteen and fourteen years old and her sons are five and eight years old. The father of the boys, Tomas, lives in the household and is aware of her HIV status. The father of the girls, José, lives nearby and is not aware of her HIV status. At the time the case was opened, the girls' father was only sporadically involved and provided no financial support.

When Mary Alice enrolled in services, she knew that she wanted her children to remain together in one household with her mother and Tomas as joint caregivers. Susan was involved in the planning process from the start and attended most meetings with the family specialist. Though the plan for all of the children was the same, the fact that two fathers were involved meant different decisions had to be made for the two sets of children. In planning for the girls, Mary Alice had to decide whether to involve their father, which in turn influenced her choice of plan. In planning for the boys, she needed to work out with Tomas and mother the details of the shared caregiving and ensure that those details were adequately documented in any paperwork put in place.

Mary Alice initially decided to include Jose in planning for the girls, but was adamant that she did not want him to know she was HIV-positive. The family specialist agreed to be present when she informed him of her intention to plan and role played with her responses if he pressured her about why. At the same time, Mary Alice stated a preference for naming her mother as the proposed legal guardian of her daughters and having the plan approved by the court before her death.

This court approval process, which in New York state is referred to as a Petition for Standby Guardianship, involves obtaining consent to the plan from all other parties recognized as having a legitimate concern in the child's well-being, including other biological parents if they can be found. It also carries a risk of disclosure during the court proceedings, inasmuch as judges often question ill parents in detail about the need for such a petition. At this point in the work, the family specialist informed Mary Alice of the possibility that her HIV status might become known to José if he chose to attend the standby guardianship court proceedings.

Over the next several months, Mary Alice continued to state her desire to speak with José and assured the family specialist that she would be setting up an appointment for them all to meet. As time went on, it became clearer to Mary Alice that the possibility that José might learn of her HIV status was too great a risk. After eight months of discussion and deliberation on the pros and cons of involving José, Mary

Alice decided against including him in the planning process despite her knowledge that it weakened the plan and could pose a problem for her mother should the plan be implemented. At this point, she decided to name her mother through a written designation of standby guardianship, using an option in New York state that does not involve the approval of the court. She also decided to write a will documenting her wishes for her children's care and stating her reasons for preferring Susan to José as caregiver for her daughters. Susan agreed to this modification and the written designations naming Susan as the proposed caregiver for both girls and a will were prepared and signed.

In terms of planning for her sons, Mary Alice decided to involve Tomas, the boys' father, in the planning process from the beginning. The family clarified their goals for the children, and both Susan and Tomas committed to jointly caring for the children, should it be needed in the future. Mary Alice, Tomas, and Susan decided that Susan also should be named standby guardian for the two boys in written designations to be used only if Tomas were unable to continue his involvement with the boys. This arrangement also was documented in a memorandum of understanding signed by all three adults, stating that Susan would become the guardian of the boys only if both Mary Alice and Tomas were unable to care for them.

This family's work with the Family Center took place over a two-year period during which numerous home visits and telephone follow up calls were made by the Family Specialist and the lawyer. The result is a plan that clearly states the mother's wishes for the care of all of her children, with agreement to the plan by the proposed caregiver and the involved father of the two youngest children. The plan remains vulnerable to change if the father of the two oldest children decides to contest the plan at the time of the mother's death. Susan and Tomas have supported Mary Alice in her decision to not involve the girls' father in the planning and will try to keep the children together in one household. The written documentation executed by the Family Center lawyer fully outlines the intentions of the plan and the wishes of the mother, further limiting the likelihood that the estranged father might significantly threaten the plan. Mary Alice, Susan, and Tomas also agreed at the last meeting with the lawyer to revisit the question of involving José if at some point he became more involved with his daughters.

This and other cases illustrate that planning is difficult but not impossible. With the guidance of trained professionals, parents and caregivers can seek and obtain the greatest protection for the future security of their children.

Summary and Implications

Planning for the future of children of parents with life-threatening illness is a complex matter that addresses health, legal, familial, economic, and social concerns. Providing services to the current and future families of these children demands a multifaceted and flexible approach that is responsive to the current circumstances within the family yet is focused on the enactment of a viable, legally sanctioned plan for the care of the children. Lessons learned by the Family Center staff in providing permanency planning services to families affected by HIV include these:

- All plans are strengthened when caregivers are involved before the death of the parent.
- Dealing directly with concerns about the noncustodial parent before the death of the parent enhances the likelihood that the plan will be secure.
- Making the caregiver aware of any potential threats or challenges to the plan and preparing the caregiver to deal with any challenges increases the chances that the parent's wishes will be upheld.
- Caregivers need assistance not only before but also after the death of the parent to adjust to the transition into their role. This assistance may include legal services, grief and loss counseling for themselves and the children, entitlement-access assistance, and guidance in reassessing their own social and professional resources in order to develop a network for support and backup.
- Older caregivers may require additional assistance in coordinating services and support because the systems in place today (schools, health care services, entitlement or social services) are more complex than when their older children were growing up.
- Finally, the need for flexibility in approach yet focus on developing a workable plan is critical to securing the future lives of children of parents with life-threatening illnesses.

References

Armistead, L., et al. 1999. Understanding of HIV/AIDS among children of HIV-infected mothers: Implications for prevention, disclosure and bereavement. *Children's Health Care* 28 (4): 277–295.

Burton, L., et al. 1995. Context and surrogate parenting among contemporary grandparents. In S. Hanson et al., eds., *Single Parent Families: Diversity, Myths and Realities,* pp. 349–366. London: Haworth.

Draimin, B. H., et al. 1998. Improving permanency planning in families with HIV disease. *Child Welfare* 77 (2): 180–194.

Draimin, B. H., and J. Hudis. 2000. Excellence in action: Creating a secure future for children whose parents have a life-threatening illness. *The Source* 10 (2): n.p.

10

Case Management Challenges and Strategies

CAROL E. DEGRAW

Older adults have been caring for spouses, partners, adult children, siblings, and close friends with HIV disease since the beginning of the epidemic. Growing numbers of grandparents have taken on primary responsibility for grandchildren who may be HIV-infected while they are also caring for dying adult children. The risks to emotional, physical, social, and financial well-being are enormous. The sheer intensity of physical care can be overwhelming as older adults in their fifties through their eighties tackle the needs of infants, toddlers, and school-age children while running a household. Older adults are frequently at risk for social isolation because of the time required by their caregiving role as well as the internalized stigma and shame of HIV/AIDS.

Social Security benefits fall short of meeting the economic needs of these caregivers and their families. Health insurance is often inadequate, especially because some insurance companies do not allow a grandparent to carry a grandchild as a dependent. Grandparents who become legal guardians are often ineligible for financial benefits received by foster parents. Ironically, these older adults, whose own lives have been irrevocably altered by HIV disease, fall through the cracks of the HIV service-delivery system because funding is directed only to the person living with HIV disease.

This chapter examines the service needs of older adults caring for grandchildren affected by HIV disease, a case-management model that was successfully piloted for this population, and policy issues that must be addressed to service these caregivers. The chapter draws on the experience of an HIV case-management agency in northern New Jersey serving one of the poorest cities in the United States.

Case Management Overview

Depending on the source, the concept of case management dates back anywhere from twenty-five to seventy years. The use of case management grew dramatically in the 1980s, especially in the areas of mental health, developmental disability, HIV disease, older adults, child welfare, and immigrants. During that time there was a shift from institutional to community-based care (Rose and Moore 1995).

Widely accepted as a valuable method of practice in health and human services, the definitions and goals of case management frequently vary depending on the field in which it is being used and the profession of the provider. Social workers, nurses, health educators, paraprofessionals, and peers, among others, have historically provided case-management services. The training of case managers therefore varies widely, from informal experience to varying degrees of professional training.

The literature agrees, for the most part, on the functions of case management. These include intake, assessment, goal-setting, care planning, resource identification, linking clients to services, advocacy, monitoring, reassessment, and evaluation (Rose and Moore 1995; Piette et al. 1992; Rothman 1991; Moore 1990).

Case Management and HIV

Case management has played a central role in the HIV/AIDS service delivery system since the mid-1980s. With earlier identification of HIV infection, people living longer from the time of diagnosis, and less need for hospitalization, social services grew in importance. The Robert Wood Johnson Foundation and the federal Health Services and Resource Administration (HRSA) began funding large-scale demonstration projects focusing on case management (Piette et al. 1992; Sierra Health Foundation 1991). By the late 1980s "policymakers and funders recognized case management might accomplish the twin benefits of reducing the spiraling cost of treating AIDS and increasing access to needed supportive services" (Sierra Health Foundation 1991).

The federal Ryan White Comprehensive AIDS Resources Emergency Act of 1990, which was amended in 1996, authorizes funding to help communities and states develop, coordinate, and operate "effective and cost efficient systems for the delivery of essential services to individuals and families with HIV disease." In 1998 more than $1 billion was appropriated for medical and social services under the act. Under this legislation, case management is an essential service in the delivery of health and support services for persons living with HIV.

Case Management with Older Adults

In the aging field, prolonged life expectancies and the change from institutional to community care settings "stimulated the emergence of case management" (Rothman 1991). The emphasis in the case-management models for older adults was on the disabled, at-risk, and frail elderly (Emlet et al. 1996; Biegel, Shore, and Gordon 1984). Interventions were geared to strengthening the support systems of the older adult, but because they were geared to the elderly most at risk, the goal was to strengthen the family's ability to provide support to the elderly member (Biegel, Shore, and Gordon 1984).

The common emphasis in the gerontological literature on case management is on service needs of the dependent older adult. The assumption is that the older adult needs a caregiver, not that the older person is providing assistance as a caregiver.

Case-Management Needs Among Older Adult HIV-Affected Caregivers

The HIV/AIDS epidemic had orphaned up to 125,000 children ages eighteen years and younger in the United States by the year 2000 (Michaels and Levine 1992). The majority of these children were taken care of by their grandparents (Roe and Minkler 1999). Although grandparents raising grandchildren is not a new phenomenon, the dramatically increasing numbers of grandparents as surrogate parents began to lead to the development of supportive services for these caregivers. Support groups that offered information and emotional support were founded in the late 1980s. Resource centers providing information and referral were developed in the 1990s (Roe and Minkler 1999). Although these beginning interventions were a positive step, many of the older caregivers who were seen in the HIV/AIDS field were not aware of these services or were too overwhelmed to even consider attending a support group. Something more was needed.

HIV case managers were seeing grandparents in HIV clinics and during home visits who had altered their entire lives to become the caregiver of their grandchildren and frequently of their own son or daughter who were dying from AIDS. These grandparents had frequently given up or lost jobs due to their caregiving responsibilities. They had not been in the social service system in the past and were not aware of the program benefits and services for which they were eligible. They frequently felt isolated because HIV in the family was kept a secret, in many cases even from the children. These were not men and women who were used to asking for help. In fact, asking for help was often seen as a weakness, an admission that they were not capable. This was sometimes accompanied by a fear of involvement from the Division of Youth and Family Services (DYFS), a New Jersey state child-welfare agency that is frequently not trusted, especially in the urban community.

HIV case managers also recognized something else. They were experienced with working with an adult population most commonly ranging in age from twenty-five to fifty. Experience with older adults was limited. Despite their inexperience, they knew that the case-management models for working with older adults, which emphasized the frail elderly, did not apply. The older caregivers encountered in the HIV service system had faced the terminal illness or death of one or more of their children, pulled the family together, cared for as many as eleven grandchildren, struggled on low incomes to maintain a household, made ends meet to have meals on the table, and frequently neglected their own emotional and health needs to do this. These were not "frail elderly." These were women and men with incredible inner strength. Any program serving these older caregivers had to begin by acknowledging and building on their strength.

The OASIS Model and Experience

In 1994, an HIV/AIDS and Aging Committee was established by the Coalition on AIDS in Passaic County, New Jersey (CAPCO), a grassroots consortium of agencies, organizations, and individuals affected by HIV disease. The purpose of the committee was to address the impact of the HIV pandemic on the aging population. One of the initial activities of the committee was a needs assessment to document the issues facing older adults raising children and adolescents who were losing their parents to AIDS. The needs assessment identified case management, transportation, and financial assistance as priority services needs. Respite and childcare were also identified as critical needs. Based on needs assessment findings, the Older Adults: Strength in Support (OASIS) Project was developed as a service intervention project to provide supportive services to these older caregivers.

With funding from the Grotta Foundation for Senior Care and the Wallerstein Foundation for Geriatric Life Improvement, the OASIS Project was implemented in July 1996 under the sponsorship of CAPCO. Before OASIS there were no comprehensive services in northern New Jersey, or in the entire state, for older adult caregivers affected by the epidemic. During its pilot year, the OASIS Project created and tested a model of supportive services for older adult caregivers in New Jersey's Passaic and Bergen counties. The project was conceived of as a "bridge" that would link older family caregivers with existing resources in the local HIV/AIDS consortium. Its ultimate goal was to bring together the HIV care and treatment network, aging services, children's services, and the volunteer network to form a safety net of services for the caregiver.

Case management was the key service component of the OASIS Project. A bilingual (Spanish/English) case manager was hired and based at CAPCO. The focus of the case management was on direct counseling, in home visiting, and coordination of services. This included entitlement assistance, advocacy, information, referral, and linkage to other community programs and resources. A direct emergency financial assistance program to assist with medications, utility bills, and other necessities supported the case management component.

During its pilot year, OASIS served thirty-three families, including fifty-one adults and ninety-two children. The vast majority (28) of OASIS clients were grandmothers. Two great-aunts, one aunt, and two grandfathers were also served. Nineteen of the caregivers reported their race/ethnicity as African American, eleven as Hispanic, two as Euro-American, and one as "other." Caregivers ranged in age from forty-six to seventy-nine, with the majority in their mid- to late fifties. In twenty-five families, representing 75 percent of the total, a grandparent or great-aunt was the sole or exclusive caregiver raising HIV-affected or orphaned children. The average number of children being raised was three, with a range from one child to ten children. The children's ages ranged from infancy to seventeen years.

Fifteen of the caregivers had lost an adult child to HIV disease. In the remaining eighteen families, the adult child was either living at home with AIDS but was too ill to parent fully or was out of the house due to drug addiction. Eight grandparents were caring for grandchildren with AIDS. Seven other grandparents were raising two grandchildren living with HIV disease.

Family income sources included earnings of the caregiver or spouse, Social Security retirement benefits, Social Security Disability (SSD), Supplemental Security Income (SSI), Social Security Survivor's Benefits, and Temporary Aid to Needy Families (TANF), previously known as Aid to Families with Dependent Children (AFDC).

The following case examples introduce the case management issues of the older adults served by this project.

Mrs. R. was a fifty-seven-year-old Hispanic female who did not speak English. The HIV coordinator at her son's substance abuse treatment center referred her to OASIS in the summer of 1996. The HIV coordinator had visited the home and was concerned about the family. When referred, Mrs. R.'s thirty-seven-year-old son was at the end stages of AIDS, living in Mrs. R.'s apartment with his fifteen-year-old HIV-negative son. His wife had died of AIDS six years before. Mrs. R. had become the primary caregiver to both her son and grandson.

Mrs. R. and her son were both receiving SSI and had Medicaid. Mrs. R. was disabled due to high blood pressure and circulation problems. Mrs. R.'s son was served by the AIDS Community Care Alternatives Program (ACCAP), a Medicaid waiver program designed to assist people with AIDS who require extensive care, to remain at home if they desire rather than be placed in a nursing home. He therefore had twenty-four-hour home health care. The fifteen-year-old had no health insurance coverage.

At the initial home visit, the OASIS Case Manager discovered there was a lack of food in the home. Mrs. R.'s son had SSI checks that needed to be cashed, but because he was not ambulatory and did not have a bank account the checks remained in a drawer while the family went hungry. Mrs. R. was requesting assistance in having a Last Will and Testament prepared. The OASIS case manager explained the need for a durable power of attorney so that Mrs. R. could cash the checks on her son's behalf. With permission from Mrs. R. and her son, the OASIS case manager elicited the help of a legal advocate. Mrs. R.'s son completed a durable power of attorney and Last Will and Testament at home. Mrs. R. was now able to cash the checks and buy food.

When this was done, Mrs. R. told the OASIS case manager that although her family was supportive and she knew they would be there for her when her son died, she felt that she needed a support group to help her. She wanted to meet other women who were facing similar issues. The OASIS case manager contacted a local

HIV mental-health program and was able to arrange for a clinician to facilitate a Spanish-speaking support group at the CAPCO office. The OASIS case manager called other Spanish-speaking clients, some of whom had also indicated an interest. The Spanish-speaking support group began. Another area community-based agency provided free transportation for the participants.

Language was an ongoing barrier for Mrs. R. Because she only spoke Spanish, she could not communicate with the English-speaking home health aides. She was very upset by this and feared that if something happened to her son, she would not be able to let the home health aide know. Requests were made for Spanish-speaking home health aides, but this was not always possible to arrange. Furthermore, the home care agency made it clear they were there to serve Mrs. R.'s son's needs, not hers. The OASIS case manager, who was bilingual (English/Spanish), became the interpreter for Mrs. R. She assisted Mrs. R. in making medical and social service appointments, as well as in applying for food stamps and for benefits for her grandson.

The heat did not come on in the building in October. It was an especially cold month, and Mrs. R. was sleeping with her son to keep him warm, waking frequently throughout the night to clean his vomit and recurring diarrhea. The same week, Mrs. R. was advised that she was being taken to court by a collection agency for medical bills.

The OASIS case manager called the lawyers, doctors, and state Medicaid office to resolve the collection issue. It was finally determined that the diagnostic firm that was pursuing the medical bill had written Mrs. R.'s Medicaid number incorrectly on the original claim two years before, and the bill had been rejected because of the typographical error. The diagnostic firm agreed to resubmit the claim and stop pursuing Mrs. R.

The OASIS case manager arranged with an area hospice for temporary quarters for Mrs. R.'s son while the heat issue was being resolved. The family refused because the son wanted to die at home. The case manager called the realtor, Board of Health, Public Service Electric and Gas, tax assessor, mayor's office, and finally a congressman regarding the heating issue. The building had recently been sold to a "shell" corporation and there were problems locating the actual owner of the building, who was responsible for fixing the problem. The utility company determined that a previous owner or tenant had taken a fixture needed to start up the boiler. The replacement cost was $1,600. After nine days without heat and with assurances that when the owner was located they would be reimbursed, the tenants pooled their money and had the fixture replaced, and heat was restored. Mrs. R.'s son died three days later.

Throughout this period daily telephone calls and frequent home visits by the OASIS case manager were made to provide Mrs. R. with emotional support. Mrs. R.

continued to attend the Spanish-speaking support group. Mrs. R.'s grandson was referred to a counselor to help him grieve the loss of both his parents.

•   •   •

Mrs. W. was a sixty-two-year-old Caucasian grandmother who was the caregiver of
her thirty-five-year-old daughter and four-year-old granddaughter, both of whom
were diagnosed with AIDS. Her daughter's HIV case manager referred her to OASIS.
Mrs. W. was reluctant to accept services because they appeared to be an acknowledgment of impending grief. In fact, it took more than six months from the time
she was first introduced to the OASIS case manager for Mrs. W. to come into the
office for an intake appointment. In the interim, the OASIS case manager would
periodically call Mrs. W. just to say hello and see how things were. This gentle act
of reaching out gave Mrs. W. the reassurance that support was there for her when
she felt ready.

Mrs. W. was employed as an office worker until her daughter and granddaughter became sick. Her job then became maintaining their home. She provided meals,
housekeeping, transportation, and other tasks. She exhausted her credit caring for
them and worried about making the mortgage payments. Family conflict arose when
the HIV diagnosis became known. Mrs. W.'s daughter felt that certain family members no longer wanted her or her daughter around. Mrs. W. acknowledged feeling
socially isolated, stating that she only related to doctors, nurses, her granddaughter
and daughter, whom she described as her best friend.

As her daughter and granddaughter became sicker, Mrs. W. would periodically
call the OASIS case manager for emotional support. Although on these occasions
Mrs. W. would acknowledge her upset and anger, she stated that she feared discussing her impending loss and preferred working it out by tending to her garden.
Mrs. W.'s daughter died the following summer.

Following her daughter's death, information was needed regarding Social Security survivor benefits and payee requirements. There was also a concern regarding
guardianship of her granddaughter. The OASIS case manager obtained the necessary
information from Social Security and accompanied Mrs. W. to her appointment. Mrs.
W.'s daughter had not been emotionally able to complete standby guardianship
arrangements. The OASIS case manager accompanied Mrs. W. to family court following the death of her daughter to petition the court for custody of her granddaughter. Mrs. W.'s granddaughter died less than two months later.

In addition to the unspeakable grief that Mrs. W. was experiencing, she was also
in serious financial trouble. Her daughter's and granddaughter's deaths brought the
end of their Social Security benefits, which had contributed to mortgage payments
on the home. Mrs. W., at age sixty-three, began to look for a job. She found part-

time paid employment, but she also found another full-time position. Her son and his daughter moved into her home. This granddaughter had a learning disability and required special attention. Mrs. W. was back in the job that she knew best. She was once again a full-time caregiver.

•   •   •

Mrs. L. was a sixty-eight-year-old African American female suffering from Parkinson's disease. Her son's HIV case manager made the referral to OASIS when Mrs. L.'s son was rushed to the hospital for a seizure, but refused admission, stating that he was concerned about leaving his mother alone with his daughters. Mrs. L. was a widow, collecting retirement benefits, and had Medicare. Her thirty-nine-year-old son was HIV-positive, an active injecting drug user, and lived with Mrs. L. and his two teenage daughters. Mrs. L.'s son's wife had died of AIDS five years earlier. The teenage daughters had been placed in foster homes by DYFS following Mrs. L.'s son's suicide attempt after his wife's death. One daughter alleged that the foster parent sexually abused her. Both daughters refused to attend school and were exhibiting acting-out behavior. Mrs. L. and her son were unable to control them.

Mrs. L.'s son and granddaughters had taken over her home. Her son's SSI check went toward his substance abuse. Whenever she bought food, Mrs. L.'s granddaughters brought home friends and fed them so there was never enough food to feed the family for the month. Mrs. L. had fallen behind on her mortgage and the bank was foreclosing on her home. The stress in the household was unbearable for her. Her health was suffering. She was nervous and cried frequently.

The OASIS case manager made daily contact with Mrs. L. to allow her an opportunity to discuss her concerns, provide supportive counseling, and prioritize the myriad of needs presented by this family. The OASIS case manager contacted the Parkinson's Disease Foundation to obtain information regarding the disease and available services. Mrs. L. felt she needed respite time away from her home and family. Mrs. L. was referred to a medical day care program and looked forward to going, but Medicare would not pay so she was unable to attend.

As the family situation continued to deteriorate, DYFS, which had been involved with the family for a number of years, called in their Family Preservation unit to provide intensive services to the family. Weekly family counseling sessions occurred. Food vouchers were provided. An attempt was made to relocate the family.

While these interventions were in progress, Mrs.'s L.'s son was hospitalized for psychiatric reasons. Mrs. L. became overwhelmed attempting to care for her granddaughters and requested psychiatric admission. After sitting in a hospital emergency room for three hours without being seen, Mrs. L. left the hospital to stay with her daughter. At Mrs. L.'s request, the OASIS case manager contacted DYFS, and Mrs. L.

relinquished her custodial responsibilities for her grandchildren. Mrs. L. left her home, which was by then days away from being padlocked following foreclosure by the bank, and moved in with her daughter. The OASIS case manager supported Mrs. L.'s decision. The HIV case manager continued to work with Mrs. L.'s son. DYFS remained involved in attempts to stabilize the living situation for her granddaughters.

Practice and Policy Issues in Case Management

These three case scenarios are but a small sampling of the myriad issues older adult caregivers served by the OASIS Project face. Caregivers frequently lacked the time for their own health needs and found it difficult to negotiate complicated service and entitlement bureaucracies. Many were living at or below the poverty line and others struggled on limited, fixed incomes. Those who felt isolated from family, friends, and traditional community supports, by the real or anticipated stigma of AIDS, were at risk of depression and self-neglect. These risks to their own well-being have implications not only for their health and independence as they age but also for their capacity to continue as the children's and adolescents' primary caregivers.

The functions of case management included assessment not only of the individual's or family's needs but also of their abilities, resources, and support systems. Assessment is a process that helps clients define their situations. Cowger (1994) emphasizes that "how clients define difficult situations and how they evaluate and give meaning to the dynamic factors related to those situations set the context and content for the duration of the helping relationship." This is important to note because the majority of the older adult caregivers served by the OASIS Project felt strongly that caring for their grandchildren took priority in their lives. It was not considered a burden, although at times it was acknowledged to be a challenge. It was a duty born out of love and family responsibility. To approach assessment from a deficit perspective would not have been beneficial for the client and may, in fact, have alienated clients who already had difficulty accepting services.

The development of the comprehensive care plan is based on this assessment. The plan includes a contract, a formal or informal partnership agreement, as to what the case manager will do and what the client will do. Moore (1990) presents a model that delineates, and a case management grid that illustrates, the relationship between "two basic dimensions of case management: enabling and facilitating" in order to maximize the potential of the individual or family and the capability of the external resources to meet the needs of the individual or family. The complexity of the case would determine the level of case management involvement. The goal of the case-management model as put forth by Moore (1990:445) "is to contribute to the achievement of a balance between individuals' capabilities and their resources."

When the client and case manager agree on a care plan, the next step is to implement it. This includes identifying resources, linking the client to services, and advocating for the elimination of barriers that may prevent a client from receiving services.

Identifying resources is frequently not given the attention it needs. Resource directories are often outdated before they are printed. Services are constantly changing. It is imperative that the case manager not only continually update resource files but also have community contacts that can be called on, network at every possible opportunity, attend meetings and community functions, and even use the Internet. Case management cannot be done behind a desk. No case manager should ever tell a client a service does not exist until a number of reliable sources have confirmed there is no such service. When that happens, the case manager's role of advocate needs to expand from client advocacy to systems advocacy, especially if this is an unmet need faced by a number of people.

In the case of Mrs. R., language was an obvious barrier for her in obtaining assistance. The impending death of her son and her need to be with him were, however, Mrs. R.'s priority. The OASIS case manager therefore took the lead in helping Mrs. R. resolve the legal and social service issues that required intervention. In attempting to resolve the heating issue, the case manager discovered that the building had been sold. Ownership and responsibility for the broken heating unit was unclear. After days of hitting dead ends, political pressure was finally brought to bear that resulted in a temporary solution until the responsible party could be identified.

When the comprehensive care plan has been developed and has begun to be implemented, it is vital that continued follow up occurs to assess whether the plan is working or whether other events have occurred that require a change in the plan.

The plan to refer Mrs. L. to medical day care for respite did not work. Simultaneously, another crisis escalated in the family. Mrs. L.'s safety became the main concern. With the support of the OASIS case manager, Mrs. L. realized that her home situation was out of control. She requested that DYFS remove her granddaughters. She left her home, which was by then in serious disrepair and later condemned, and moved in with her daughter. For the first time, this woman, who had been battered for years by an alcoholic husband before his death and who then lived in fear of her son and granddaughters, had some peace.

Sometimes, despite the best interventions, families are so dysfunctional and destructive to each other that the best plan is for the family members to separate. There were at least six social service, mental health, and state agencies involved in an attempt to stabilize Mrs. L.'s family. Weekly case conferencing between the agencies and family set goals, coordinated responsibilities, reviewed progress, and most often identified more problems. No one, including Mrs. L., could control the effects of the substance abuse that had permeated this family. The OASIS case manager was able to help Mrs. L. recognize this and to support her as she worked through her guilt about not being able to care for her family. The case manager, in effect, gave Mrs. L. the permission she needed to leave.

Mrs. L.'s son was subsequently committed to a long-term psychiatric hospitalization. There he finally detoxed from drugs completely for the first time since he was age eight, when he had begun drinking and smoking marijuana with his father. Today he is doing well. DYFS placed one of Mrs. L.'s granddaughters in a distant relative's home, and she returned to school. The other granddaughter moved in with her boyfriend and became pregnant. Mrs. L. continues to live with her daughter and has reestablished relationships with her son and granddaughters.

Case Manager as Counselor

Frequently overlooked in the literature is the case manager's role as counselor. The functions of case management related to assessment and linkages to service are what are most typically emphasized. In fact, in developing the OASIS Project, the initial focus was on the concrete services needed by the families that would be served. The supportive counseling component, which became the most utilized and valued aspect of the project, had been greatly underestimated.

Rothman (1991) defines counseling as "not highly intrapsychic" and involving "problem solving, reality testing, socialization skills, and practical help." He also distinguishes the difference between long-term therapy with a focus on "deep-seated personality problems" and short-term therapy with a focus on "immediate living problems" (Rothman 1991). Soares and Rose (1994:145) acknowledge that even experienced, competent social workers "deny or devalue the clinical aspects of what they do" when they are in a case-management role, despite the fact that frequently they are providing "enormously effective clinical interventions."

Because the key to any therapeutic intervention is the relationship, it seems obvious that a case manager is ideally positioned to provide counseling. As Soares and Rose (1994) point out, the case manager typically begins his or her work during a crisis, usually around concrete issues. The relationship develops around the concrete issue and service. Trust and a supportive relationship develop, and gradually the clients begin to discuss their feelings.

This was the experience of the OASIS case manager. By entering the relationship as a helper in accessing needed concrete services, she was less threatening to the families. As a trusting relationship developed, older adults, who would have never accessed the mental health system, readily spoke with the OASIS case manager about issues such as grief, loss, fears, and anxieties. These discussions occurred over coffee, on the phone, in the office or in their home. The location did not matter. Neither did the time. Some conversations lasted for five minutes—enough for the client to know that the case manager was there for him or her. Some conversations lasted for hours, as the hurt of a lifetime was poured out to a trusted "friend." The fact that these were not structured therapy sessions did not make them any less therapeutic. It was what made the "therapy" possible.

Issues in Developing a Case Management

HIV is a family disease. It affects not just those diagnosed with HIV, but all family members whose lives are irrevocably altered because of HIV. Unfortunately, the social service delivery system and public funding of HIV care does not support this concept.

Ryan White CARE Act funds can only be used for the benefit of the person living with HIV disease. The only time that CARE Act funding can be used for an "affected" family member is to assist the "affected" member in becoming a better caregiver to the family member with HIV. Similarly, the Housing Opportunities for People with AIDS (HOPWA) Program, funded under the Department of Housing and Urban Development, provides housing assistance only to families that include a person living with HIV disease.

When that family member dies, families typically have until the end of the lease or six months to move or to find a way to pay the rent they were unable to pay when the family member with HIV disease was alive. So, at a time when a family is grieving the loss of a loved one, they must also face the potential loss of their home.

In defense of the CARE Act and HOPWA, the legislation that created these programs was emergency legislation to authorize federal funding to assist states and local communities in meeting the crisis created by the HIV epidemic. Neither program was developed to support people with HIV disease or their families permanently. What HIV has done, however, is expose the inadequacies of our social service system and public policies. HIV has demonstrated how economically fragile many families are when a catastrophic illness invades their homes. Because it is not likely that there will be major health and social service reforms that will address these needs in the very near future, it is vital that opportunities to maximize limited resources are sought. This may include seeking private funds to support demonstration programs and forging alliances across funding streams.

The OASIS Project was successful because it was created and implemented with the support of an entire coalition of service providers who saw the need and wanted to do something to meet the need. Turf issues were pushed aside in the interest of the mission and providers offered what they could to accomplish the common goal. The OASIS case manager's community outreach during the program development phase was essential to strengthening the service base as well as developing referral sources.

Through these outreach efforts, the mental health department of a large teaching hospital provided a Spanish-speaking clinician to run a support group in Spanish. An area hospice provided a clinician to run an English-speaking support group. A transportation provider provided transportation assistance. A legal services agency provided guidance and an attorney when necessary to address legal needs such as powers of attorney, custody issues, advanced directives, and even a divorce.

Outside the Coalition network, project outreach and community education extended the service base to include respite/baby-sitting, art therapy for bereaved children, and donations of food and holiday gifts. Organizations providing these services included a county office on aging, a senior services program, childcare programs, churches, and a local university. Even a local restaurant got involved and provided food for funeral repasts.

An additional gain from community outreach was the greater awareness by community agencies of HIV/AIDS and its impact on older adults. Presentations were given at offices on aging, community centers, nutrition sites, geriatric assessment programs, hospice programs, mental health agencies, senior membership programs, churches, and synagogues. Some of these programs had turned down requests in the past to discuss HIV. Now they welcomed the discussion on older adults as caregivers. In doing so, they learned something about HIV. And those in the HIV field began to learn more about aging.

Several important issues in client recruitment and referral were identified by the OASIS Project. First, given the nature of HIV disease, agency staff serving families where the adult child or grandchild is living with HIV/AIDS are often focused on that individual and less likely to give attention to the needs of the older caregiver. Second, HIV/AIDS programs may lack experience working with older adults. Skill development in assessment and engagement may be required. Third, HIV/AIDS-related stigma made it especially difficult for more middle-class and suburban families to be recruited by the program. Service agencies, including hospitals, home care, and senior programs in more suburban areas often believe that HIV/AIDS does not affect families or older adults in their area. Isolation of suburban grandparents raising grandchildren orphaned by HIV/AIDS was a key outreach issue identified by the project.

Older adults raising children orphaned by HIV/AIDS have been overlooked by both the aging and HIV service systems. In serving this neglected population, the OASIS Project identified several client-related service delivery issues. Families affected by HIV, including the caregivers to AIDS orphans, are often isolated from community resources. Caregivers may be reluctant to seek and accept services for themselves, fearing or dreading another agency intrusion into an already distressed household. Some caregivers believe that seeking help, even admitting to a medical problem, demonstrates that one may be unfit as a surrogate parent. Some grandparents are fearful that DYFS will "discover" them and snatch the children away. Other caregivers have internalized the shame and stigma of HIV and continue to maintain the secrecy rather than disclose a diagnosis that can cause social ostracism and rejection. As noted in the case of Mrs. W., acceptance of services can also mean accepting the reality of death. Isolation is also associated with the overwhelming tasks involved in managing HIV treatment regimens, side effects, medical appointments, negotiating the social service system, and coping with the emotional distress of death and loss. Client recruitment required persistent and sensitive outreach to a broad range of agencies in order to encourage referral of potential clients and encourage caregivers to use the OASIS Project.

Additional frustrations arose in service providers who wanted to refer older adult caregivers, but because the parent had not disclosed their HIV status, assistance from a program geared only to caregivers of children affected by HIV was not possible. This raised the question as to whether a project such as this belongs in an HIV service agency. In one instance, the mother living with HIV disease actually wanted the OASIS case manager to tell her parents of her status because she did not feel able to do so. This mother knew she was nearing her death and wanted her parents to have the assistance being offered by OASIS. This was not, however, a common occurrence. Because strict confidentiality laws apply to disclosure of HIV status that extend to after death, a number of families in need of services could not be served.

Systemic Barriers

Although the case-management model piloted in the OASIS Project was successful, project implementation identified unmet needs that were beyond the scope of the project. These unmet needs call for advocacy initiatives to address the policy issues. Many older relative caregivers and uninfected children lacked health insurance. Some uninsured caregivers were no longer employed or otherwise had no job-related health insurance because they worked part-time or spousal coverage did not extend to them. Their income did not allow them to afford private or dependent group insurance, but it prevented them from meeting the eligibility requirements for Medicaid. Many of the grandparents were not yet sixty-five, and so were ineligible for Medicare.

As new treatments continue to extend the length and quality of life, those living with HIV disease are not always in a state of catastrophic illness. With greater chronicity of the disease, there has been a narrowing of the definition of "medical need" for publicly funded home care. This in turn limits the availability of support services that can assist caregivers. Tighter restrictions allow fewer hours of home care, thereby reducing the in-home assistance that give caregivers some respite and the household greater stability.

The lack of adequate childcare, especially after-school programs, summer programs, and programs for adolescents, was a major concern of caregivers.

When an already overburdened grandmother, raising four young grandchildren under the age of eight, approached her local school district for an afterschool program for one of the school-aged children, she was advised that for the child to be accepted she would need to volunteer her time to the program. In addition to the lack of programs, school personnel need to become more sensitive to the issues of older relative caregivers.

Safe, affordable housing was a major concern for many of the caregivers. Some families coped with a lack of adequate space for new household members. Some feared eviction from public housing or senior housing because of regulations governing minors or number of tenants. Others feared the safety of the neighborhood and of outdoor play areas.

Conclusion

Older adults raising children orphaned by HIV/AIDS have been overlooked by both the HIV/AIDS and the aging service delivery systems. In serving this neglected population, the OASIS Project tested a model of supportive services. The project demonstrated the value of case management as the core service component. Individual supportive counseling provided by the case manager was the project's most used and valued service.

The project also identified unmet service needs that extended beyond the OASIS service capacity. Long-term funding of supportive services is needed to reduce the risks to caregivers' own physical and emotional well-being. Public policy initiatives are called for to address broader service needs and service delivery issues, such as the lack of health insurance for caregivers and uninfected children, safe and affordable housing, continued denial that HIV/AIDS affects older individuals, and the financial needs of these caregivers and their families.

References

Abramowitz, S., N. Obten, and H. Cohen. 1998. Measuring case management for families with HIV. *Social Work in Health Care* 27 (3): 29–41.

Biegel, D. E., B. K. Shore, and E. Gordon. 1984. *Building Support Networks for the Elderly*. Beverly Hills, Calif.: Sage.

Burnette, D. 1999. Custodial grandparents in Latino families: Patterns of service use and predictors of unmet need. *Social Work* 44 (1): 22–34.

Cowger, C. D. 1994. Assessing client strengths: Clinical assessment for client empowerment. *Social Work* 39 (3): 262–268.

Emlet, C. A., J. L. Crabtree, V. A. Condon, and L. A. Treml. 1996. *In-Home Assessment of Older Adults.* Gaithersburg, Md.: Aspen Publishers.

Joslin, D., C. Mevi-Triano, and J. Berman. 1997. Grandparents raising children orphaned by HIV/AIDS: Health risks and service needs. Paper delivered at the Annual Scientific Meeting of the Gerontological Society of America, Cincinnati.

Jue, S., and C. D. Kain. 1989. Culturally sensitive AIDS counseling. In C. D. Kain, ed., *No Longer Immune: A Counselor's Guide to AIDS,* pp. 131–148. Alexandria, Va.: American Association for Counseling and Development.

Meyer, C. H., ed. 1986. *Social Work with the Aging.* Silver Spring, Md.: National Association of Social Workers.

Michaels, D., and C. Levine. 1992. Estimates of the number of motherless youth orphaned by AIDS in the United States. *Journal of the American Medical Association* 268:3456–3461.

Moore, S. T. 1990. A social work practice model of case management: The case management grid. *Social Work* 35 (5): 444–448.

Mullahy, C. M. 1995. *The Case Manager's Handbook.* Gaithersburg, Md.: Aspen Publishers.

Piette, J., J. A. Fleishman, V. Mor, and B. Thompson. 1992. The structure and process of AIDS case management. *Health and Social Work* 17 (1): 4756.

Poindexter, C. C., and N. L. Linsk. 1999. HIV-related stigma in a sample of HIV-affected older female African American caregivers. *Social Work* 44 (1): 46–61.

Roe, K. M., and M. Minkler. 1999. Grandparents raising grandchildren: Challenges and responses. *Generations* 22 (4): 25–32.

Rose, S., and V. Moore. 1995. Case management. In Richard L. Edwards et al., eds., *Encyclopedia of Social Work,* pp. 335–340. 19th ed. Washington, D.C.: NASW Press.

Rothman, J. 1991. A model of case management: Toward empirically based practice. *Social Work* 36 (6): 520–528.

Sierra Health Foundation. 1991. Challenges for the future coordinating HIV/AIDS care and services in the next decade. Report of the National Symposium on Case Management and HIV/AIDS, December 16 and 17, 1991.

Soares, H. H., and M. K. Rose. 1994. Clinical aspects of case management with the elderly. *Journal of Gerontological Social Work* 22 (3–4): 143–156.

Thorn, K. 1990. *Applying Medical Case Management: AIDS.* Canoga Park, Calif.: Thorn Publishing.

11

Caregivers and the Educational System

MATHILDA BRACEROS CATARINA

Sara R. called the community-based family therapy clinic to see if she and her family could get help because of her grandchildren's school-related problems. She had become familiar with the hospital's community services during her daughter's various HIV-related illnesses and, ultimately, during the final stages of her daughter's losing battle with AIDS. When her daughter died, the care of Sara's four grandchildren became her responsibility. The father of the children had died two years earlier in a drug-related fight. Sara had no other children and her few remaining elderly relatives lived down south.

When Sara, her spouse, and her four grandchildren came to the small therapy room, their presence overpowered the tiny surroundings. It was a cold winter evening and everyone was bundled up in scarves, sweaters, and coats. The two husky grandsons, ages fifteen and sixteen, crowded into a two-seated plastic couch, the thirteen-year old granddaughter took a single chair, and the grandparents sat on the couch with the three-year-old granddaughter.

The two young men declined an invitation to take off their heavy jackets, which increased the bulk of their presence. Neither the grandfather nor the grandsons made eye contact with the therapist, and the teen-aged girl glanced nervously around the room. However, the grandmother appeared to the therapist to be eager to begin. The baby remained the center of attention for much of the beginning of the session, with each grandparent taking turns trying to hold her or distract her from touching the few things in the room. Even the boys reacted to her. She was talkative and playful; enjoying the attention that she appeared quite used to.

The grandmother was well dressed and appeared to be the organizer and head of the household. She had worked for the same company for more than twenty years and had received another promotion in middle management a year earlier. She had been looking forward to retiring in two years. Her husband had retired a little more than a year ago.

Despite her neat and careful dress, her face was drawn and haggard. She looked as if she had not been sleeping well, an observation that she later confirmed. Although she looked very tired, she wanted to begin the session. Sara described herself as feeling as if she were at the end of her rope. She said she had been severely drained during the course of her daughter's terminal illness, and she described herself as feeling helpless and hopeless throughout her illness and its aftermath. Now she said that she felt chronically fatigued and depressed.

Sara stated that she did not know what to do about her grandchildren. The two boys would not talk about their mother to anyone, yet they were obviously troubled by her dying and by the cause of her death. They were morose, hostile, and uncommunicative. They were manifesting behavioral problems in school and their academic performance was suffering.

Sara felt that school counselors were unconcerned with the children's emotional distress from their mother's death. They had been assigned a counselor by the hospital's community services agency but had stopped attending counseling sessions. The boys were frequently truant, and when they did go to school they were often involved in fights. Their previously satisfactory grades were declining to the point that they were now failing, and they did not indicate any great degree of concern over this negative turn of events.

The teenage girl attended school regularly, but Sara described her as "in a daze most of the time." She had been diagnosed as learning disabled two years previously, but since her referral to special education, her attention and memory problems had gotten worse. Sara did not feel that an appropriate individualized educational plan had been developed, but she did not feel qualified to discuss these issues with the special education personnel or the school administrators. Although she was a manager in her own professional life, the professionals in the school intimidated her.

Sara said that the teachers, counselors, and administrators in the school were not particularly helpful. She complained that she had great difficulty getting to school for parent-teacher meetings. Going to school during school hours required that she take time off from work, which was very difficult for her to do. However, the school personnel were not at all flexible regarding times when they could meet. In addition, the teachers and guidance counselors seemed unable to coordinate their meeting times to enable her to deal with the issues of more than one of the grandchildren on a single trip to the school.

Sara did not feel that her children's needs were being addressed adequately by the school, and she felt that her issues as a surrogate parent were being ignored. Interactions with school personnel tended to be stressful, anxiety-provoking, and even humiliating. She felt that teachers and counselors were often condescending in their tone and dismissive in their attitude.

During subsequent sessions, in which the therapist met only with the grandparents, other unresolved family issues were brought out. Her husband was not the father of the daughter who had died. He and Sara had married when her daughter was in her teens. Sara's husband was very resentful of his new role as a caregiver to Sara's grandchildren, having looked forward to retirement after thirty-five years in a factory. Now that he was home all day he had assumed responsibility for much of the care of the three-year-old (whom he favored), as well as for the supervision of the three teenagers (whom he did not favor).

Whereas before he could look forward to fixing special dinners for his wife and spending quiet evenings together, the situation now was completely turned around. He had lost his dreams for his wife's impending retirement when they could travel a little and live a moderately comfortable life. Even worse, he felt guilty. He loved his wife and little Kyeisha, yet he hated the turn of events that changed his world.

Sara's dreams, too, were shattered. Not only did she lose her only child, but now she also had a very different future, not one of retirement, but rather one of raising her grandchildren under extremely trying economic and emotional circumstances. Sara feared that her health and stamina might not hold out.

To make matters worse, Kyeisha had recently been diagnosed as HIV-positive, and she had not yet told her husband and her other grandchildren. In addition to her immediate concerns of informing them, Sara was overwhelmed at the possibility that Kyeisha might become seriously ill. She dreaded the prospect of following her granddaughter through a terminal illness as she had her daughter. She was also apprehensive regarding the manner in which the news of Kyeisha's HIV-positive status might affect the child's relationships with her siblings and peers, how it could impact on the child's access to day care, and how it might ultimately impact on Kyeisha's own experience in school.

Sara's story illustrates some of the key issues that grandparents face when they become responsible for raising grandchildren. They may be physically exhausted, emotionally drained, and psychologically shattered. They may also be angry at their children, whose behaviors precipitated their assumption of the caregiving role. They may feel lonely and isolated, and often feel totally inadequate to play the role of advocate for their grandchildren in the school and community.

This chapter will focus on the educational system and older caregivers of HIV-affected and infected children and adolescents. After a brief review of the magnitude of custodial grandparenting and caregiver needs, the chapter will discuss the special problems of both infected and affected children being raised by grandparents including psychosocial needs related to grief, depression and anxiety, behavioral problems, and special educational issues. Responses by school staff and the educational system as a whole are discussed, with attention to current interventions and supportive programs.

Custodial Grandparents: Trends and Caregiver Needs

Fuller-Thomson, Minkler, and Driver (1997) noted that the 1990 census reported a dramatic increase of 44 percent in the number of children living with grandparents or other relatives. Approximately 5 percent of all American children under the age of eighteen were living in their grandparents' homes in that year, and in approximately one-third of these homes, neither parent was present. Based on data from the National Center for Health Statistics, Saluter (1996) estimated that nearly four million children under the age of eighteen were living with their grandparents, representing 5.4 percent of this age cohort. The trend was most pronounced among African American children, 13 percent of whom were living with grandparents. The proportions were lower among white children (3.9%) and Hispanic children (5.7%). Factors cited most often in connection with the most recent increases in the number of custodial grandparents are parental substance abuse, related child abuse and neglect, drug-related incarceration, and the impact of HIV/AIDS (Edwards 1998; Fuller-Thomson, Minkler, and Driver 1997; de Toledo and Brown 1995; Burton 1992).

With respect to the AIDS epidemic, women of childbearing age comprise the fastest growing group of HIV/AIDS infected individuals (Centers for Disease Control and Prevention 2000). Wodrich et al. (1999) argue that schools will have increasing responsibilities toward children and adolescents who are either HIV-positive themselves or have been directly impacted by AIDS through the loss of a parent. They suggest that these trends will manifest themselves in HIV-infected young children surviving and entering school as well as increased numbers of HIV-positive adolescents and young adults in the school and community. African American and Latino youth are overrepresented in this cohort.

These trends indicate the need for a greater working knowledge of the medical, psychoeducational and demographic implications of HIV/AIDS for school personnel. For example, children with HIV progress to symptomatic AIDS in less time than do adults, although this progression is not uniform. Other medical sequelae of HIV-positive status are discussed later in the chapter.

Another concern is that high-risk sexual behavior and drug use is placing middle-school children and adolescents at greater risk for HIV/AIDS (Centers for Disease Control and Prevention 2000). These youngsters were not exposed to the extensive educational campaigns of the 1980s and early 1990s. Because HIV/AIDS can have a very long incubation period, the effects may not show up for years, making the younger part of the cohort particularly vulnerable.

These trends suggest that the number of grandparents raising grandchildren is not likely to decline. They also suggest that educational intervention in the schools may play an important role in the reduction and prevention of HIV/AIDS.

Psychosocial and Developmental Needs of Grandchildren Being Raised by Their Grandparents

De Toledo and Brown (1995) suggest that "every case of grandparents raising grandchildren is somehow about loss . . . whether a parent is absent owing to death or drugs, these children suffer a profound sense of loss, abandonment, and rejection" (p. 74). They point out that children may manifest this grief in nightmares and confusion, but they may also manifest grief through anger. Moreover, as bad as the situation is where one or both parents have died, the situation where the parents are in and out of jail, rehabilitation, or the street is potentially worse, inasmuch as the child harbors the hope that they will return and/or get their act together, a hope that is periodically dashed.

These grandchildren need reassurance, nurturing, and consistency. They need their custodial grandparents to reassure them that they will not abandon them as well. This need may be problematic, for we have seen that the grandparents themselves may be resentful and needy. Furthermore, exhausted older grandparents may genuinely fear for their own health and may not be altogether convinced that they will live long enough to see their grandchildren achieve adulthood.

These grandchildren are characterized by a tendency to blame themselves for what has happened in the family, and because of this self-blame they may suffer from poor self-esteem. Their peer relations and support system are also negatively affected. They require support and encouragement from family members who are providing care, and they frequently are in need of professional counseling.

The specific psychosocial adjustment problems displayed by these grandchildren include sleeping problems, eating disorders, regressive infantile behavior, excessive clinging, angry acting-out behaviors, defiance, and school-related problems. These psychosocial needs directly and indirectly affect school and academic performance. Many youngsters displaying these adjustment problems become truant; they may find that they cannot deal with pressures of school while their issues of confusion and loss are their major concerns. If they do attend school, they often get into fights and perform poorly in the classroom. Grandparents report that discipline, particularly with their adolescent grandchildren, is a major problem. Given the emotional and behavioral problems manifested by these youngsters, it is no surprise that academic problems usually follow.

Pinson-Millburn et al. (1996) point out that grandchildren whose parents were involved with substance abuse are at increased risk for birth defects and fetal alcohol syndrome, which may be manifested ultimately in mental retardation or learning disabilities or even in such disorders as cerebral palsy. It is clear that these children have an elevated incidence of attention deficit disorder and attention deficit disorder with hyperactivity, and they are more likely than other children to be evaluated for special education. They are also more likely than other children to become substance abusers themselves and to demonstrate precocious and/or risky sexual behavior.

Grandchildren whose parents have been in and out of rehabilitation facilities and those who have been in and out of prison may experience shame and embarrassment among peers and family members alike. Members of the community and school and social service professionals may adopt stereotypical attitudes toward the children, assuming that they are the products of "bad seeds." These children may also suffer from post-traumatic stress as a result of witnessing violent family disputes, finding out that a parent has been injured or killed through violence, or seeing a parent being arrested by the police.

Special Needs of the Uninfected Child

Lewis (1995) describes a population of children whose needs are often unaddressed, those who are not infected with HIV/AIDS but who are nonetheless seriously affected by the consequences of the disease. These are children whose parents or siblings have died from the disease or are ill from HIV/AIDS. These children are exposed to major psychological risk factors—"stigma, secrecy, exposure to acute and chronic illness, death of parents and /or siblings, separations, losses, orphanhood, and foster home placements—all of which are often experienced in an environment of poverty, drugs, alcohol, violence, abuse, and prostitution" (Lewis 1995:50). He discusses the developmental tasks that children of various ages must accomplish and the unique risk factors that HIV/AIDS add to the picture. He also describes how the secrecy that often surrounds AIDS in a family often results in intense anxiety and anger, which may be expressed by depression and disruptive behaviors.

For children of HIV/AIDS-affected parents who are not themselves HIV-positive, there is still a strong likelihood of experiencing feelings of shame and embarrassment, due to the social stigma attached to the disease (Herek 1999). In addition, those outside the family will very likely not know whether a particular grandchild is HIV-positive or not. Thus grandchildren who are not HIV-positive may experience isolation for the same reasons as those who are HIV-positive.

Gomez, Haiken, and Lewis (1995) have suggested that children of HIV-affected parents can benefit greatly from peer support groups. These groups can help children and adolescents deal with grief and bereavement, feelings of shame and guilt, social stigma, and issues surrounding their own developing sexuality.

As Lewis (1995) says, it is imperative that "accurate information about AIDS and its prevention is provided to children in pedagogically sound ways, consistent with the child's cognitive stage of development and emotional state" (p. 62).

HIV-Infected Children

Infected children have an additional set of problems and special needs (see chapter 7). This situation requires a rigorous medical response, along with which come the concomitant time management and financial problems. Wodrich and his associates (1999) point out that children with HIV tend to progress to symptomatic AIDS in far less time than adults. Children exposed to the HIV virus in utero typically manifest the most problematic course, often expressing full-blown AIDS and debilitating encephalopathy that lead to death during the preschool years. Rutstein, Conlon, and Batshaw (1997) have pointed out that this poorer course for children infected in utero is the result of the immaturity of the fetal immune system.

Antiretroviral medication, including AZT taken by mothers during pregnancy, diminishes the rate of mother-to-child transmission and tends to improve the child's prognosis. Later exposure to the HIV virus, such as that which may occur during the birth process, may allow the baby's more mature immune system to ward off infection altogether. Moreover, if infection does occur at this time, there may be a long asymptomatic period before the symptoms of full-blown AIDS appear.

Nevertheless, several studies have pointed out that even in cases where AIDS does not develop immediately or at all, it is possible that HIV infection may be accompanied by subtle deficits in the central nervous system which may be associated with later learning and attention problems (Mayes et al. 1996; Landau, Pryor, and Haefli 1995; Colegrove and Huntzinger 1994).

It should be noted, however, that some of the learning problems that characterize HIV-positive students may not be the result of the HIV infection itself, but rather of related environmental factors. For example, Landau, and his associates (1995) point out that HIV-positive infants are more likely to have been exposed to deficient prenatal and postnatal care and a lack of social supports. These babies are also far more likely than other babies to have been exposed in utero to heroin, crack, cocaine, alcohol, and nicotine, any one of which could account for deficits in the infant's neurological development.

Although Landau et al. (1995) admit that although environmental factors may potentially confound etiological hypotheses, they indicate that the literature finds that HIV will impede the healthy development of the nervous system in pediatric cases and subsequently will negatively affect the attainment of motor, intellectual, and developmental milestones. Younger children tend to show deficits in language development and other major developmental phenomena, whereas older children tend to exhibit deterioration in cognitive functioning. Some young children regress and lose milestones previously attained.

Wodrich et al. (1999) state that children with HIV, even without signs of encephalopathy, show higher rates of expressive rather than receptive language problems. Those with encephalopathy, as demonstrated by CT scans, show even greater language deficits. In addition to verbal problems, they may demonstrate motor and emotional expression limitations. These motor problems may involve fine motor deficits as well as impairments of muscle tone or gross motor control affecting balance and gait. Whatever the etiology of the learning problems that characterize HIV-positive children, the prevalence and importance of these problems is such that Wodrich and his colleagues recommend that school psychologists should regularly assess these children to identify difficulties and assist in remedial and supportive planning.

In addition to the physical and neurological problems that frequently affect HIV-positive children, they also tend to encounter adverse social environments that may contribute to poor psychosocial adjustment. For example, HIV-positive children may encounter discrimination from those who have not learned or accepted the fact that AIDS is not spread through casual contact (Herek 1999). One manner in which such discrimination has been manifested is by denying the admission of HIV-positive children to public school. Ginzburg (1992) notes that such action is clearly illegal, but he also makes it clear that the stigma associated with AIDS can be a powerful force with which the legal system may sometimes be unable to cope.

The Right of HIV-Positive Children to an Education

Ginzburg (1992:134) notes that the due process clause of the Fourteenth Amendment to the Constitution guarantees all persons equal protection under the law. When a state establishes a public school system and requires that children within a specified age range attend school, then every child in that age range "has a constitutionally protected right to a public education."

In addition to this constitutional protection, two major pieces of federal legislation directly address the rights of children with handicapping conditions, including HIV infection, to attend school. The Education of the Handicapped Act of 1982 and its amendment, the Handicapped Children's Protection Act of 1986, require states to provide a free and appropriate education to handicapped children. Additionally, section 504 of the Rehabilitation Act of 1973 provides that no otherwise qualified individual should be excluded from participation in any program receiving federal financial assistance solely because of a handicap. The Supreme Court has ruled that individuals with contagious diseases are covered by section 504, arguing that the purpose of the act was to ensure that handicapped individuals are not denied an education (or employment) because of the prejudice or ignorance of others.

Unfortunately, the prejudice or ignorance of others can be extremely powerful. Ginzburg (1992) notes that the presence of HIV-positive children in schools "has been associated with concern, frustration, anger, and violence in the local populations" (p. 133). Ginzburg relates the stories surrounding several landmark court cases concerned with the right of HIV-positive children to an appropriate education. For example, the Ray brothers were hemophiliacs who were HIV-positive but asymptomatic. In 1986, when their family voluntarily informed the school board in Arcadia, Florida, of their HIV infection, the school removed the three brothers (and their HIV-negative sister) from the classroom and began home instruction. The family responded by moving to Alabama and enrolling the children in school there. However, when the school authorities in the new Alabama town learned of their HIV-positive status, the boys were also removed from the classroom in the new school district.

This prompted the family to return to Arcadia, where they obtained health department certificates indicating that the boys were able to attend school. However, the school again refused them admission. When the case came to court, the judge first permitted a "separate but equal full-time, isolated instruction" at home (Ginzburg 1992:138), but then she granted an injunction to the school ordering that the school return the children to an integrated classroom setting. In her ruling the judge cited signs of psychopathology in the boys that were directly attributable to the stress of being excluded from the classroom, and she reasoned that the actual ongoing injury to the brothers outweighed the potential harm to others. She recognized the concern and fear of the community, but she also noted that the court could not allow itself to be influenced by community fear, parental pressure, or the threat of additional lawsuits. Her ruling further ordered the school district to provide educational programs for local parents and their children regarding the realities HIV infection and the modes of transmission of the disease.

Unfortunately, the court's ruling did not have the desired effect. When the brothers began to attend classes, many parents boycotted the school. Numerous threats of physical violence were directed toward the family. Finally, the Ray family home was burned to the ground. The family was forced to leave the community once again, this time settling in a different county in Florida, where the boys were able to enroll in school without the benefit of a court order. In Arcadia, the school board hired an AIDS consultant to educate the community about AIDS and HIV infection. However, the community refused to attend the lecture.

Regrettably, the problems of ignorance and prejudice may manifest themselves not just with respect to the public, but with respect to school personnel as well. Many schools have not provided adequate in-service education in this area, and attitudes regarding HIV/AIDS may be particularly difficult to change.

Herek and Glunt (1988) suggest the existence of two parallel epidemics, one of HIV infection and one of the resultant stigma. After the Atascadero, California, school board voted to exclude Ryan Thomas, an HIV-infected kindergartner, from school, the federal government (Thomas v. Atascadero Unified School District 1987) extended the definition of disabilities in the 1973 Rehabilitation Act to cover individuals with AIDS symptoms as well as those who were asymptomatic and HIV-positive (Pyle 1992).

Landau et al. (1995) describe confidentiality and the right of privacy as one of the most daunting issues for school officials. The CDE guidelines (1985) urge all school personnel to exercise sensitivity to confidentiality and privacy needs. The Education for All Handicapped Children Act (EHA, 1975), Individuals with Disabilities Act (IDEA, 1991) and the Family Education Rights and Privacy Act (FERPA) further protect families and children's rights to confidentiality and privacy. Katisiyannis (1992) found that, in addition, all of the states that he surveyed had policies on disclosure of HIV status for school children. Disclosure continues to be a difficult decision for families to make. The Agency for Health Care Policy and Research (1994) sees positive benefits of disclosing students' HIV status in the family, such as having greater access to entitlement resources.

Disclosure also allows for greater social support. Wodrich et al. (1999) see the teachers of HIV-positive students as important members of the assessment and monitoring team working with the school psychologist. Because teachers see children on a daily basis, they can detect changes in behavior and motor skills and learning problems before they are apparent in medical and psychological tests. They can also inform caregivers when illnesses are circulating the classroom so that children with suppressed immune systems can be kept home. Currently teachers are not informed if a child is HIV-positive.

However, disclosure has serious possible negative effects such as housing discrimination, loss of employment or child custody, a reduction or cessation of health benefits, and social ostracism (Agency for Health Care Policy and Research 1994), all of which can impact the HIV/AIDS-infected or affected child.

Although many sophisticated school policies are in place, in reality, many problems still exist regarding confidentiality. According to Pyle (1992), the most likely source of a breach of confidentiality lies with the child, parent, or other caregiver. In some instance, acts of violence have been committed to prevent children with HIV/AIDS from attending school (Landau et al. 1995). Researchers (Wodrich et al. 1999; Schmitt and Schmitt 1990) see the school as the most likely place to educate children and their parents about HIV/

AIDS and prepare them for dealing with HIV-infected individuals realistically and humanely.

Proactive school-based curricular interventions need to be designed and implemented. These programs would address differing needs, cognitive development, and experiences. Britton, de Mauro, and Gambrell (1992) found that all fifty states mandate or recommend AIDS education programs in the school. Although most programs reflect sexuality education for students who have reached the age of potential sexual activity, the curriculum design may not have been timed to address those at higher risk. For example, Holtzman et al. (1992) found that although 82.3 percent of surveyed districts provided HIV education to seventh graders, only 37.3 percent of twelfth-grade students were receiving this curriculum. AIDS education programs have been declining, overshadowed in part, by greater focus on academic issues of standards and assessment.

Caregiver Needs and Implications

Pinson-Millburn et al. (1996) emphasize the diversity of the population of grandparents raising their grandchildren. They observe that "some grandparents are 40 years old, others 50, some 80. . . . There is no single age that represents grandparents" (p. 549). Similarly, there is no single pattern of household arrangements. More than one million households are headed by a single grandparent, and in these households the median income is $18,000 a year.

Some grandparents have legal custody of their grandchildren, while others have no legal rights. Where the grandparents are not the legal guardians of the children, they often experience difficulties getting their grandchildren registered for school and activities within the community. Some schools do not routinely invite grandparents who do not have legal custody to parent-teacher conferences, and some schools will not disclose confidential information to grandparents regarding their grandchildren. When grandparents are not legal guardians, they often experience substantial anxiety regarding the prospect that their grandchildren's parents will undermine their efforts to help the grandchildren, or even take the grandchildren away. When the parents are not in the picture, grandparents may worry that the courts will take the grandchildren from them. In some cases caregiving for grandchildren lasts until the children become adults, while in other households the caregiving is temporary and/ or intermittent.

According to Pinson-Millburn et al. (1996), assuming the parenting role "changes everything about the grandparents' lives: leisure, friendships, work, health, and finances" (p. 549). The grandparents frequently feel that they have been cheated out of their most cherished aspirations, and on top of this they may blame themselves for what has happened. They no longer share activities with their age peers. Grandparents who used senior centers for recreation and support no longer attend senior center functions because they no longer have sufficient free time. In some instances, they feel that they no longer have anything in common with their peers or are embarrassed by their new circumstances. They are at risk of impaired psychosocial functioning themselves, and the resentment they may feel toward both their children and toward the grandchildren for whom they must care places the grandchildren at risk for adjustment problems as well. Many custodial grandparents express a need for help with discipline issues. The "rules" for raising children often are different from those of a generation ago. Some report that as the children grow, so do their discipline problems. In fact, a number of grandparents have requested classes on discipline.

Clearly, these grandparents have a need for contact with peers in support groups with whom they can share their anxieties and fears. They also have a need for access to adequate mental health services, should stresses reach the point, as they did with Sara, where depression sets in. It is important to realize that grandparents' physical health needs may reduce their stamina for active interaction and household chores. Fully one-third report observable declines in their personal health (Minkler, Roe, and Price 1992). In addition, anxiety, depression, and isolation affect not only their own well-being but also their ability to provide an adequate psychosocial environment for their grandchildren.

Those grandparents who lack legal guardianship of their grandchildren are also in need of legal advice and representation. They need to know what their rights are with respect to the children, and they may need help in securing legal guardianship.

Dealing with the educational system on behalf of their grandchildren is likely to be a particularly problematic area for grandparents who provide care to their grandchildren. Like Sara, such grandparents may not feel qualified to discuss their grandchildren's academic program or progress with teachers. They may feel that time has passed them by and that they are out of the loop. Like Sara, they may feel embarrassed or even threatened by school personnel who are not particularly helpful and who speak unintelligible technical jargon while providing little effort to explain. It is also possible that the frustrations grandparents experience in dealing with school personnel contribute to increased disharmony in their interactions with grandchildren at home.

These grandparents may need counseling to develop assertiveness and advocacy skills. It goes without saying that these grandparents would benefit greatly from school-based outreach programs and from programs aimed at increasing the sensitivity and communication skills of educational professionals.

One can see that caregiver and grandchildren needs interact and can result in negative implications for both. The caregivers may have increased problems with disciplining their grandchildren. Their own anxiety, lack of energy, and, sometimes, lack of educational skills may make them unable to help with homework and attend school meetings and activities. In turn, the negative psychosocial environment resulting from caregivers' unmet needs and support contributes to increased stress and emotional problems for the youngsters.

Programmatic Responses

The school-related needs of custodial grandparents demand a vigorous response from the educational system. This response includes creating an awareness of the nature of the grandparent caregivers' needs, why schools should and can respond and developing and testing programmatic interventions.

Professional Awareness of Caregivers' Needs

Recent articles in professional journals addressed to educators and policy makers have documented custodial grandparent needs and recommended responses by school systems. Because society and schools have changed markedly since grandparents first performed the parenting role, Schwartz (1994) recommends that schools develop special procedures for involving grandparents and explaining critical educational issues in terms that older individuals can easily understand.

In her study of black grandparents raising the children of drug-addicted parents, Burton (1992) notes the frustration of a sixty-eight-year-old grandfather trying to help his granddaughter with her homework: "I don't know nothing about this new arithmetic. I can't help her at all. I am too embarrassed to go to her teacher and tell her that I can't help" (p. 749). Burton calls for schools to provide tutorial assistance to children whose grandparents are overwhelmed, including outreach programs to overcome the type of embarrassment mentioned by this grandparent.

Also addressing the intergenerational differences that custodial grandparents confront in contemporary schools, Strom et al. (1996) recommend that schools institute grandparent classes to make grandparents "aware of changes in schools, the difficulties students experience, and ways families can cooperate with teachers to facilitate academic achievement" (p. 129). Also recommended are grandparent education councils to identify ways in which custodial grandparent needs can be addressed. Including both grandparents and educators, these councils help to bridge the gap between the two groups.

School policy changes are needed to reflect the role of custodial grandparents by recognizing the importance of including them in the school process and culture and by becoming more aware that their needs may differ from the traditional parent figure. Providing for these needs and differences create a more positive situation for all concerned.

Rothenberg (1996) and Morrow-Kondos et al. (1997) recommend that schools alter regulations regarding enrollment and the disclosure of confidential information to accommodate grandparents who are raising grandchildren but are not actually legal guardians. Rothenberg (1996) also recommends that school administrations notify grandparents raising HIV-infected children of childhood illness epidemics so that children with weakened immune systems might be kept home at grandparental discretion.

Rothenberg (1996) suggests that schools maintain a store of helpful information that can be made available for grandparents, including information on parenting the second time around and information on support groups and grandparenting classes that may be available in the community. She further advises school administrators to provide before- and after-school activities for students to provide grandparents with short-term respite. She also suggests that school policy should support appropriate referrals for educational, health, and social services and proposes "family-friendly" strategies to encourage surrogate parents to take an active role in their grandchildren's education. These include the use of inclusive language on home-school communications, including the use of such salutations such as "Dear Parent/ Guardian," as opposed to simply "Dear Parent," scheduling extra time for grandparent-teacher conferences, letting grandparents know how to reach the teacher not just when there is a problem but at any time, and encouraging grandparents to volunteer at school to become more comfortable with the system.

Edwards (1998) criticizes schools for not recognizing that grandparent-raised children tend to display learning and behavior problems in school. He argues that nonparental caregivers and teachers tend not to communicate well with each other. Caregivers assume that their grandchildren are behaving appropriately in school, but the teachers consider the children to be behavior problems. Edwards suggests that schools take steps to improve communication between school personnel and custodial grandparents. Edwards also suggests that school personnel frequently manifest negative attitudes toward children being raised by grandparents, including the belief that these children take up too much of their time.

Pinson-Milburn and associates (1996) recommend that schools (1) provide training and development to all school personnel on the issues facing grandparent households, (2) conduct awareness training for counselors and teachers to assist them in working with grandparent families in school conferences, (3) conduct a schoolwide assessment to determine the number of grandparent-headed families and needs, (4) conduct school-based support groups, (5) support teachers who are having classroom difficulties with children raised by grandparents, and (6) promote a schoolwide inclusion policy by having teachers seek out grandparent custodians to involve them in school activities.

Wodrich et al. (1999) argue that school psychologists must become sensitive to the issues associated with HIV as a chronic illness, such as school absenteeism and adjustment to medication regimens, the prospect of encephalopathy as the disease progresses, and HIV stigma and social ostracism. School psychologists should also educate teachers with respect to the particular problems faced by HIV-positive students, such as addressing "the educational and psychosocial stressors experienced by the infected child" (p. 234). "Appropriate and accurate education about HIV/AIDS and related issues in the schools" (p. 236) is needed to decrease or halt the spread of the disease and to reduce discrimination against and increase understanding of children with HIV/AIDS.

Educators at the high school level should acknowledge the need for supportive school-based interventions for grandparents of older children where issues of autonomy and rebellion and high-risk behaviors are more likely pronounced. Upper levels of school tend to be less supportive of families, which are viewed as irrelevant except when there are problems. Grandparents raising older children especially need informed, sensitive, and trained staff that can also identify psychosocial problems, find community resources, and make referrals.

Jones and Kennedy (1996) describe Project GUIDE (Grandparents United: Intergenerational Developmental Education). This is a comprehensive service program administered by the Neighborhood Service Organization (NSO), a Detroit social service agency. This program was designed to reduce caregiving stress among grandparents by assessing the grandparents' needs, providing individual and family counseling, reducing social isolation, enhancing the life skills of both the grandparents and the grandchildren, helping to meet basic human needs such as food and clothing, assisting grandparents seeking custody of their grandchildren, educating family members about substance abuse, and stimulating positive communication between grandparents and grandchildren. Nowhere in this article is there any mention of the problems that grandparents may encounter in dealing with schools, and nowhere is there any reference to any actions that might be taken by schools to help these families.

Taylor-Brown et al. (1998) describe a program in Rochester, New York, to provide children who have lost a parent to AIDS with case-management services, mental-health services, medical care, child-welfare services, and legal services. This article similarly contains no reference to the schools.

Program Interventions

Several interventions aimed at meeting the school-related needs of custodial grandparents are found in the literature. Gross (2000) describes a program created and taught by Carole Cox, a professor of social work at Fordham University, which acts as an adjunct to support groups for grandmothers. Working with a handpicked group of grandmothers, she teaches them skills to help raise their grandchildren. They, in turn, will go out to help other grandparents in the community. The curriculum is rigorous, and the grandmothers are discouraged from using the time as gripe sessions (they can do that in a separate support group). At each session a topic such as behavior problems, grief, sex, social services, legal issues, or advocacy skills is discussed. They learn to cope with grandchildren at different age levels and to differentiate between discipline and punishment. They learn skills of persistence and assertiveness to deal with various agencies. They learn how to deal more efficiently with politicians and bureaucracy. The goal is to empower them to cope with their problems and to become peer educators.

Strom, Beckert, and Strom (1996) developed the "Becoming a Better Grandparent" course. This course consists of twelve weekly one-hour lessons centering on "ways to keep up with the times, how to give and seek advice, acquiring group process communication skills, and respecting the individuality of family members" (p. 641). The course was evaluated with a group of twenty-nine grandparents (who participated along with twenty-nine grandchildren and twenty-nine of the grandchildren's parents). The course took place at a church, but it could be conducted in other settings as well.

Before and after the course, the grandparents completed the Grandparent Strengths and Needs Inventory (GSNI) (Strom and Strom 1993), a sixty-item test that measures six dimensions: (1) satisfaction with the grandparent role, (2) success in performing the grandparent role, (3) guidance and reinforcement of goals, (4) difficulties encountered in trying to fulfill obligations to the family, (5) frustration with the behaviors of their grandchildren, and (6) information required to understand the grandchild as an individual. Study results indicated that the grandparents' scores rose significantly from pretreatment to posttreatment on four of the six GSNI subscales: satisfaction, success, providing guidance and information.

Grant, Gordon, and Cohen (1997) describe a school-based program to provide medical care, mental-health services, and social services to custodial grandparents and their grandchildren in East Harlem. The program was used by twenty-three grandparent-headed families. The participants demonstrated a willingness to use the medical care provided by the program despite the fact that their prior use of medical services had been very low. The participants also took advantage of counseling and legal services. Social workers helped several families obtain appropriate special education classifications for grandchildren. Several other grandparents were assisted in their efforts to become the legal guardians of their grandchildren. Still other families received referrals for daycare. The authors did not conduct a formal pretreatment to posttreatment evaluation study, but their descriptions strongly suggest that the school-based program was at least well used.

A school-based, psychoeducational, small-group intervention was reported by Burnette (1998). Participants were ten African American grandmothers and one Latino grandfather whose grandchildren were attending a public elementary school in Brooklyn. About one-third of these grandchildren had special physical, social, emotional, and/or educational needs. The intervention consisted of eight weekly ninety-minute sessions led by a school-based social work practitioner and the study investigator. Each session began with a half-hour presentation of a specific topic followed by an hour of discussion. Topics presented included issues facing grandparents raising children, social supports, stress and coping, interpersonal family issues, parenting skills, legal and social services, and community-based initiatives. Interestingly, advocating for grandchildren in the school was not included as a specific topic.

During the hour-long group discussions, members focused on such issues as their sense of stigma, feelings of isolation, concerns for the future of their grandchildren, and their feelings of guilt and anger regarding their children, most of whom were struggling with drug addiction or HIV/AIDS.

Pretreatment and post-treatment measures indicated that participants' scores on depression decreased significantly over the course of the intervention, as did coping via distancing. Problem-solving and coping through seeking social support increased significantly. Burnette (1998) interprets the results of the study as indicating that "small groups offer a promising means to educate grandparent caregivers about the availability and accessibility of much-needed services to support this demanding, "off-time" parental role" (p. 25). She also suggests that "because grandparents tend to be in contact with child-related institutions such as schools and pediatric health care providers . . . these normative social settings may be natural places to offer support groups" (p. 25).

The Grandfamily School Support Network (GSSN), provides "a structured social and academic support system for grandfamilies" (Edwards 1998:178) that begins when the school's registrar notifies a member of the student services staff that a "grandkin" has entered the school. The school psychologist or school counselor makes contact with the grandparent(s) and teacher to determine if there is a need for services at school or at home. A classmate serves as a "peer partner" to grandchildren, helping the child adjust to school and serving as a peer tutor and "homework buddy." A teacher, paraprofessional, or other student staff member serves as a surrogate parent on site. The GSSN also provides group counseling and grandparent effectiveness training for caregivers.

Summary and Recommendations

There are large numbers of grandparents in this nation who are raising their grandchildren, and who experience particular stresses associated with the school system in this role.

Priority should be given to continued efforts to determine the needs of custodial grandparents, and efforts should now be directed toward influencing policy makers to provide funding for grandparent support and education programs. It appears that such programs can appropriately be linked with existing community organizations, including churches. The use of such existing organizations may help to overcome any reluctance that grandparents may feel regarding the prospect of interacting with professionals in medical, mental health, or school settings. However, the school-based pilot program described by Grant and his associates (1997) indicates clearly that, with proper sensitivity and planning, professional venues may also be employed effectively.

An additional recommendation would be to increase the frequency and intensity of in-service education for professionals, particularly in the schools. Recent informal focus groups of educators conducted by the author indicated that they had received little training regarding the needs of grandparents. They had received some training with respect to HIV-positive children in the schools. However, the group members indicated that even this training had diminished in recent years. Wodrich et al. (1999) offer a comprehensive school based program combining child-, teacher-, and system-centered services related to HIV/AIDS. They feel that school psychologists should take a proactive role in designing and implementing these services.

There are serious concerns that policy makers and educators have concluded that the AIDS epidemic has passed its peak (Centers for Disease Control and Prevention 2000). This idea has been fueled by new medical technologies that have reduced the number of individuals dying of AIDS, and by reports that safe sex education programs have been effective. What is less generally known is that the fastest-growing population of AIDS patients is women of childbearing age. Another group that is growing in numbers for greater than their representation in the population is gay and bisexual adolescents of color. They missed the intensive safe sex education of the late 1980s and early 1990s. Unfortunately, they are lulled by reports of new medications and are unaware that HIV-infected individuals who are on medication and symptom free are not necessarily risk-free for transmitting AIDS. It seems clear that the AIDS epidemic is not over among children and adolescents, and schools will continue to bear responsibility for meeting the needs of HIV-positive students and HIV-affected children.

References

Agency for Health Care Policy and Research. 1994. *Quick Reference Guide for Clinicians.* Washington, D.C.: CDC National Clearinghouse.

Anderson, V. 1998. HIV infection and children: A medical overview. *Child Welfare* 77 (2): 107–114.

Britton, P. O., D. de Mauro, and A. E. Gambrell. 1992. HIV/AIDS education: SIECUS study on HIV/AIDS education for school finds states make progress, but work remains. *SIECUS Research Report* 21:1–8.

Burnette, D. 1997. Grandparents raising grandchildren in the inner city. *Families in Society: The Journal of Contemporary Human Services* 72:489–499.

——. 1998. Grandparents rearing grandchildren: A school-based small group intervention. *Research on Social Work Practice* 8 (1): 10–27.

Burton, L. (1992). Black grandparents rearing children of drug-addicted parents: Stressors, outcomes, and social service needs. *The Gerontologist* 32 (6): 744–751.

Centers for Disease Control and Prevention. 1985. Education and foster care of children infected with HTLV-III/LAV. *Morbidity and Mortality Weekly Report* 34:517–521.

——. 1999. Status of prenatal HIV prevention: US declines continue. http:www.cdc.gov/hiv.

Colegrove, R. W., and R. M. Huntzinger. 1994. Academic, behavioral, and social adaptation of boys with hemophilia/HIV disease. *Journal of Pediatric Psychology* 19:457–473.

De Toledo, S., and E. E. Brown. 1995. *Grandparents as Parents: A Survival Guide for Raising a Second Family.* New York: Guilford Press.

Edwards, O. W. 1998. Helping grandkin—grandchildren raised by grandparents: Expanding psychology in the schools. *Psychology in the Schools* 35 (2): 173–180.

Fuller-Thomson, E., M. Minkler, and D. Driver. 1997. A profile of grandparents raising grandchildren in the United States. *The Gerontologist* 37 (3): 406–411.

Ginzburg, H. 1992. The right of an HIV-infected child to an education. In M. L. Stuber, ed., *Children and AIDS,* pp. 133–146. Washington, D.C.: American Psychiatric Press.

Gomez, K. A., H. J. Haiken, and S. Y. Lewis. 1995. Support groups for children with HIV/AIDS. In N. Boyd-Franklin, G. L. Steiner, and M. G. Boland, eds., *Children, Families, and HIV/AIDS: Psychosocial and Therapeutic Issues,* pp. 156–167. New York: Guilford Press.

Grant, R., S. G. Gordon, and S. T. Cohen. 1997. An innovative school-based intergenerational model to serve grandparent caregivers. In K. Brabazon and R. Disch, eds., *Intergenerational Approaches in Aging: Implications for Education, Policy and Practice,* pp. 47–61. New York: Haworth.

Gross, J. 2000. Childraising 201: A graduate course for grandparents. *New York Times,* March 8, 2000.

Herek, G. M. 1999. AIDS and stigma. *American Behavioral Scientist* 42 (7): 1106–1116.

Herek, G. M., and E. K. Glunt. 1988. An epidemic of stigma: Public reactions to AIDS. *American Psychologist* 43:886–891.

Holtzman, D., B. Z. Greene, G. C. Ingraham, L. A. Daily, D. G. Demchuk, and L. J. Kolbe. 1992. HIV education and health education in the United States: A national survey of local school district policies and practices. *Journal of School Health* 62:421–427.

Jacobson, S. 1993. Selling depression to the old folks. *Atlantic Monthly* (April): 46–51.

Jones, L., and J. Kennedy. 1996. Grandparents united: Intergenerational developmental education. *Child Welfare* 75 (5): 636–650.

Katisiyannis, A. 1992. Policy issues in school attendance: A national survey. *Journal of Special Education* 26:219–226.

Kelley, S. J. 1993. Caregiver stress in grandparents raising grandchildren. *IMAGE: Journal of Nursing Scholarship* 25 (4): 331–337.

Landau, S., J. B. Pryor, and K. Haefli. 1995. Pediatric HIV: School-based sequelae and curricular interventions for infection prevention and social acceptance. *School Psychology Review* 24 (2): 213–229.

Lewis, M. 1995. The special case of infected children. In S. Geballe, J. Gruendel, and W. Andiman, eds., *Forgotten Children of the AIDS Epidemic,* pp. 50–63. New Haven: Yale University Press.

Mayes, S. D., H. A. Handford, J. H. Schaefer, C. A. Scogno, S. R. Neagley, L. Michael-Good, and L. E. Pelco. 1996. The relationship of HIV status, type of coagulation disorder, and school absenteeism to cognition, educational performance, mood and behavior of boys with hemophilia. *Journal of Genetic Psychology* 157:137–151.

Minkler, M., and K. M. Roe. 1996. Grandparents as surrogate parents. *Generations* 22: 34–38.

Minkler, M., K. M. Roe, and M. Price. 1992. The physical and emotional health of grandmothers raising grandchildren in the crack cocaine epidemic. *The Gerontologist* 32:5752–5761.

Morrow-Kondos, D., J. A. Weber, K. Cooper, and J. Hesser. 1997. Becoming parents again: Grandparents raising grandchildren. In K. Brabazon and R. Disch, eds., *Intergenerational Approaches in Aging: Implications for Education, Policy and Practice,* pp. 35–46. New York: Haworth.

Pinson-Millburn, N. M., E. S. Fabian, N. K. Schlossberg, and M. Pyle. 1996. Grandparents raising grandchildren. *Journal of Counseling & Development* 74:548–554.

Pyle, C. R. 1992. AIDS and government responsibility and/or liability. Paper presented at the National College of District Attorneys, San Francisco.

Rothenberg, D. 1996. Grandparents as parents: A primer for schools. http://eric.ps.ed.uiuc.edu/eece/pubs/digests/1996.

Rutstein, R. M., C. J. Conlon, and M. L. Batshaw. 1997. HIV and AIDS: From mother to child. In M. L. Batshaw, ed., *Children with Disabilities,* pp. 163–181. 4th ed. Baltimore: Paul H. Brookes.

Saluter, A. 1996. *Marital Status and Living Arrangements, March 1994.* U.S. Bureau of the Census, Current Population Reports, Series P20-484. Washington, D.C: U.S. Government Printing Office.

Schmitt, T. M., and R. L. Schmitt. 1990. Constructing AIDS policy in the public schools: A multimethod case study. *Journal of Contemporary Ethnography* 19:295–321.

Schwartz, L. L. 1994. The challenge of raising one's nonbiological children. *The American Journal of Family Therapy* 22 (3): 195–207.

Strom, R. D., and S. K. Strom. 1993. Grandparents raising grandchildren: Goals and support groups. *Educational Gerontology* 19:705–715.

Strom, R. D., T. Beckert, and S. K. Strom. 1996. Determining the success of grandparent education. *Educational Gerontology* 22:637–649.

Strom, R., S. Strom, P. Collinsworth, P. Strom, and D. Griswold. 1996. Black grandparents: Curriculum development. *Internal Journal Aging and Human Development* 43 (2): 119–134.

Taylor-Brown, S., J. A. Teeter, E. Blackburn, L. Oinen, and L. Wedderburn. 1998. Parental loss due to HIV: Caring for children as a community issue—the Rochester, New York experience. *Child Welfare* 77 (2): 137–160.

Thomas v. Atascadero Unified School District, No. 886-609 AHS (BY) (C.D. Cal. 1987).

Wodrich, D. L., M. E. Swerdlik, T. Chenneville, and S. Landau. 1999. HIV/AIDS among children and adolescents: Implications for the changing role of school psychologists. *School Psychology Review* 28 (2): 228–241.

12

Immigrant and Migrant Families

TERENCE I. DORAN, HOWARD LUNE, AND RACHEL DAVIS

Since the identification of HIV/AIDS in the early 1980s, people who work with individuals with HIV/AIDS have recognized that the disease affects many who are not infected (Bayer and Oppenheimer 2000; Schneider and Stoller 1995; Gostin 1990). The "affected" population includes spouses and sexual partners, children, parents, siblings, and other family members as well as the friends, schoolmates, workmates, and neighbors of those with HIV/AIDS. Often the stigma and related fear of consequences of disclosure will limit the number of people who share the knowledge of one's sero-status (Siegel, Lune, and Meyer 1998). This frequently places an extra burden on the few people who are aware of that status as they become responsible for the emotional, financial, and physical support of the people living with HIV/AIDS. The elderly grandmothers described here constitute an overlooked and overburdened population of those affected by HIV and its aftermath.

In this chapter we consider the experiences of elderly Hispanic caregivers from poor immigrant and migrant families living in the South Texas border region. (The term *Latino* is rarely used among the Mexican Americans of the region, except among the college-educated or those who have lived in other regions.) These families are all patients at the South Texas AIDS Center for Children and their Families, where one of the authors is the director. Although South Texas has its unique features, the families here share crucial features with immigrant families throughout the United States. These include combinations of poverty, low education, substandard housing, lack of health care, and fear of the Immigration and Naturalization Service (which extends to a fear of most government agencies), on top of the AIDS-specific concerns pertaining to health, social stigma, and disruption of family dynamics. And although the border region is more isolated than many urban centers, the support systems for people with AIDS that exist in the cities rarely extend to the elderly caregivers who survive their infected children.

The experiences of those affected by HIV/AIDS in the United States are shaped by a host of social factors such as race, gender, and socioeconomic status, and of personal factors such as the availability of networks of social support and access to knowledgeable health-care providers. For immigrant and migrant families, most of these factors impair the health and well-being of those affected. Such families tend to be poorer, seasonally employed or underemployed, often without insurance, and separated from their extended families and communities of origin. They also tend to be nonwhite, undereducated, and frequently lacking fluency in English, all of which have associated barriers to necessary care and services. Many migrant workers enter the United States illegally, and they would not qualify for most state-supported health assistance programs if they even dared to apply for them. Finally, under welfare reform initiatives since 1996, many fewer benefits are available even to legal immigrants (Skilton-Sylvester and Garcia 1998; Mullen 1996).

Migrant populations of color and temporary immigrant labor pools are at greater risk for HIV than the national population and have considerably less access to both routine and extraordinary medical care (Goicoechea-Balbona 1997). Poor rural people of color die sooner from HIV/AIDS than the national average, in part due to cultural barriers between patients and medical-care providers (Goicoechea-Balbona 1997). An additional factor exacerbating the costs of HIV/AIDS among migrant populations is the "coming home" phenomenon (Verghese, Berk, and Sarabbi 1989; Selwyn 1986). People from small communities often travel to larger cities where the risk of exposure to HIV may be greater. In some cases, substance use or anonymous sexual encounters, both of which may be prohibitively difficult in the smaller towns, may be more acceptable or available in the cities. Even if an HIV diagnosis is subsequently made in the city, as the infected individuals become ill or terminal they often return to their families. Yet the medical expertise, support services, and other resources that are available in the largest cities with the highest HIV/AIDS rates are rarely available in small towns where these individuals may face discrimination from laypersons and health-care professionals alike. The already skimpy HIV/AIDS resources of the local communities may be wiped out by the hospitalization of one or two very sick patients or by the large medication expenditures for people who lack the ability to pay for them. Likewise, the return home of the sick family member often causes the families to confront their own fears and prejudices concurrent with the cost and other burdens of care.

Numerous studies have documented the negative consequences of poverty, minority ethnic status, poor education, and relative social isolation for those living with HIV/AIDS (Cohen 1999; Weitz 1991). Less well understood are the consequences of these same issues for caregivers, particularly elderly ones, who may acquire the simultaneous burdens of caring for their adult sons and daughters with HIV/AIDS and their children's children (Joslin and Harrison 1998; Joslin, Mevi-Triano, and Berman 1997; Brabant 1994). When the infected parents die, it often falls to the extended family to care for the children. This may include uncles and aunts, but most often it is the grandmother who becomes the guardian, surrogate parent, and primary caregiver to the surviving children.

These grandmothers often face their own medical problems in addition to poverty. Diabetes is rampant among the Hispanic population of the border region, and many of the elderly suffer the consequences of that disease. Hypertension, arthritis, and other conditions of the elderly may be untreated or poorly controlled. Many of these women have performed physical labor for much of their lives, in the home or in the fields, with subsequent wear and tear on their bodies. With few financial resources, little education about health care in general or HIV in particular, and little awareness of available HIV-related help, the elderly of the border region are stepping forward to care for their children and grandchildren infected and affected by HIV disease.

The South Texas Border

The U.S. border with Mexico extends nearly two thousand miles from the Gulf of Mexico to the Pacific Ocean, bordering four U.S. states and six Mexican states. The Rio Grande forms the entire 1,254-mile border between Texas and Mexico, which measures 889 miles if the serpentine curves are smoothed out. The river is spanned by numerous bridges between sister cities in Mexico and the United States and is shallow enough in some places to be crossed on foot. Except for the verdant agricultural area of the lower Rio Grande valley at the southern tip of Texas, where the river empties into the Gulf of Mexico, much of the land extending on both sides of the border is flat, semiarid scrub brush.

The South Texas border region has a unique culture, language, music, history, and geography. "The Border" is often described as a distinct region or a "third country." The region draws on the languages and cultures of both the United States and Mexico but differs from both. English and Spanish are both spoken, separately or in local blendings called "Spanglish," "Tex-Mex," or simply "Border Spanish." The border region has been described as "a liminal area where creative energies are released, creating signs and identities that are born outside of the national projects of the two nations which presume to control identities in this zone" (Kearney 1991:70). The national allegiances associated with these "border identities" are often unclear, as are the responsibilities of the different states to the families living there.

The border unites as well as divides. The economies of the border communities are closely linked though dramatically distinct, and residents of one side often cross to the other to work or shop. The geographic perimeter has always been more of a sieve than a barrier to crossing. Reinforcement of language and culture is sporadic. Immigrant and migrant communities exist literally, symbolically and culturally at the nexus of two worlds. Yet, where the border as a metaphor often serves to break down boundaries and erase "a host of binary oppositions—center-periphery, global-local, assimilation-ethnic-purity" (Smith 1992:517), such ambiguity itself may call for a renewed investment in the definition of sides by those who have an interest in the contrast. Maintaining strong ties to Mexico, along with ongoing reinforcement of the "home" language, culture, and values, these immigrant families often remain as separate from the dominant culture of the United States as they are physically separated from Mexico. Similarly, it is only in those states with the largest Spanish-speaking populations that we find laws defining English as the official language. As Gupta and Ferguson point out, "Territoriality is . . . reinscribed at just the point it threatens to be erased" (1992:11). Thus, neither the U.S. government nor that of Texas is anxious to make itself accountable for the lives of the families residing in this region.

Life on the border is often harsh. The Texas-Mexico border region is one of the most impoverished areas of the United States. Of fourteen Texas counties that are contiguous with the Border, twelve had poverty rates of more than 35 percent and eight had rates greater than 50 percent in 1994 (Texas Kids Count 1994). The average poverty rate for the border region defined by the Texas Comptroller of Public Accounts was 29.5 percent, higher than any state in the United States. Per capita personal income was $15,570 in 1995, less than any state. Substandard housing, poverty, and low educational levels are common. Diseases such as tuberculosis, hepatitis A, and measles occur at rates well above the U.S. averages, and there are periodic reports of more exotic diseases such as rabies and dengue fever. Unemployment is chronically high, averaging 8 percent in 1997, again ranking it first in the nation if the region were treated as a separate state. Even so, this figure masks the seasonal affects of the local agricultural industry. Several counties chronically report unemployment rates of 15–20 percent off-season (Bureau of Labor Statistics 2000; U.S. General Accounting Office 1998).

Many of the poorest families live in impoverished rural communities called *colonias,* unincorporated neighborhoods usually found close to the border. Many lack electricity, running water, garbage service, adequate sewer systems, and other infrastructure mandatory for recognized residential areas in the United States. In these communities, homes may be one- or two-room shacks with blankets instead of doors. It is not uncommon to see a garden hose running from one home to another to serve as the water source for a family, or similar jerry-rigging for electricity. Shallow wells are at risk for contamination from the homemade septic systems installed by many families, as well as by raw sewage and factory discharge into the Rio Grande and agricultural chemicals prevalent in the area.

Hidalgo County in the lower Rio Grande valley has an estimated eight hundred colonias housing hundreds of thousands of migrant farm workers and their families, along with large numbers of undocumented individuals. In Cameron, Hidalgo, and Starr counties, which comprise the lower Rio Grande valley, between 83.2 percent and 97.6 percent of the population is Hispanic American, or Mexicano (U.S. Bureau of the Census 1999). The exact size of the population is impossible to calculate because it is in a constant state of flux. More than 160,000 people from Mexico were granted permanent resident status in 1996 (U.S. General Accounting Office 1998), in addition to a comparable number estimated to have entered the country illegally. (Approximately 1.5 million undocumented immigrants were apprehended in the Southwest Region by the U.S. Immigration and Naturalization Service in 1998 [U.S. General Accounting Office 1998].) These Mexicano families are often perceived as placing undue strain the local resources dedicated to schools, medical facilities and other social services, particularly as Texas already invests less in such services than any other state in the nation (Flores, Douglas, and Ellwood 1998).

Documented and undocumented immigrants enter the United States in tremendous numbers annually, reinforcing Mexican traditions, culture, and language in the border region, but also lending a certain wariness of authority and existing institutions. Many colonia residents rely on family and community, with a distrust of governmental, medical, educational, and other mainstream American institutions. For their part, the institutions and authorities of the border region are at least equally wary of the immigrants. Migrant families are allowed to live in dangerous and unhealthy conditions, all but ignored by state and society. This lack of oversight contrasts sharply with the nearby Border Patrol, which spends millions each year on "a sophisticated high-tech surveillance program that also includes motion sensors, searchlights, television cameras, helicopters, spotter planes, and patrols in various kinds of boats and ground vehicles, all coordinated by computers and radio communications" (Kearney 1991:57). Aid to Families with Dependent Children benefits, the primary source of formal support for the grandparent caregivers in the border region, are considerably lower in Texas than in neighboring states (Mullen 1996:513). The resulting message is mixed. "Foreign labor is desired, but the persons in whom it is embodied are not desired" (Kearney 1991:58).

Absent routine interactions with formal service providers, the border communities lean heavily on family and local resources. Hispanic cultural norms favor allocentrism, the reliance on community support (Burnette 1999b). Researchers have also used the term *familismo* to refer to the strong sense of family identity in many Hispanic cultures (Diaz 1997). Burnette describes the "preference for natural helping networks over the formal service sector" as a "core cultural value" among elder Hispanics (1999b:51). Studies of numerous Hispanic families in both urban and rural regions throughout the United States have indicated that "older persons are frequently relied on to provide assistance with child care and thus are likely to be called on to assume primary responsibility for raising grandchildren when parents are incapacitated or absent" wherein "turning to formal agencies for assistance may be perceived as not adhering to traditional values and expectations" (Cox, Brooks, and Valcarcel 2000:221).

Although it is dangerous to overgeneralize across all Hispanic populations, the reliance on extended family and elder relatives as caregivers, noted among numerous Hispanic communities in the United States, has been particularly documented among Mexican Americans (Black, Ray, and Markides 1998). Furthermore, and in contrast to the cultural explanations, prior research has identified numerous structural barriers that lead such communities to rely on informal care. Such factors include language barriers, lack of transportation, poverty, low levels of integration into the mainstream culture, and "difficulty comprehending the serious nature of illness or disease" (Goicoechea-Balbona 1997:172). "Nonwhite elderly people from ethnic minority groups tend persistently to underuse formal services for which they are eligible" due in part to difficulty with registration procedures, lack of knowledge about available benefits and lack of assistance (Burnette 1999a:24). Each of these factors plays a role in border life.

HIV on the South Texas Border

HIV was slow to be recognized on the Texas-Mexico border. Its occurrence was more familiar in the large urban centers of the east and west coasts of the United States, and it was popularly described as a disease of gay men and drug users. For a variety of reasons, neither drug use nor sexual behavior is discussed much in the border region, and many doctors remained relatively ignorant while HIV entered the population. Geographic distance, a largely rural environment, and traditional cultural values further conspired to shield HIV/AIDS from view. Yet this lack of attention did not reflect the reality of the situation. By the end of the 1990s, Texas had a cumulative total of 50,158 reported AIDS cases, ranking fourth among the states (Centers for Disease Control and Prevention 1999).

South Texas is considered to be a low-moderate area of HIV prevalence. In Texas, females comprise 18 percent of AIDS cases but 28.2 percent of HIV cases, the latter representing more recent infections (Texas Department of Health 1999). This is indicative of the continued spread of HIV among women in recent years. In Texas, as in much of the United States, the burden of AIDS in women is highest among African Americans (61.5%) (Texas Department of Health 1999). Hispanic women comprise 14 percent of HIV cases among women in Texas. The figure is much higher along the South Texas border; approximately one-fourth of the patients now receiving care at HIV service organizations in South Texas are female.

Cumulatively, 43.6 percent of adults with AIDS in Texas and 31.7 percent of adult HIV cases have been men who have sex with men. People with HIV that has not yet advanced to AIDS generally have more recent infections than those with AIDS. Injected-drug use and heterosexual transmission account for 17.1 percent and 19.3 percent of HIV cases. Injected-drug use accounts for 30.8 percent of cumulative AIDS cases, but only 20.8 percent of HIV cases among women. Heterosexual transmission accounts for 53.1 percent of female AIDS cases and 45.1 percent of HIV cases. This is somewhat misleading however, in that 33.3 percent of women had an unknown risk. The Centers for Disease Control and Prevention has found that most cases of unknown risk in women ultimately are shown to be heterosexual transmission cases. Thus, well over half of new cases are likely to have resulted from sexual activity. Eighty-five percent of women with HIV are of childbearing age.

Because AIDS cases represent the advanced stage of HIV disease, the true prevalence of HIV in South Texas is unknown. This question becomes more complicated because of the population movement back and forth across the Rio Grande, which also complicates epidemiology and prevention interventions. Although Texas law since January 1, 1996, has required that women be offered HIV testing during prenatal visits and at delivery, population mobility undermines this mechanism. Many women receive no prenatal care at all, or none in this country, and often disappear before receiving their test results.

Residents of the border are at considerably greater risk for HIV/AIDS than the popular discourse on gay, white urbanites would suggest. Worldwide, HIV/AIDS is closely associated with what we may refer to as secondary risk factors. These include poverty, minority ethnicity, lack of formal education, and lack of access to health care, all of which are abundant problems on the border (Organista and Organista 1997; National Commission to Prevent Infant Mortality 1993). People often have no accurate information about HIV/AIDS. Communities in the region have little contact with the kinds of prevention education sources that are used in urban areas. Often men who engage in same-sex relationships do not identify as gay or bisexual, so education aimed at those populations does not reach them either (Organista and Organista 1997).

The cases examined in this chapter come from case histories of patients at the South Texas AIDS Center for Children and their Families (STAC). STAC was formed in 1988 with support from a Pediatric AIDS Demonstration Project grant from the Bureau of Maternal and Child Health (HRSA/PHS) of the U.S. Department of Health and Human Services, and it is operated as part of the Department of Pediatrics of the University of Texas Health Science Center at San Antonio (UTHSCSA). STAC provides medical care, case management, counseling, and developmental testing for minors. It is the only center of its kind within the forty-seven counties served by the organization. The Texas Department of Health estimates that almost all known pediatric AIDS cases in the region receive treatment from the STAC. Medical care is provided by physicians from the UTHSCSA Departments of Internal Medicine and Pediatrics.

The Hispanic representation among patients at STAC is considerably higher than for the state of Texas overall (U.S. Bureau of the Census 1999; Doran 1993, 1995). Women and children evaluated at STAC were previously shown to be predominately Hispanic (58.8%), with lesser numbers of African American (16.5%) and white, non-Hispanic (24.7%) individuals (Doran 1993). In that study it was noted that Hispanic women were predominately infected by sexual transmission (73.3%) compared to African American (33.3%) and white (31.3%) women who had higher levels of injected-drug use than Hispanic women. Only 16.7 percent of Hispanic women had a history of injected-drug use, more than half of whom also had HIV-infected partners. In contrast, more than half of African American and white women had a history of drug injection, and some had HIV-infected sexual partners as well.

Since that initial article was published, the percentage of women of Hispanic heritage has increased slightly to 59.7 percent, while the percentage of women who are African American (21.3%) has continued to increase and now exceeds that for white women (19%) (Doran, unpublished data). The percentage of women who have been infected by heterosexual transmission has increased to more than 73 percent for all women and 81 percent for Hispanic women. Strikingly, African American and white women have had a dramatic increase in HIV infection by injected-drug use to 66.7 percent and 55.3 percent (Doran, unpublished data). Women infected by injected-drug use or who have both HIV-infected sexual partners and a history of drug injection account for approximately one-fourth of the women, including 18.8 percent of Hispanic women, 33.3 percent of African American women, and 44.7 percent of white women (Doran, unpublished data).

Most of the women have husbands or sexual partners who also prove to be infected, if they are willing to be tested. Some of the men refuse or consent reluctantly. Many men blame the women, who tested positive first. All too often both parents come to medical attention long after HIV seroconversion, when their chances for long-term survival are greatly reduced. When the parents become sick, caregiver responsibility typically rests with the mothers. When they become sick or die it often falls to the extended families rather than to the fathers to care for the children. Most often, the children are given over to their grandmothers.

The new caregiver role creates dilemmas for these elderly women of the border region. On one hand, there is the traditional valuation of *familismo.*

When a child is orphaned, the expectation is that a family member will step forward to provide care. Similarly, elderly relatives are rarely placed in nursing homes. Instead a daughter, granddaughter, or daughter-in-law will take their relative into their home or move in to provide care. On the other hand, the death of the mother means that these elderly relatives often lose their own source of family support even as they acquire responsibility for the children. They must also confront their fears of HIV and its associated stigmas.

When the infected person in need of care is a gay son, a drug user, or a child with open sores, the caretaker will have to resolve many role conflicts before deciding how to respond. Not everyone is able to accept such a burden. It would be misleading if at the end of this chapter the reader has the impression that all of the families have responded with selfless generosity.

The Children and Their Elderly Caregivers

Most newly diagnosed HIV-infected women in South Texas are tested during pregnancy and receive treatment with antiretroviral drugs to decrease the risk of transmission to their infants. Nevertheless, for various reasons some women and their infants have not benefited from such treatment. Problems that have occurred include systematic errors such as failure to act on the results of a serologic test in a timely manner, failure to refer the women to treatment or to provide medications in a timely manner, and mistakes in medication prescriptions. In addition, the legal requirements to inform the women in advance that the HIV serologic test will be performed and to provide pre- and post-test counseling have often been ignored or poor (Doran, unpublished data).

Half of the infected children referred to our clinic in the past five years were from Mexico and other Latin American countries. Most were misdiagnosed or did not have a diagnosis until just before referral. Opportunities to intervene with medications during pregnancy have been not been available in such cases. Other failures have occurred with women who are unable to adhere to a regimen of medications because of substance abuse, mental retardation, or adolescence (denial or hiding of pregnancy). Despite these failures, approximately 85–90 percent of pregnant HIV-infected women and their offspring who were referred to STAC have taken all or part of the Zidovudine protocol.

In the past, most of the children with HIV/AIDS from the lower Rio Grande valley were diagnosed only when they became seriously ill, often with disease that was quite advanced. Almost all acquired HIV by vertical transmission from their mothers. In many cases, the mothers were oblivious to risk factors and knew nothing about HIV/AIDS. Many of the women were unaware of their HIV status until their children became ill, at which time both the children and their mothers were diagnosed. It is still not uncommon for women to have never heard of HIV or AIDS at the time of diagnosis.

Ernesto was first referred to us in August 1991 at the age of twenty-two months by his pediatrician. He had been born to Sylvia, a mentally retarded twenty-one-year-old woman who was subsequently diagnosed with HIV. Ernesto's maternal grandmother, Ms. Martinez, has been the care provider for him and his mother for all of their lives.

On his initial physical exam, Ernesto was already quite ill and advanced with his disease. He was found to have failure to thrive, massively enlarged liver, spleen and lymph nodes, oral yeast infection (thrush) severe delays in development and small head size (microcephaly) consistent with an AIDS-defining condition called HIV encephalopathy. He was unable to walk, stand, or pull himself up, or, at his first visit, to perform even the simplest of gross motor or verbal skills. He demonstrated no ability to speak and had no recognizable words of consistent vocalization. He was very passive, interacted poorly with others, and simply smiled, though not at the time of that visit. He was reportedly able to crawl, but only with difficulty. He was treated for his infections, given antibiotics to prevent *Pneumocystis carinii* pneumonia, and begun on the zidovudine, the only antiretroviral medication available at the time.

By the second visit, Ernesto had already showed some improvement in his HIV-related symptomatology, though he remained developmentally significantly below average. He was noted to have "no evidence of intelligible expressive language" and only "jabbered expressively." By the time this exam was done, Ernesto had already been referred to an early childhood intervention program and was making slow but noticeable improvements.

Ernesto, his grandmother, mother, and several aunts and uncles live in a humble home in a town on the Texas-Mexico border. Ms. Martinez is the caretaker for the entire family. Sylvia provides almost none of Ernesto's care. She and Ernesto are completely dependent on Ms. Martinez. Ms. Martinez herself has limited education and also appears to have somewhat below average intelligence. Despite almost ten years of repeated attempts to educate her about HIV, the purpose of the medications, and her daughter's and grandson's guarded prognosis, she has never displayed any more than a superficial understanding of these issues. Neither Sylvia nor Ernesto has any concept of the disease or need for medications. Ernesto has had problems adhering to his medication regimen, and he is frequently uncooperative with the administration of medications. Ms. Martinez had little success in giving some of the newer regimens of medications due to palatability and the complexity of administering multiple medications to him. Despite all of the difficulties achieving the necessary adherence to medical regimes, she has significant and at times naive confidence in the ability of health care providers to keep her daughter and grandson alive and well indefinitely.

On the positive side, Ms. Martinez rarely misses a clinical appointment. She has worked to provide a safe and nurturing environment for her family. She tries to assure that medications are given and that clinical appointments are kept. That her daughter and grandson are alive is a testament more to her general care than to the medications, which are clearly given on a somewhat erratic basis.

Ms. Martinez is a caretaker whose own health has suffered because her attention is focused on the needs of her family. She was recently hospitalized for coronary-artery bypass surgery. She expressed concerned about the care Ernesto would receive during the time of her absence and recovery as he presents quite a challenge to anyone caring for him. Arrangements were made to provide respite care for Ernesto in San Antonio, but this meant he would be about four to five hours away from his home and family. Fortunately, his new step-grandfather and an aunt were able and willing to care for him during this time, and he was able to remain at home.

This situation shows the precariousness of Ernesto's situation. As long as his grandmother is able to care for him he will do fairly well; after all, he has surpassed our expectations. But we are concerned about what would happen to him if she became unable to provide care for him. Through coordination with her case manager we are working on permanency planning him and his family.

There are many reasons why people living with HIV/AIDS choose not to disclose their status to others. In some cases they are able to make an exception with family; in other cases it is from the family that they most wish to hide (Siegel, Lune, and Meyer 1998). In such cases, there will be little or no opportunity to prepare the caregivers, emotionally or otherwise, for the complexity of their new responsibilities. As difficult as it is for people with HIV/AIDS to find the necessary medical and social support to protect their own lives and well-being, permanency planning for their children represents yet another hurdle that they may not be able to clear.

Ms. Gomez obtained custody of her grandchildren Lupe and Pablo on the death of her daughter, who had been living in another state. Lupe was ten and her brother was thirteen when Ms. Gomez first brought her to our clinic. Ms. Gomez did not know that her daughter had died of AIDS-related complications and discovered this only three years later when she requested a copy of the birth certificate. On reading this, she contacted the HIV/AIDS agency in her community to inquire about the risk to the children. They were tested at the agency, and subsequently referred to STAC when Lupe's test came back positive.

Lupe is clinically well, but her grandmother was understandably distraught. Much of their initial visits were dedicated to HIV/AIDS education for Ms. Gomez, who elected not to tell her granddaughter about her HIV status at that time due to her own emotional turmoil. Lupe was begun on medications, though somewhat less than the ideal regimens. In order to forestall difficult questions, the grandmother has told Lupe that the medications are for asthma, which she also has.

When Lupe reached the age of twelve, Ms. Gomez agreed to tell her about her HIV status. This was a very emotional experience for both child and grandmother, but it has improved our ability to provide medical care for the child. The grandmother is able to provide the stability and love that Lupe and Pablo need. However, this has continued to take an emotional toll because she is in fear of losing her granddaughter. She has been able to use a local Ryan White Care Act-funded AIDS organization for transportation and other assistance. Nobody outside of the family or the local AIDS providers is aware of her status. Before the disclosure to Lupe, Ms. Lopez had nobody with whom to discuss the disease. Ms. Lopez and Lupe are reliant on each other for emotional support, but, as is common for many border families dealing with HIV, there is little support other than the medical staff and case management staff.

Once elder caregivers step into the breach, they often find that they have no idea what services are necessary or available or how to access them. They may have no knowledge about HIV/AIDS, or worse, they may be considerably misinformed. They often are unaware that helping agencies exist, if such agencies are even available to them. In many rural areas and small towns there may be no local resources at all.

Juan was diagnosed with HIV in a San Antonio at four months of age after he developed a serious opportunistic lung infection. His parents were diagnosed shortly after that. At that time they lived in a small border town 150 miles from San Antonio. Soon after, the father left for a job more than five hundred miles from their home. Subsequently, the mother was deported to Mexico, where she lived in the sister city on the Mexican side of the border. She chose to leave the child in the care of the child's maternal grandmother, Mrs. Hernandez, who resided on the U.S. side. This allowed the child to get medical care, but took him from his mother.

Mrs. Hernandez was ill prepared to provide care for an infant. She had no income and little money, no automobile, and elementary-level education. Her understanding of HIV was poor despite efforts to explain the illness and medications. Instructions for medications were written in simple Spanish and explained verbally, but mistakes were made in dosing. She was very reliant on the understaffed local AIDS organization, whose staff of four people provides AIDS education, testing, and prevention services for a nine-county rural area. They provided transportation to San Antonio for Mrs. Hernandez and Juan, sometimes as often as weekly when the child became ill.

Mrs. Hernandez made periodic trips to Mexico to allow Juan to visit with his mother, who received little or no medical care for herself. There was a large emotional toll for Mrs. Hernandez following the initial diagnosis of HIV in her daughter, grandson, and son-in-law. She had anger for her son-in-law for infecting his family members and sorrow for her daughter and grandson, both of whom eventually died of HIV complications.

Discussion

It is not universal that older family members embrace caregiver roles or place the needs of others above their own. Fear of HIV/AIDS can be extreme, as can the moral taint that many people associate with it. Nonetheless, many people, reluctantly or not, overcome the negatives and accept the caregiver role. Sometimes the HIV-infected adult will reveal his or her status early in the clinical course, when the grandmother can be educated along with the children. Some women will reveal or discover their status during pregnancy, allowing the family to know of the child's status from birth. In such cases, the grandmothers' transitions to caregiver are often made easier. They have the chance to learn about the disease and its treatment and may develop a relationship with the case management team. Whether it is through love, duty, spiritual beliefs, family expectation, or social norms or some combination thereof, many elder women have come forward to do their best to care for their families. Yet this phenomenon has been little remarked upon, even by the families involved, in part due to the expectation that they are merely fulfilling their obligations.

In the first case, Ernesto and his mother had been in Ms. Martinez's care since birth due in part to the mother's mental retardation. Ms. Martinez knew of Sylvia's HIV status and of Ernesto's condition from the start. There was no transition beyond the HIV-specific education that must be given to any parent providing care for an infected child. In this case, she had two generations of infected people to care for with a number of additional complications. As difficult as the situation was, Ms. Martinez did what she could to shoulder all of the burdens for her family.

In sharp contrast, Ms. Gomez found out her daughter's status several years after her death and had to initiate testing for her grandchildren on her own. She was emotionally devastated by the combined discoveries of her daughter's and granddaughter's diagnoses. She required a tremendous amount of education in a short time. Yet there was never any question that she would care for the child. The question, for her, was how.

As the third case demonstrates, there are many other barriers between elderly caregivers and the services that their infected children and grandchildren need. Many family members are unwilling to involve themselves in AIDS care. In other cases, many older women do not want to attend facilities that seem to serve a predominantly young, gay male population. These agencies frequently display posters and other explicit sex- or drug-related materials. Older women commonly tell us that they find such displays embarrassing or that they do not want the children to see them. Additionally, children may not be aware of their own infection status or the status of their parents. The frank and open discussions and displays that are the hallmark of many community-based HIV/AIDS organizations are incompatible with the caregivers' desire to shield the children from issues with which they themselves are still coming to terms.

Yet the caregivers and surviving people with HIV/AIDS in the border region are critically dependent on the few clinics and community-based organizations in their area. Antiretroviral medications, while sometimes available in Mexico, are realistically only available to the small percent of the population with wealth. They are beyond the reach of virtually all of the immigrant populations, colonias, and most of border inhabitants without specific AIDS-related government insurance, such as ADAP. Because many of the border families have a history of avoiding contact with state agencies for legal and personal reasons, it becomes far less likely that they will discover the help they need.

When medications are made available to the HIV patient, the grandmother's lack of formal education and possible illiteracy often complicate the caregiver burden. It is difficult for some elder caregivers to understand the concept of a viral disease when they lack the germ theory of disease to build on. Medical instructions, medication doses, and warnings of side effects are written as well as given orally, but compliance can not occur if neither the patient nor the caregiver can read the materials. Simple pictures, color-coded medication boxes, and similar devices help, but misunderstandings and errors are common despite the caregivers' best efforts.

Finally, the caregiver's abilities to manage the complex and multifaceted issues of HIV disease are complicated by their limited relationships with medical personnel. Access to medical care is limited, and the use of *curanderos* (traditional Mexican folk healers) is widespread throughout the border region. Patients use the traditional system of care either in addition to or in place of the western tradition of scientific medicine. When money is limited, or when a respected elder suggests it, family members may rely on a curandero or may alternate between the systems of care. Patients sometimes use various herbs and other treatments with limited or unknown value and unknown interaction effects with prescribed medications. It is not unusual for families to conceal the use of these alternatives from their physicians. In some cases, the inability or unwillingness of physicians and nurses to accept these traditional methods as legitimate only serves to alienate patients further from medical-care providers.

Conclusion

The social, medical, and cultural barriers faced by elderly caregivers in the South Texas border region are not unique. Most immigrant families in the United States and many American families of color face cultural barriers to comprehensive health care, social services, and insurance. Even where primary difficulties such as language are not involved, doctors and service providers often lack sufficient understanding of the patients' social and economic lives to give meaningful advice. Written instructions for medicines may be unclear to caregivers who have had little exposure to such things in their past. For patients and families who have never had a primary care physician or routine medical contact, the idea of regular follow-up exams may be elusive. And, of course, such practices are generally based on the assumption that the patients have insurance with which to pay for them.

Immigration policies greatly exacerbate the difficulties faced by the affected families. Immigration into the United States is occurring at higher rates than ever, with the majority now coming from Latin America and the Caribbean (Skilton-Sylvester and Garcia 1998:58). Coincident to this, recent legal changes have reduced the entitlements of legal aliens, and fear of deportation discourages many immigrants from seeking accurate information. Even in cases where the surviving children are citizens, their grandparents may avoid applying for aid to which they are entitled. The result is a growing population of older and younger people in need, increasingly isolated, and increasingly dependent on informal means of support.

Elderly caregivers everywhere in the United States lack the support mechanisms necessary for the burdens of HIV/AIDS care or even childcare. Many of them lack the support necessary to take care of themselves (Mullen 1996). Elderly Latinos, the largest population category among older immigrants, also have higher morbidity rates and less insurance coverage than other elderly populations in this country (Cox, Brooks, and Valcarcel 2000). Getting legal benefits is often difficult for the first generation of youth of immigrant families. The problems are far greater for the elderly immigrant population (Skilton-Sylvester and Garcia 1998). Insurance is limited, and although ADAP can help a person living with AIDS to receive medical attention it does nothing for surviving children and their surrogate parents.

The same patterns described here among Mexican American families in the border region have been observed among Latino and African American families in New York City (Joslin and Brouard 1995). As drug use, HIV/ AIDS, and incarceration thin the ranks of parents, the children and grandparents are increasingly thrown together. In New York, HIV/AIDS among women is already the leading cause of children becoming orphans, and the rates are highest for children of color (Working Committee on HIV, Children and Families 1996). Nationwide, the occurrence of skip-generation households has been increasing faster than any other household type (Pruchno 1999:209). Formal systems of care have yet to accommodate the unique needs of these families.

Caregiver burdens for those affected by HIV/AIDS have been particularly demanding even for those with greater support systems. Many researchers have been surprised and impressed by the degree of innovation and the range of activities dedicated to providing care in the wake of HIV/AIDS among organized communities (Altman 1994; Chambré 1991). Yet these efforts are often beyond the reach of or unknown to elderly family members unaccustomed to dealing with community-based organizations. In the absence of formal sources of care and support, and with limited contact with informal and community-based sources, both the youngest and the oldest generations of people affected by HIV/AIDS remain relatively uncounted, unaided, and left to their own devices.

We have achieved some understanding of HIV/AIDS in individuals and in communities. We must now turn our attention to the effects of HIV/AIDS on families, for it is changing the shape of the family before our eyes.

References

Altman, D. 1994. *Power and Community: Organizational and Cultural Responses to AIDS.* London: Taylor and Francis.

Bayer, R., and G. M. Oppenheimer. 2000. *AIDS Doctors: Voices from the Epidemic.* Oxford: Oxford University Press.

Black, S. A., L. A. Ray, and K. S. Markides. 1998. The prevalence and health burden of self-reported diabetes in older Mexican Americans: Findings from the Hispanic established populations for epidemiologic studies of the elderly. *American Journal of Public Health* 89 (4): 546–552.

Brabant, S. 1994. An overlooked AIDS affected population: The elderly patient as caregiver. *Journal of Gerontological Social Work* 22 (1–2): 131–145.

Bureau of Labor Statistics. 2000. Metropolitan area at a glance. http://stats.bls.gov/eag.

Burnette, D. 1997. Grandparents raising grandchildren in the inner city. *Families in Society* 78 (5): 489–499.

——. 1999a. Custodial grandparents in Latino families: Patterns of service use and predictors of unmet needs. *Social Work* 44 (1): 22–34.

——. 1999b. Social relationships of Latino grandparent caregivers: A role theory perspective. *The Gerontologist* 39 (1): 49–58.

Centers for Disease Control and Prevention. 1999. *HIV/AIDS Surveillance Report 1999* 11 (2): 1–47.

Chambré, S. 1991. The volunteer response to the AIDS epidemic in New York City: Implications for research on volunteering. *Nonprofit and Voluntary Sector Quarterly* 20:267–288.

Cohen, C. J. 1999. *The Boundaries of Blackness: AIDS and the Breakdown of Black Politics.* Chicago: University of Chicago Press.

Cox, C. B., L. R. Brooks, and C. Valcarcel. 2000. Culture and caregiving: A study of Latino grandparents. In C. Cox, ed., *To Grandmother's House We Go and Stay: Perspectives on Custodial Grandparents,* pp. 218–232. New York: Springer.

Diaz, R. M. 1997. Latino gay men and psychological barriers to AIDS prevention. In M.

Levine, P. Nardi, and J. Gagnon, eds., *In Changing Times: Gay Men and Lesbians Encounter HIV/AIDS*, pp. 221–244. Chicago: University of Chicago Press.

Doran, T. I. 1993. HIV/AIDS in women and children in South Texas: Experience at a family AIDS clinic. *Pediatric AIDS and HIV Infection: Fetus to Adolescence* 4:204–210.

——. 1995. Factors contributing to delayed diagnosis of HIV-infected women and their children in South Texas. *Pediatric AIDS and HIV Infection: Fetus to Adolescence* 6: 206–210.

Flores, K., T. Douglas, and D. A. Ellwood. 1998. The children's budget report: A detailed analysis of spending on low-income children's programs in 13 states. http://Newfederalism.urban.org/html/occal14.html.

Goicoechea-Balbona, A. M. 1997. Culturally specific health care model for ensuring health care use by rural ethnically diverse families affected by HIV/AIDS. *Health and Social Work* 22 (3): 172–180.

Gostin, L. O., ed. 1990. *AIDS and the Health Care System*. New Haven: Yale University Press.

Gupta, A., and J. Ferguson. 1992. Beyond "culture": Space, identity, and the politics of difference. *Cultural Anthropology* 7 (1): 6–23.

Joslin, D., and A. Brouard. 1995. The prevalence of grandmothers as primary caregivers in a poor pediatric population. *Journal of Community Health* 20 (5): 383–401.

Kearney, M. 1991. Borders and boundaries of state and self at the end of empire. *Journal of Historical Sociology* 4 (1): 52–74.

Mullen, F. 1996. Welcome to Procrustes' house: Welfare reform and grandparents raising grandchildren. *Clearinghouse Review* (September): 511–520.

National Commission to Prevent Infant Mortality. 1993. *HIV/AIDS: A Growing Crisis Among Migrant and Seasonal Farmworker Families*. Washington, D.C.: National Commission to Prevent Infant Mortality.

Organista, K. C., and P. B. Organista. 1997. Migrant laborers and AIDS in the United States: A review of the literature. *AIDS Education and Prevention* 9 (1): 83–93.

Pruchno, R. 1999. Raising grandchildren: The experiences of black and white grandmothers. *The Gerontologist* 39 (2): 209–221.

Selwyn, P. A. 1986. AIDS: What is now known. *Hospital Practice,* June 15, 1986.

Schneider, B. E., and N. E. Stoller. 1995. *Women Resisting AIDS: Feminist Strategies of Empowerment*. Philadelphia: Temple University Press.

Siegel, K., H. Lune, and I. Meyer. 1998. Stigma management among gay/bisexual men with HIV/AIDS. *Qualitative Sociology* 21 (1): 3–24.

Skilton-Sylvester, E., and A. Garcia. 1998. Intergenerational programs to address the challenge of immigration. *Generations* 22 (4): 58–64.

Smith, M. P. 1992. Postmodernism, urban ethnography, and the new social space of ethnic identity. *Theory and Society* 21 (4): 493–531.

Texas Department of Health. 1999. *Texas AIDS/STD Surveillance Report*. December.

Texas Employment Commission with Bureau of Labor Statistics. 1997. *Economic Research and Analysis*. Austin: Texas Employment Commission.

Texas Kids Count. 1994. *The State of Texas Children: 1994: A County by County Fact Book*. Austin: Center for Public Policy Priorities.

U.S. Bureau of the Census. 1999. *Statistical Abstract of the United States 1999*. 119th ed. Washington, D.C.: U.S. Bureau of the Census.

U.S. General Accounting Office. 1998. *Report to the Honorable Lloyd Bentsen U.S. Senate. Health Care: Availability in the Texas-Mexico Border Area*. October.

Verghese, A., S. L. Berk, and S. Sarabbi. 1989. *Urbs in rure*. Human immunodeficiency virus infection in rural Tennessee. *Journal of Infectious Disease* 160 (6): 1051–1055.

Weitz, R. 1991. *Life with AIDS*. New Brunswick, N.J.: Rutgers University Press.

Winer, L. S., A. Septimus, and C. Grady. 1998. Psychosocial support and ethical issues for the child and family. In P. A. Pizzo and C. M. Wilfert, eds., *Pediatric AIDS: The Challenge of HIV Infection in Infants, Children and Adolescents*, pp. 703–727. Baltimore: Williams and Wilkins.

Working Committee on HIV, Children and Families. 1996. *Families in Crisis: Report of the Working Committee on HIV, Children and Families*. New York: Federation of Protestant Welfare Agencies.

13

Policy Implications for HIV-Affected Older Relative Caregivers

NATHAN L. LINSK, CYNTHIA CANNON POINDEXTER, AND SALLY MASON

Lacy Jones[1] is a sixty-one-year-old African American woman from Mississippi who lives in a duplex on the northwest side of Chicago. She lives with and cares for five of her grandchildren, one of whom, Adam, age six, has AIDS. In addition, she provides occasional care for Adam's mother Jen, who also has AIDS and lives elsewhere in the city. Both Jen and Adam take prophylactic medicine to avoid opportunistic infections. Both are cared for by a Ryan White CARE-funded Title IV Women and Children's project at the county hospital, which means they obtain medical care, have a case manager, and receive HIV information. Lacy also is designated by the state as primary caregiver for her forty-year-old daughter Susan, who lives upstairs and has been impaired by a stroke. Lacy provides personal care in addition to the case management and home care Susan receives. Lacy receives a monthly care stipend for caring for Susan. The remaining four grandchildren are not HIV-infected and are placed with her through kinship foster care. Lacy has not told Adam that he has HIV because she is afraid he will tell others and will then be shunned. He has been told that his mother is sometimes sick and that is why his grandmother is caring for him.

Although Lacy states that she is in good health when asked, she adds that she has hypertension and diabetes, which are primarily controlled by diet and medication. She is adamant that it is her job to take care of her "own" and embraces the duty of caregiving for her loved ones. She says that she is sustained by her family's need for her and by her religious faith. She says that when HIV came into her life it made her stronger and has increased her empathy for others' pain and sadness. She receives most of her support from the church and her family, and she states that caring for the children and attending church make up her social life.

Older adults providing care to HIV-positive or affected children in their families do so within the context of varied care and services networks, including senior service programs, child welfare services, and HIV services. As in Lacy's case, the confluence of many care needs in one family context indicates the need for outside help in the form of direct services and service coordination. However, most services are population-specific and are not designed to encompass multiple recipients and caregivers of services within the home. In fact human problems occur in diverse circumstances regarding family norms, cultural constraints, and individual patterns and preferences. Our policy responses must be sufficient and flexible enough to support the range of care needs, at the same time avoiding penalizing families for their strengths in caring for each other.

Lacy's story suggests a number of questions with policy and practice implications. These questions are typical of those facing older relatives who are caregivers for HIV-affected children. In Lacy's case we must consider that multiple systems are overseeing this care. The Ryan White CARE Title IV HIV service system provides primary care and case management; the Department on Aging and Disability supports the family by paying a care stipend for Susan and sending home health staff to the home; and the state child welfare department oversees Lacy as a foster parent and provides some specific services for both Adam and the other grandchildren. In addition, the family accepts some assistance from their church volunteer committee, and Jen has been involved with a needle-exchange research project that includes education, support, and linkages to medical care. These systems clearly do not communicate with each other.

Lacy has developed strategies to try to protect her benefits. She is reluctant to share any information because she believes that if other agencies knew that her family receives benefits elsewhere she would lose services. She knows that the foster care program she is in limits the number of people in the home and fears she will not be able to care for them without the foster-care stipend. She feels she needs the home-care stipend for Susan and the foster care payments to "hold house together."

Is she robbing Peter to pay Paul by using benefits from one program to help other family members? This raises both ethical issues and questions about how to frame policies to ensure that people can creatively obtain what they need in an open way without abusing the system. Lacy is "working the system" by applying for all the benefits she can and managing information that might be used to limit her services. This can be seen as heroic or manipulative. From a policy perspective, Lacy's situation may be seen by case managers or program administrators as noncompliant with program rules, as a violation of clearly stated policy, or as a necessary arrangement outside the usual rules that supports this family despite the variation from stated policies.

Finally, who is caring for Lacy? It appears there are no services in home to meet her own needs, even though she may qualify for some senior support services. How can policies be framed that assure us that the caregiver also receives the necessary services and supports?

HIV Caregiving as a Policy Issue

Although caregivers and families of persons infected by HIV often are seen as a determining factor in whether a person can be maintained in home- or community-based surroundings, there are few national or state-specific caregiver policies. Most home- or community-based long-term care programs tend to determine eligibility and successful outcomes based on the "identified client" rather than see the client and caregiver together in a family context. This may be problematic because not all HIV-affected older caregivers are caring for HIV infected children. Policy needs to include relative caregivers raising HIV-*affected* children, those whose parents are dead or unavailable to care due to their HIV status. Policies for families vary within and between states, and their consequences may, in effect, be a disincentive for older adults providing family care. The result is that family or other caregivers are often overlooked regarding services, policy, and planning.

The impacts of policy on grandparent caregivers include a mix of policy areas, based on the juncture of various populations involved in grandparent care. Caregiving always involves at least two stakeholders, the caregiver and the care-receiver, and may involve others in varying supporting or even non-supportive roles. Table 13.1 shows some examples of policy fields, beneficiaries, funding sources, services provided, and potential consequences. In varying systems of care the older adult may be viewed as client or patient, care provider, or primary responsible relative, or be marginalized because programs may not address caregivers at all.

Our consideration of policies that relate to HIV-affected children and their caregivers includes three assumptions.[2] First, we assume that care in the home is an underlying value for policymakers, service providers, and families as the best choice for at least some HIV-affected children and families. Our

Table 13.1 Policy Fields, Clients, and Program Consequences

Policy Field	Beneficiary Who is the Client?	Funding Source	Services	Outcome Caregiver Gaps
Child Welfare	Children or Adolescents	State child welfare programs	Income support case management permanency planning	Needs of caregiver not a focus of services Systems pressures toward permanency (adoption, guardianship)
Aging Services	Older adults	Older Americans Act	Information and referral, legal assistance, employment programs, transportation, case management, nutrition services, etc.	Programs generally are designed to address needs of people who live in single generation households Age criteria may limit participation
HIV/AIDS services	Focus on the infected person or person at risk	Ryan White CARE, Housing Programs People with AIDS (HOPWA)	Examples (based on local plans) Primary care, case management, housing assistance, mental health	Caregivers may not be be eligible for benefits
Health Policy	Eligibility for adults and children based on income or contributiions	Medicare, Medicaid, Primary care, Specialist care, HMOs	Home and community based care, medical care	Managed care may limit service access Support services may not be available and may limit access Family may end up with care at diverse sites or diverse providers

second assumption is that care policies should be client-, family-, and community-based and should exist to benefit the clients rather than primarily to solve administrative problems or contain cost. Third, we assume minimum criteria of at least not excluding caregivers from services and benefits.

Societal values are "legitimized" through the political process, which then affect the kind of policies we expect and how we treat and define both "social problems" and people involved in those problems. Policy and program approaches generally focus on individual deficits and how to address them, as well as on eligibility for benefits. These policy values may function as barriers to care and services for older adults caring for HIV-affected children. Caregivers for HIV-affected children are people at risk, particularly given that HIV remains a highly stigmatized condition and that older women are the usual caregivers.

The role of women in the family and the expectations that women would give up other roles to provide family care, particularly in minority communities, suggests another critical value, which is often not made explicit. It is therefore not surprising that the needs of the caregiving older women are often overlooked, or, worse, that they have unrealistic demands placed on them navigating differing social and health service programs on behalf of those they care for or themselves. Older women are often called on to provide care within the family, sometimes even when they need care themselves. This "invisible labor" includes financial, social, and personal costs that need to be addressed in policies and programs to sustain quality of care and life. This added burden on the caregiver is an invisible cost until the care systems are overwhelmed and break down, to be replaced by more expensive alternatives (Minkler and Roe 1993; Abramowitz 1988; Osterbusch et al. 1986).

In considering the varying federal policies affecting older family members as caregivers for HIV-affected children, we have developed a framework suggested by the work of Gilbert and Specht (1986). The framework considers the beneficiaries of services, the policy dimensions involved, and the outcomes.

How the beneficiaries of services are defined predicts who receives or is excluded from services. Possible beneficiaries are the older adult caregiver, the child who receives care, other informal supports in the social context, or the family as a whole. Our perspective is that some services should meet the needs of each and when possible should be integrated to maximize access and convenience.

Three interrelated policy dimensions are considered: the services or benefits, the funding source, and access. For any given set of beneficiaries specific benefits or services are available, with corresponding eligibility requirements. For each the source of funding also may influence who can take advantage of the service and is influenced by the structure of the policy and administrative rules that limit or invite utilization.

Program outcomes are conceived of as positive and/or negative for the children, caregivers, and others in the family. We consider both intended and unintended effects of policies on family support and function and on the lives of the people affected by HIV or by aging.

These assumptions and components will be used to discuss the policies throughout the rest of this chapter, which addresses existing programs and policies within the context of care provided by older relatives to HIV-affected children. We primarily address federal policies and consider how these manifest at the state and local levels. First we will consider the aging service system and related issues. We then address HIV-related services and programs. Finally, we consider an array of child welfare-related programs. After these three fields of policy and programs are reviewed we will consider current and emerging policy issues, including welfare reform, health care arrangements, and future trends and directions.

Aging Programs

As caregivers age, they are increasingly likely to need and qualify for various types of senior services relating to aging policies. Preliminary research (Mason and Linsk 1999; Joslin, Mevi-Triano, and Berman 1997; Poindexter 1997) has suggested that older caregivers are less likely to consider their own service needs than they are to search for services to support the children for whom they are providing care. The consequences of putting oneself last include neglect of health, increased vulnerability, poorer coping duration, and crisis-oriented care. Policy and program responses need to emphasize outreach, case finding, accessibility, and information sharing in the community of older adults so that caregivers will know about services and be encouraged to use them. A number of programs created to address the service needs of elders are discussed in the context of older caregivers. Note that Medicare and Medicaid are included here although they are available across the age span; however, both may have particular impacts for older adults who are caregivers.

Older Americans Act and Social Services Block Grants

The Older Americans Act of 1965 (OAA) funds a continuum of care for persons over age sixty, creating an "aging network" to support elders and their caregivers that does not specifically focus on elders who are providing care to younger ill persons. The OAA supplements the help families provide for older adults (DiNitto 2000) through educational programs in senior centers, family-oriented case management, information and referral, advocacy, legal services, outreach, and nutrition and home-delivered meals. These could all be vehicles to disseminate information to older persons about the needs of HIV-affected families, link them with appropriate support services, and plan for an array of supports for the HIV-affected caregiver. In the past, funds have been allocated through Title IV of the OAA for training of and information dissemination to service providers and planners. The OAA creates several mechanisms for input from the community into this network of services, including the Area Agency on Aging Advisory Councils (DiNitto 2000) and training forums to educate aging-network members about how they might address the needs of this population.

Social Services Block Grants (formerly Title XX Amendments to the Social Security Act) offer additional community-based and home-based services, especially for those who receive Supplemental Security Income. Social Services Block Grants (SSBGs) are the largest federally funded social services program, capped at $2.5 billion annually (DiNitto 2000). These goals are state-specific, and grants are determined by population size on the premise that "economic and social needs are interrelated and states know best what services their residents need" (DiNitto 2000:323).

However, these services are discrete from services that may be provided to other family members. For example, in one of our research interviews a grandmother caregiver stated, "You can't get your kid on the Council on Aging van! How can you get your kid to the doctor if you don't drive?" What may appear as an administrative necessity for the program may not take into account that multiple family members require needed care.

Older adults caring for children affected by HIV are reluctant to use services for which they are entitled for a number of reasons including the demands of child care precluding time to consider their needs as older adults. Given that service access is decreasing, older caregivers who do seek services are too often disappointed. As recommended by the 1995 White House Conference on Aging, AFDC, food stamps, and programs funded by the Administration on Aging should be more accessible to caregiving grandparents, not less so (White House Conference on Aging 1996).

Supportive services, such as support groups or respite and daycare, and some direct services such as food services, are needed to support varying family members. The lack of integration or coordination across target populations for the various services creates inequities and may be confusing and complex when viewed in the family relative care context. The SSBG programs are not an aging program per se and are flexible enough so states can decide on services and beneficiaries. Because they are not age prescribed or diagnostically designated, SSBGs could in fact fund a full array of services for HIV-

affected older caregivers. These grants should be a target for advocates to influence SSBG priorities to benefit older caregivers of HIV-affected children.

Older caregivers for HIV-infected children may be reluctant to use services available within the aging network both because of fear of disclosure and
the time and child-care constraints imposed by the care situation. For example, while nutrition programs available in on-site congregate dining programs
often associated with senior centers could help with socialization and be a
source of social support and information, older adults caring for affected
grandchildren may be unlikely to participate unless these services are designed
to provide grandchild care. Home-based services including home meal programs and homemakers may be available through the aging network only if
the older adults level of functional ability is inadequate to provide this care.
Although this is less likely for older adults who take on caregiving, it would
be important to ascertain that others in the home who do qualify for these
supports utilize them, possibly reducing the care burden, if this is consistent
with the desires and values of the family. Our example of Lacy shows that
older adults may become involved as caregivers for several family members;
she received payments for providing care for another adult family member,
which provided support to home-based disabled adults. The state units on
aging and area agencies on aging may well consider how they can provide support for older family members who in turn care for others and ascertain that
their programs eligibility criteria are sufficiently broad to encompass an array
of family care configurations.

Senior Housing Programs

A range of housing options exists for older adults and disabled persons including independent housing, congregate housing, assisted living, and government
programs, including section 202 housing loans for moderate-income older
people and disabled people and section 236 and section 8 programs that use interest reduction or rent supplements to make housing available to those who
meet income tests. The Housing Program for People with AIDS (HOPWA)
is discussed later.

Relative caregiving families may be eligible for housing services based on
overall family income or the aging/disability status of specific family members. Income, however, may make the family ineligible for these services. Unfortunately, these programs are generally very limited in terms of availability
and access. Section 8, which provides rent supplements, generally uses a cer-

tificate mechanism; only a limited number of certificates may be available in a specific community. Programs are generally not designed to incorporate multiple family members in need, although this may be possible.

Grandfamily housing may be incorporated into existing or developing programs to establish a housing option that specifically is designed for grandparent care. The history of innovation around intergenerational programs and a focus on multigenerational families is a promising prospect. However, housing communities may be reluctant to open their doors to diverse populations. HIV may be viewed by the family as so stigmatizing as to be kept private or by the community as so fear-generating that it can lead to overt discrimination.

Medicare

Medicare offers an insurance mechanism to provide for the cost of hospitalization, nursing home care, and physicians for individuals who are disabled or are age sixty-five or older. Part B, enrolled in electively by participants, offers some physician and hospital outpatient services, limited home health care including personal care, diagnostic and x-ray services, and miscellaneous services.

Medicare is potentially accessible to all adults over age sixty-four; 99 percent of the older population is enrolled in Part A (Hospital Insurance), and 97 percent is enrolled in Part B (Supplemental Insurance) (Hooyman and Kiyak 1996:525). It is to great extent universally accessible to this population. However, Part B is not accessible to those who cannot afford to pay for it and covers only 80 percent of the cost of services. Younger grandparents caring for grandchildren generally do not have access to health care, which is a significant policy gap related to the uninsured in the United States. Grandparents and other caregivers generally have limited financial resources in the face of high costs to pay for the children's needs, and many cannot provide the co-payment to enroll in the supplemental insurance provisions (Part B).

HIV-infected children may also be eligible for Medicare and may receive benefits due to their disability status. The complexity of the Medicare program may be challenging to the caregivers, who not only must keep track of their own benefits, related bills, and reimbursements but also must do this for grandchildren. Older adults over age sixty-five who provide relative care are insured for medical services, but these are not always accessible and the cost is shared with the recipient. Recent proposals to expand Medicare to include prescription drugs would offer substantial help to older caregivers who are now at risk of skimping on their own medications to be sure their children's needs are met.

Medicaid

Medicaid is a federal and state means-tested welfare program of medical assistance for the categorically needy regardless of age. Medicaid is administered based on state regulations through local welfare departments. The possible stigma of receiving public assistance may combine with the stigma of caring for an HIV-affected child and discourage the older adults from seeking help for themselves.

It is unknown how many relative caregivers are themselves eligible for Medicaid due to their own financial status or health needs or how many are also caring for other older adults who are eligible. For Lacy, whose story begins this chapter, Medicaid may have been a source of care for herself as an older adult in addition to several of her dependents through their status as HIV-positive or disabled home- and community-based waivers. It is likely that affected grandchildren who are not HIV-positive themselves will lack access to coverage.

The outstanding policy dimensions for Medicaid are the use of eligibility criteria that can include both a means test and a functional assessment of need. This can require a grandmother to go through complicated exhausting recertification process, adding to their stress, lack of time, and attention to own needs (Daphne Joslin, personal communication). As noted with regard to Medicare, case management may be very important, but if not offered in a manner to encompass the entire family, may add to rather than decrease the complexity.

Medicaid community-care programs require a functional assessment for the identified client (older or disabled adult or child). These assessments either ignore the amount of stretching of one's financial and psychological resources the older adult may need to do to provide care, or subtract social supports from the scores. The fact that older adults are caring for others may be used as a criterion to exclude them from services, reasoning that if they can help others, they do not need help themselves. Although our research and practice have shown older caregivers to be quite resourceful, this resourcefulness does not come without stress and family strain. The result is that the services may not be available until the family support network is exhausted and is no longer able to provide the needed support. Consequently, the policy requirements act as a disincentive for families to provide care or to request help with care.

HIV-Related Services

HIV-related services emanate out of both specific HIV-related legislation and HIV components of federal programs for housing and medical care for indigent people. We will briefly discuss the Ryan White Comprehensive AIDS Resources Emergency (CARE) Act of 1990, Housing Opportunities for Persons with AIDS (HOPWA), and Medicaid Home and community-based waivers.

The Ryan White CARE Act

The passage of the Ryan White Comprehensive AIDS Resources Emergency Act of 1990 (CARE) was the result of a variety of forces—community-based advocacy, professional coalition building, bipartisan congressional support—and redefined HIV as affecting people from all socioeconomic levels, ethnic groups, and sexual orientations (Poindexter 1998). The federal legislation sets up a national network of care and services including highly affected cities (Title I); statewide programs and drug reimbursement (Title II); early intervention at federally funded clinics (Title III); women and children's programs (Title IV); programs for health provider education (AIDS Education and Training Centers); and demonstration/evaluation programs (Special Projects of National Significance). Through local and state planning councils and consortia, communities choose to fund services such as case management, medical clinics, drug-assistance programs, transportation, nutrition support, complementary therapies, home-based care, mental health and substance use services.

The CARE Act contains diverse possibilities for responding more effectively to family caregivers, but most of these are not explicit. Title I planning councils and Title II consortia are charged with assessing and meeting community needs; these bodies are often concerned about caregivers of people of all ages with HIV, but may not be aware of the hidden population of older caregivers and how they may provide better outreach and support to them.

The fact that the CARE Act funds vital medical, pharmaceutical, and social services for children with HIV is of enormous help to HIV-affected grandparent caregivers; this benefit should not be minimized. Without the services the CARE Act makes possible, HIV-affected grandparent caregivers would have little recourse when the HIV-infected care recipients need medical and social services. However, in households with both HIV-positive children and noninfected children, medical care may come from several providers for the children and additional providers for the older caregiver, making obtaining medical care very burdensome. Efforts to develop "one-stop shopping" programs (e.g., in Title III and IV of the CARE Act) may not succeed in meeting the entire family's needs unless both older and younger family members are taken into account.

The intervention target of this Act is, understandably, persons with HIV. However, there are opportunities within the scope of this Act to address some of the concerns of caregivers. Title IV provides comprehensive health and support services to HIV-positive children, youth, and women and to the families of these individuals. "Title IV grantees provide family-centered care, meaning that services are designed to meet the needs of whole families affected by HIV. Although the number of grandparents in Title IV services is unknown, the primary caregiver for over 25% of children in Title IV is a family member other than a parent. Family support services provided by Title IV projects include family case management and counseling, logistical support, respite care and day care, parenting education and permanency planning" (Moore 2000). Although Title IV is already organized to provide family centered care, the definition of families may not be broad enough to encompass the range of older relatives who are caring for HIV-affected but uninfected children. The services should become more sensitive to the unique needs of older families.

The national AIDS Education and Training Centers are expected to teach professionals in all disciplines about HIV and the needs of clients and patients, as well as widely disseminate new information. The AETC network is an important outlet for raising the psychosocial and support issues of isolated and stressed caregivers. SPNS projects are specifically designed to reach minorities, low-income persons, prisoners, and drug users; again, the older caregivers who are living in the wake of these crises should be better served through these programs. These areas of the CARE act could be the basis for assessing, planning for, and implementing services that grandparent caregivers may need, such as respite, daycare, transportation, food, education, and individual and group counseling. These set-asides and demonstration projects should include those older care providers and guardians who are struggling to provide personal care and to hold together parent absent families.

Because the CARE Act is targeted to persons with HIV, when the HIV-infected adult or child dies or leaves the home the caregiver no longer has access to these services. Losing one's supportive contacts with case managers as well as service coordination and advocacy can be emotionally difficult at a time of grief.

Housing Opportunities for People with AIDS

HOPWA is authorized through the AIDS Housing Opportunity Act (42 U.S.C. 12901) as amended by the Housing and Community Development Act of 1992 (Pub. L. 102-550, approved October 28, 1992). Funds were appropriated starting in fiscal year 1992. Persons with HIV who meet financial and medical criteria are eligible for monetary support for their housing costs.

The HOPWA program provides housing assistance and supportive services for low-income persons with HIV/AIDS and their families, especially those who are homeless or at great risk of becoming homeless. HOPWA also funds three activities that can serve persons with HIV at any income level: housing information, community outreach, and education. HOPWA funds may be used for a broad range of housing, including emergency shelter, shared housing, apartments, single-room occupancy units (SROs), group homes, and housing combined with supportive services. Agencies may also use HOPWA funds for a variety of housing-related expenses, social services, and program-development costs such as housing information and resource identification; purchase, rehabilitation, conversion, lease, and repair of housing; new construction for SROs and community residences; paying rent, mortgages, and utility payments; operating costs; technical assistance; administrative expenses; and supportive services (such as health care, mental health services, chemical dependency treatment, nutritional services, case management, and help with daily living). Each household receiving rental help or living in housing funded under the program pays rent based on their income (under the same formula as tenants of public housing or Section 8–assisted housing, 30 percent of their adjusted income). HOPWA programs can be designated to target disabled, homeless, and large families as long as they also respond to the greater needs of HIV-infected persons. There are provisions to fund housing units with a larger number of bedrooms to serve large families, for instance. When a person with AIDS dies, however, the family is no longer eligible for HOPWA and must find other housing.

HOPWA was an outgrowth of the recognition that homelessness and substandard housing are linked to the lack of adequate medical care. Although

HOPWA does not specifically target grandparent caregivers, it has the goal of housing at-risk, HIV-affected families. HIV-affected families may live together in a HOPWA-supported housing arrangement. Caregivers are supported directly when they and their HIV-infected family members are supported with safe and appropriate housing. The same situation is true in HOPWA as is the case for the CARE Act: when the adult or child with HIV is absent or deceased, HIV-negative caregivers cannot receive HOPWA support.

HIV-Specific Medicaid Waivers

In addition to information about Medicaid discussed earlier, states can request Medicaid waivers from the federal government to provide home-based and community-based services to persons who may be at risk for institutionalization, including persons with HIV. The waiver program affords flexibility to develop and implement creative alternatives to institutionalizing Medicaid-eligible individuals and to enhance their independence and maintain ties to family and friends. The waiver program expands Medicaid eligibility so that states can make home- and community-based services available through Medicaid to individuals who would otherwise qualify for Medicaid only if they were in an institutional setting. Seven services may be provided: case management, homemaker, home health aid, personal care, adult day health, habilitation, and respite care. Others, such as transportation, in-home support services, meal services, special communication services, minor home modifications, and adult daycare, may be provided subject to Health Care Finance Administration approval. To receive approval to implement a waiver, a state Medicaid agency must assure the HCFA that on average it will not cost more to provide home- and community-based services than providing institutional care would cost and that there are safeguards to protect the health and welfare of service recipients. Although Medicaid waivers are for persons with HIV, not their caregivers, they are important for grandparent caregivers because home-based services can help them provide personal care to the children and adults in their families when they become incapacitated with HIV disease.

The Child Welfare System

Kinship care is the "full-time care, nurturing, and protection of children who must be separated from their parents by relatives" (Child Welfare League of

America 1994:2). Until recently, most children in a relative's care were provided for informally, outside of the child welfare system (Hegar and Scannapieco 1995; Hill 1977). Kinship care consists of formalized kinship arrangements with the relative fulfilling the role of foster parent for the state. Although the relatives may be aunts, uncles, cousins, godparents, stepparents, or any person who has a kinship bond to the child, grandparents provide at least half of relative care. These caregivers are also more likely to be people of color, to have lower incomes, and to have less education than traditional or nonrelative foster parents (Child Welfare League of America 1994). Reasons for the increase in formal kinship care including: increased reporting of abuse and neglect; increased drug abuse, especially crack cocaine; increased levels of poverty; and HIV/AIDS (Child Welfare League of America 1994).

The Adoption Assistance and Child Welfare Act of 1980 reformed the child welfare system by preventing the removal of children from their own homes and facilitating placement of children who enter substitute care in permanent family homes, either by reuniting them with their families of origin or through placement in adoptive homes (Stein 1991:37). By federal law each state designates a single agency to operate its child welfare programs, either in one centralized agency or decentralized to local units.

Nonrelative foster parents are carefully screened and trained before having a child placed in their home. The child may receive a monthly board payment rate determined by the state agency and a medical insurance card to cover health needs and allowances for food or furniture. The caregiver receives, on the child's behalf, case management from a caseworker who is part of a public or private child welfare agency. The caseworker is the foster parent's link to the resources of the larger system and is generally responsible for monitoring the care of the child in the foster parent's home. The intent is for the child to achieve legal permanence again, through adoption or guardianship, possibly by the foster parent or through returning to the parent's home.

Relatives, on the other hand, take children into their home because they are kin and often take on the care of the child with little notice. Relative foster care builds on a tradition of families caring for each other, especially in African American families (Stack 1974). Family care is generally considered the best option for children, based on the assumption that remaining within the kin network reduces trauma for children and maintains important relationships (Child Welfare League of America 1994). For example, research suggests that relative care is less likely to disrupt and to last longer then traditional foster care (Testa 1997; Wulczyn and Goerge 1992; Goerge 1990). Before the increased attention to kinship care, relative foster family members—caregivers, children, and children's birthparents—were not monitored as closely nor did they receive as many services as traditional foster parents. In most states, as the number of formal kinship placements increased, kinship care came under closer scrutiny.

The Adoption and Safe Families Act of 1997 mandated aggressive action toward permanency for all children, including those in formal relative care. An emphasis on legal permanence has taken on special meaning in kinship care because kin are encouraged to adopt children, which terminates the rights of parents and severs the foster parent's relationship with the child welfare agency. Other legal options, such as guardianship, do not require termination of parent rights but guardianship does not have a subsidy attached to it while adoption does. Kinship care families, as mentioned earlier, are often low income. They may have difficulty taking on the permanent care of children without some financial support, so guardianship may not be a realistic option. Eleven states are currently demonstration sites for a new permanency option—subsidized guardianship. With subsidized guardianship, children obtain legal permanency through guardianship and the relative may receive a subsidy for the care of the child, but the child welfare system no longer has monitoring or case-management responsibilities for the child and family.

The tension between private and public responsibility has increased with the greater numbers of kin foster parents and has affected policies about reimbursement and oversight for the children in kin care. Some states view kin placement as a way to divert children from the child welfare system. Others view kinship care as a form of family preservation. The majority of states view kin care as a foster placement, however, and relatives are supported at different levels depending on how they meet licensing standards (Gleeson and Craig 1994).

In the mid-1980s child welfare systems, especially in large urban areas, responded to the HIV epidemic as infected children entered the child welfare system because families could not or would not care for them (Boland et al. 1988). Child welfare agencies across the United States developed specialized foster care units to support foster homes where an infected child was placed (Taylor-Brown 1991; Gurdin and Anderson 1987).

HIV-infected children are defined as having "special needs," which entitles them to a higher monthly allowance from the state to support those needs. At least one child welfare agency in Illinois has developed a unit that specializes in relative placements of HIV-infected children; many of these caregivers are older women. In these cases, the children receive the same benefits as other HIV-infected children. In addition, caseworkers are trained to be attentive to the unique aspects of relative care, including family dynamics and role changes.

The child welfare system, by definition, is intended to meet the best interests of children and thus, the benefits, such as board payments or case management, focus on the well-being and safety of the child who is the ward of the state. In HIV child welfare services, the emphasis has also been on the infected child and his or her special physical and mental health needs. Increasingly, child welfare providers are being urged to provide services that meet the caregiver's needs as well as those of the children (Child Welfare League of America 1994). For example, as many relative caregivers are older, many have more health problems, and often have fewer financial resources (Berrick, Barth, and Needell 1994; Le Prohn 1994; Dubowitz, Feigelman, and Zuravin 1993; Thornton 1991).

Titles IV-B and IV-E of the Social Security Act are the main sources of federal funds that provide matching funds to the states for child welfare services, including board payments and related administrative and training costs. Families providing formal kinship care must meet certain standards to receive the board payments, depending on the state where they reside. Unlicensed kin caregivers, or those who cannot meet those standards, are often eligible to receive income support from the state's department of public assistance, rather than receive board payments or allowances from the child welfare system. In some states, the unlicensed caregiver can receive a foster care board payment that is lower than licensed foster care but higher than public assistance.

As formal kinship care has replaced informal care, the state and the federal governments are paying for more care through foster board payments, adoption subsidies, and human resources such as caseworkers. As kinship foster children have been less likely to reach legal permanency—adoption or guardianship—the children stay in the state child welfare system longer than do traditional foster children and use more resources than traditional foster care. In addition, foster board payments for HIV-infected children are based on-special needs reimbursement rates, making their costs to the system considerably higher than for noninfected children.

Legal permanence—adoption, guardianship, or return home—is the main goal of child welfare. Using legal permanence as a desired outcome, kinship care appears less successful than traditional foster care. Children in relative homes are less likely to be adopted and less likely to return home, thus remaining in the child welfare system longer. On the other hand, children in kin placements are also less likely to reenter the child welfare system once they leave and their placements are less likely to change or be disrupted (Courtney and Needell 1997; Berrick, Barth, and Needell 1994). These data suggest that stability may be an important outcome for children in kinship care, even if legal permanency is not. In addition, some recent data indicate that adoption of children in kinship care may be more prevalent or more likely than once thought (Testa et al. 1996). Research on relative care is only now catching up in response to the increasing need (Gleeson 1999).

Outcome data on infected children in foster care are nonexistent. Research and scholarly work has most often focused on the infected person rather than on the caregiver or siblings. There is a growing body of scholarly clinical work on the impact of HIV on the family; preliminary data suggest that HIV-affected relative caregivers have special needs related to stigma, loss, and support (Linsk and Poindexter 2000; Poindexter and Linsk 1999; Joslin, Mevi-Triano, and Berman 1997). Relative caregivers also report more severe emotional and behavioral problems with the HIV-affected children in their care (Mason and Linsk 1999). As the child welfare system develops its response to kinship care, we have an opportunity to advocate for services and polices that are responsive not only to infected children, but also to their affected relative caregivers.

Impact of Welfare Reform on Older Caregivers

Studies of grandparents who are raising grandchildren due to drug use (Minkler and Roe 1993) and incarceration (Dressel and Barnhill 1994) show that poverty is often a serious problem for many of these families. Poverty is also an issue for many grandparent caregivers where HIV has been identified in the home (Burnette 1999; Joslin, Mevi-Triano, and Berman 1997). Therefore, recent changes in policies pertaining to government cash and medical assistance to low-income families will affect this population.

The Personal Responsibility and Work Opportunity Reconciliation Act of 1996, usually referred to as "welfare reform," transformed the federal family assistance program to state block grants, which allowed individual states to determine which families receives assistance and under what circumstances. With welfare reform, Aid to Families with Dependent Children (AFDC) was repealed and replaced with Temporary Assistance to Needy Families (TANF) (Smith 1996). The new law ends the federal guarantee of cash assistance for children in low-income families (Darnell and Rosenbaum 1997). This legislation also ended the automatic link between cash assistance and health insurance (Medicaid) (Ellwood and Ku 1998; Darnell and Rosenbaum 1997). In 1993, AFDC assisted almost five million families, which included 9.8 million minor children (Darnell and Rosenbaum 1997). The Welfare Reform Information Center and Poverty Law Project (National Clearinghouse for Legal Services 1996) estimated that welfare reform would put 1.1 million children into poverty.

In terms of outcomes, on the positive side, there is a remnant of a safety net for poor children and families. The welfare reform law contains requirements that states cover anyone with Medicaid who is eligible through the old AFDC standards on July 16, 1996 (Darnell and Rosenbaum 1997). The State Children's Health Insurance Program (CHIP) of 1997 extends health insurance coverage for uninsured children, although it is not known whether states will be able to successfully and adequately address this need (Weissman et al. 1999). In addition, many children will receive Medicaid under an existing law phasing in guaranteed coverage for low-income children through 2002, although what happens after 2002 is unclear (Smith 1996).

Policies extending coverage for uninsured children but not adults demonstrates that as a society we have made a choice that may have unintended consequences for children. Having an HIV-positive adult family member who is without insurance and getting inadequate medical care affects resources available to both the children and grandparent caregivers. In addition, there are several reasons why welfare reform will likely decrease the financial well-being of some HIV-affected grandparent guardians.

First, receiving assistance is now tied to mandatory requirements to secure paid employment within two years of receiving aid; families can suffer reductions in their monthly checks as penalty for not meeting this requirement (Aaronson and Hartmann 1996; National Clearinghouse for Legal Services 1996), and the back-to-work requirement may not be reasonable for older adult caregivers (Mullen 2000). Many older parental surrogates are not receiving TANF because they are not legal guardians or foster parents, but for those who are on the TANF roles, these work requirements may be very difficult due to parenting responsibilities, their own health concerns or functional limitations, or caring for ill family members. In addition, there is no guarantee of childcare for working guardians (Aaronson and Hartmann 1996).

Second, there is a time limit of five years total in entitlement programs (Aaronson and Hartmann 1996), which generally will not support persons with HIV over the course of an illness that becomes more rather than less debilitating with time, thus putting an increased financial burden on the older caregivers. Mullen (2000) makes the important point that in households headed by older adults, including grandparents, where the child's parent is not present, there may be advantages of applying for "child-only benefits," which do not have the sixty-month time limit. She notes that "grandparents must weigh their family's need for additional cash assistance they would receive as part of the assistance unit against their grandchild's need for benefits beyond the time limits" (p. 118). Similarly, grandparents over age sixty-five should not be part of the assistance unit as they can apply for SSI benefits based on their own age.

Third is the problematic mandate that adolescent parents must live with their parents or in another adult-supervised setting (National Clearinghouse for Legal Services 1996), which sometimes forces conflicted families into the same household. This can negatively affect the grandparent caregiver who is struggling to maintain a problematic relationship with an HIV-positive adolescent parent of an HIV-infected or HIV-affected child.

Fourth, welfare reform has narrowed the eligibility criteria for Supplemental Security Income (SSI) for children with disabilities (Smith 1996; National Clearinghouse for Legal Services 1996), which affects grandparents raising children who have HIV.

Fifth, SSI and SSDI (Social Security Disability Income) have been eliminated for persons with substance use histories. In addition, persons who have been convicted of drug-related felonies will be barred for life from receiving TANF or food stamps unless the particular state opts out of this requirement (National Clearinghouse for Legal Services 1996). Obviously, the HIV-infected population intersects with the drug-using population, so multigenerational families with HIV who might have been supported on government assistance are ineligible in some cases due to these rules.

Sixth, the new requirement that paternity disclosure and the pursuing of child support be a prerequisite for receiving aid (National Clearinghouse for Legal Services 1996) is a potential disaster for HIV-affected grandparents who may not know who or where the fathers of their grandchildren are (Mullen 2000). Finally, immigrants who are not citizens usually are not eligible for SSI or food stamps (National Clearinghouse for Legal Services 1996), so grandparent caregivers who are newcomers cannot get financial support for their childrearing duties (Mullen 2000).

The health of children may suffer the most from welfare reform because Medicaid is attached to SSI and SSDI, and Medicaid is cut off one year after TANF is lost (Pappas 1998). With shifting state-determined eligibility requirements for Medicaid, children, parents, and families who have previously been able to rely on this source of medical coverage may lose their only insurance (Darnell and Rosenbaum 1997; Smith 1996).

States can now decide to terminate medical insurance for persons whom they say are refusing to work (Smith 1996). Previously, Medicaid did not require a separate application process and standards. Medicaid enrollment may be affected because of the added paperwork and effort required. People will probably wait until they have need for medical intervention, rather than enroll for primary care and prevention (Darnell and Rosenbaum 1997). In addition, there are questions about whether poor families losing cash assistance will know that they can still apply for Medicaid, and whether states will do outreach to them and try to insure coverage (Ellwood and Ku 1998). These reductions in Medicaid eligibility and the increased red tape of applying will make it more difficult for disabled HIV-infected children and adults to receive medical care, which will directly affect the already stressed, frightened, and frustrated grandparent caregivers.

Managed Care Impacts on Older HIV Caregivers

The health of children with HIV is of great concern to their caregivers, as is their access to medical and mental health services. One of the recent policy trends affecting grandparent caregivers grew out of the Managed Care Act of 1973, which gave legal sanction to Health Maintenance Organizations (HMOs) and repealed all existing measures preventing prepaid medical care (Gallagher 1999). Although managed care is more of a delivery mechanism than a policy per se, it was developed through legislative policy and as such is discussed here. As of 1995, more than 11 percent of people on Medicare and 32 percent of people on Medicaid were under a managed care system (Gamliel, Singer, and Marconi 1998). Analysis by the Center for Health Policy Research indicates that in purchasing managed care services, relatively few state Medicaid agencies either address HIV or AIDS specifically or require collaborative partnerships between the plans and state and local agencies responsible for communicable disease control (Wehr and Rauch 1998). More and more, managed care is affecting persons with HIV and therefore their caregivers. The number of privately insured persons with HIV who are in HMOs is growing, as is the trend of states moving Medicaid recipients into managed care plans (Katz et al. 1997).

Managed care systems were developed to contain health care costs, an outcome that theoretically benefits all of society. However, with the trend toward delivering health care by for-profit organizations, we are seeing a shift from quality of care to cost containment as the primary focus. Several aspects of managed care reflect issues are problematic for HIV-infected children and their caregivers as well. Strom-Gottfried (1998) outlines these general concerns: capitation of costs, gatekeeping, financial incentives, and ethical compromises by providers.

On the positive side, the cost-containment trend in managed care could be used as an advantage for programs that promote early intervention, health maintenance, functioning, and rehabilitation for persons living with HIV (Montoya et al. 1997). Several successful models for HIV-related managed care are more responsive to HIV-affected families and operate with HIV specialists. These programs tend toward centralized care systems and specialty HIV clinics with multidisciplinary teams, which are accessible and responsive to HIV-affected families (Melchior, De Veauuse, and Huba 1998; Havens et. al 1997). Some include a more realistic and higher rate of reimbursement, called a risk-adjusted capitated rate, based on historic data for costs for persons who have AIDS (Burr 1999; Bartlett 1996).

However, many of the consequences of managed care are of concern to HIV-affected grandparent caregivers. For example, because of managed care, there is a trend to close down or downsize inpatient and outpatient units, which serve adults and children with HIV. Community health centers are therefore attracting more HIV-affected families and thus doing more hospital rounds, but not getting more financial compensation for their increased workloads (Gallagher 1999), a fact that is likely to affect quality of care. Managed care may weaken the health-care system's ability to diagnose and treat tuberculosis, sexually transmitted disease and HIV; conduct public health disease surveillance and outbreak control; provide sexual and drug contact tracing; and offer health education (Rutherford 1998). Gamliel et al. (1998) found that managed care's capitated payment system creates incentives to limit services and to avoid caring for people at high risk or requiring high care. People with disabilities or chronic impairments, including adults and children with HIV, are therefore at greater risk of losing coverage, and those with coverage may receive limited access to care, care of lesser quality, or inappropriate care. They conclude that we need systems that adequately reimburse providers and have standards for quality of care. Kocurek (1996) warns that there is a danger that the practitioner in managed care will lost sight of the whole person when doing HIV care and focus on micro-management, the difficulties with complex new therapies, and the financial aspects of care. In a study of satisfaction with medical care in a sample of 593 HIV-infected men identified as gay or bisexual (Katz et al. 1997), men with fee-for-service insurance were significantly more satisfied with their interpersonal relationships with care providers than those in managed care organizations, but they were less satisfied with the financial aspects of their plans. This fits with findings from the general population.

Managed care usually does not operate on a family-centered model. HIV-affected families often experience frustration and bewilderment with truncated and uncoordinated medical care that involves various sites, physicians, and case managers. The lack of a family-focused approach is exacerbated when the definition of family is not a mother and her children, as is the case of grandparent and other kin care. Children with HIV may not as easily go outside the provider group for second opinions or specialists. Persons on Medicaid and/or Medicare in some states will get no choice about provider groups, so families will be limited in access to choice in care. With Medicaid and Medicare managed care, the burden shifts to the family to negotiate changes in programs, policies, and eligibility status. In addition, managed-care groups may discontinue Medicare recipients, which means a sudden change and the loss of a trusted provider. Managed care systems may limit access to appropriate, state of the art, aggressive treatments; sabotage the vital patient-provider partnership; dilute consumer-centered care; and make it more difficult to access supportive counseling, which usually requires a mental-health diagnosis and may be severely time limited. All of these consequences for children and adults with HIV directly affect the grandparent caregivers, who are focused on the well-being of their family members and who have taken on the responsibility for coordinating their care and negotiating difficult service systems. Given combination therapies and drops in the death rate, there may be less emphasis on HIV and related support systems as HIV becomes defined by a poorer, often substance-abusing population and populations of color.

Policy Issues for the Future

Systems of Care

In reviewing these opportunities to address needs of older caregivers caring for children affected by HIV, we offer some policy suggestions. Our first suggestion is the need for a system of care that does not create obstacles for older caregiving families. The confluence of older adults caring for children with special needs defines the need for at least two care receivers per family, the child and the older adult, yet most of our care systems are categorical and often age-specific. This can create burdens for the caregiving family regarding travel, expense, coordination, and added stress and paperwork. Without this more inclusive definition of client, providers may face limits in offering case management, counseling, transportation, or other needed services. We suggest that policies seek to create communication mechanisms that integrate the care plan across involved systems of care, insuring that care is delivered to all family members and the needs of both older caregivers and younger care receivers is included in the overall plan. Care coordination across service networks would assure child welfare or HIV service agencies that they do not need to take sole responsibility for specific families.

Although this issue transcends location, one improvement would be to develop one-stop shopping for all family members versus specialized care services, either in a family medicine context or by offering geriatric and child-related services under a single organizational auspice. Although clinics may occasionally be co-housed in the same location, this remains an exceptional situation and should be applied wherever possible.

Family-Based Services

Related is a concern about how to create policies that ensure that services are integrated or at least complimentary when both caregiver and care receiver need medical and social support. Policy makers and program managers need to find policies that honor and validate these families. This will require modifying reimbursement and funding mechanisms to broaden the definition of the client and the scope of services. Caregivers are likely to advocate and accept care for their childcare receivers rather than for themselves. Offering help to help the children may be an effective way to engage caregivers in helping find ways to be more responsive to families.

In addition, policy makers need to find ways to insure that caregivers also receive care for themselves. When program developers and case managers consider the needs of persons with HIV, the whole family system should be taken into account. Policy makers may consider how to support the caregiver as well as the persons with HIV and be aware of the tendency of overburdened older caregivers to neglect their own needs, because this neglect could lead to a rapid physical and mental burnout. Finally, care to the family should be flexible enough to extend a specific amount of time past the death of an infected member.

Practitioners in the aging network, clinics and hospitals, and AIDS service organizations should be more aware of the older vulnerable caregivers who are silently and secretly supporting family members with HIV. Targeted outreach to caregivers is needed so that respite care, benefits advocacy, support groups, counseling, case management, bereavement support, transportation, financial and nutritional assistance, and information on resources, HIV disease, and how to provide personal care can be obtained for the family (see Joslin and Nazon 1996). In addition, practitioners have an advocacy role on a number of levels to include older caregivers in legislative authorization for HIV programs and older adult programs and ensure that organizations address older adult caregivers as part of the family of the clients that are served.

Recognizing the Benefits of the Care Relationship to the Caregiver

Current policies all too often neglect the caregivers in determining care needs of the care receivers. As noted earlier, in functional assessment programs the existence of the caregiver is either ignored or their presence is calculated as "social support," which then means that the care recipient is assessed as needing less service. No current programs outside of Ryan White CARE Title IV seem to address this issue. Family care can be primary in terms of its centrality to the needs of the recipient, it can be secondary or adjunctive to care provided by professionals or subprofessionals, or it may be complementary to other care provided.

How would these suggestions change the life of a caregiver like Lacy, whose story introduced the chapter? We can consider the following as a possible scenario:

As an older adult providing family care to several relatives, Lacy has come to the attention of service providers in the HIV service network as well as the aging and disability service arena. These providers recognize that because she is growing older and taking on the burden of care for multiple family members, she may have particular care needs. She is sent to a caregiver support agency that completes a full family assessment of the care she is providing, how the benefits and regulations between them can be integrated to maximize the care for all, the role of various family members in supporting the care, and what supports she will need to sustain care. She is offered a number of support services to sustain her. These include a one-stop, family-based medical care facility at which primary care for all of the family members can be obtained, with referrals to specialists as needed. She is referred to a support network that includes telephone support, Internet discussion groups, and face-to-face support groups with caregivers that include transportation and childcare. She also is made aware of a variety of respite services that can give her a break. In fact, due to the variety of care she provides, the care manager nominates her for a caregiver of the month award, which includes recognition for her work as well as some nominal prizes and a certificate recognizing her efforts. She is encouraged to come in for a semiannual caregiver assessment that will include examining her changing caregiving needs as well as her own needs for care and support.

Conclusions

The current availability of more effective medical treatment that may greatly extend the quantity of life and enhance the quality of life for HIV-infected citizens coincides with a political climate that may diminish access to care and services. Current policy proposals, laws, and political trends tend to exacerbate rather than relieve the problems of children with HIV and their elder caregivers.

Policies and programs need to address the need for more information and awareness about this population. Practitioners in the aging network, in hospitals, and in AIDS service organizations should be more aware of the needs of vulnerable grandparent caregivers who are silently supporting family members with HIV. If policies address the caregiver as well as the care receiver, they may encourage providers to consider families as a unit.

Policies would best equip practitioners to aggressively seek and deliver care, information, and supportive services to older HIV-affected caregivers and to help them enhance their naturally occurring sources for social, emotional, and practical support. Policies need to ensure that support groups, information, advocacy, counseling, and case management must be confidential, trustworthy, and accessible to this population. Caregivers need access to respite care, home health and hospice services, counseling for emotional support, education about providing personal care to someone who is critically ill, bereavement support, transportation, and financial and nutritional assistance.

These will only be available if policies support assessment of caregiver needs and how to ensure they receive needed services.

Given that the older adult has elected to provide ongoing care to raise the child, policies should first be directed to the child's needs in terms of eligibility and the forms of the benefit. Care provided by older adults may be unlike caregiver services for dependent elders and for parents of disabled children, where caregivers are presumable competent adults. Grandparents or older caregivers might also have significant age related needs that require attention and may qualify for service among the federal or local programs described above and in earlier chapters. The caregiver should not be penalized for providing family care.

Our programs need to address the unique aging needs of older caregivers and help them to feel connected, supported, and recognized for their contributions. This is particularly a challenge given the complexity, stigma, and uncertainties of HIV, whether one is affected as a person living with HIV or as a family member. Our responsibility as practitioners, researchers, and policy makers is to find a way to facilitate their care, sustain that care, and care for them as well as those for whom they provide vital support and assistance.

Acknowledgments

The authors thank Regina Kulys and Elizabeth Essex for their useful comments that contributed to this chapter.

Notes

1. All names are changed to protect confidentiality.
2. The following discussion reflects earlier work by Linsk et al. (1992).

References

Aaronson, S., and H. Hartmann. 1996. Reform, not rhetoric: A critique of welfare policy and charting of new directions. *American Journal of Orthopsychiatry* 66 (4): 583–598.

Abramowitz, M. 1988. *Regulating the Lives of Women: Social Welfare from Colonial Times to the Present*. Boston: South End Press.

Bartlett, J. G. 1996. HIV managed care through a hospital system of care: The Johns Hopkins HIV care program. Paper presented at American Public Health Association 124th Annual Meeting.

Berrick, J .D., R. P. Barth, and B. Needell. 1994. A comparison of kinship foster homes and foster family homes: Implications for kinship care as family preservation. *Children and Youth Services Review* 16:33–63.

Boland, M. G., T. J. Allen, G. I. Long, and M. Tasker. 1988. Children with HIV infection: Collaborative responsibilities of the child welfare and medical communities. *Social Work* (November–December): 504–509.

Burnette, D. 1999. Custodial grandparents in Latino families: Patterns of service use and predictors of unmet needs. *Social Work* 44 (1): 22–35.

Burr, C. 1999. The AIDS-friendly HMO. *Poz* (August): 36–37.

Child Welfare League of America. 1994. *Kinship Care: A Natural Bridge*. Washington, D.C.: Child Welfare League of America.

Courtney, M. E., and B. Needell. 1997. Outcomes of kinship care: Lessons from California. *Child Welfare Research Review* 2:129–159.

Darnell, J., and S. Rosenbaum. 1997. Welfare reform: Unanticipated but inevitable consequences for health insurance coverage for the poor. *Nutrition* 13 (5): 490–491.

DiNitto, D. M. 2000. *Social Welfare: Politics and Public Policy*. 5th ed. Boston: Allyn & Bacon.

Dressel, P. L., and S. K. Barnhill. 1994. Reframing gerontological thought and practice: The case of grandmothers with daughters in prison. *The Gerontologist* 34 (5): 685–690.

Dubowitz, H., S. Feigelman, and S. Zuravin. 1993. A profile of kinship care. *Child Welfare* 72:153–169.

Ellwood, M. R., and L. Ku. 1998. Welfare and immigration reforms: Unintended side effects for Medicaid. *Health Affairs* 17 (3): 137–151.

Gallagher, D. M. 1999. The era of managed care: The struggle of cost containment and compassionate, effective care of persons with HIV/AIDS. *Nursing Clinics of North America* 34 (1): 227–235.

Gamliel, S., B. Singer, and K. Marconi. 1998. HIV healthcare delivery and managed care: Applications and implications from the special projects of national significance program. *Home Health Care Services Quarterly* 17 (1): 101–109.

Gilbert, N., and H. Specht. 1986. *Dimensions of Social Welfare Policy*. 2d ed. Englewood Cliffs, N.J.: Prentice Hall.

Gleeson, J. P. 1999. Kinship care as a child welfare services: What do we really know. In J. P. Gleeson and C. F. Hairston, eds., *Kinship Care: Improving Practice through Research*, pp. 3–34. Washington, D.C.: Child Welfare League of America.

Gleeson, J. P., and L. C. Craig. 1994. Kinship care in child welfare: An analysis of states' policies. *Children and Youth Services Review* 16:7–31.

Goerge, R. M. (1990). The reunification process in substitute care. *Social Service Review* 64:422–457.

Gurdin, P., and G. R. Anderson. 1987. Quality care for ill children: AIDS-specialized foster family homes. *Child Welfare* 66:291–302.

Havens, P. L., B. E. Cuene, D. Waters, J. Hand, and M. J. Chusid. 1997. Structure of a primary care support system to coordinate comprehensive care for children and families infected/affected by human immunodeficiency virus in a managed care environment. *Pediatric Infectious Disease Journal* 16 (2): 211–216.

Hegar, R. L., and M. Scannapieco. 1995. From family duty to family policy: The evolution of kinship care. *Child Welfare* 74:200–216.

Hill, R. B. 1977. *Informal Adoption among Black Families*. Washington, D.C.: National Urban League Research Department.

Hooyman, N., and H. A. Kiyak. 1996. *Social Gerontology: A Multidisciplinary Perspective.* Boston: Allyn & Bacon.

Joslin, D., and M. Nazon. 1996. HIV and aging networks. In K. M. Nokes, ed., *HIV/AIDS and the Older Adult,* pp. 129–141. Washington, D.C.: Taylor and Francis.

Joslin, D., D. Mevi-Triano, and J. Berman. 1997. Grandparents raising children orphaned by HIV/AIDS: Health risks and service needs. Paper presented at 50th Annual Scientific Meeting of the Gerontological Society of America, Cincinnati.

Katz, M. H., R. Marx, J. M. Douglas, G. A. Bolan, M. Park, R. J. Gurley, and S. P. Buchbinder. 1997. Insurance type and satisfaction with medical care among HIV-infected men. *Journal of Acquired Immune Deficiency Syndromes and Human Retrovirology* 14:35–43.

Kocurek, K. 1996. Primary care of the HIV patient: Standard practice and new developments in the era of managed care. *Medical Clinics in North America* 80 (2): 375–410.

Le Prohn, N. S. 1994. The role of the kinship foster parent: A comparison of the role conceptions of relative and non-relative foster parents. *Children and Youth Services Review* 16:107–122.

Linsk, N., S. M. Keigher, S. L. Rusinowitz, and S. E. England. 1992. *Wages for Caring: Compensating Family Care of the Elderly.* Westport, Conn.: Greenwood.

Linsk, N. L., and C. C. Poindexter. 2000. Older caregivers for family members with HIV or AIDS: Reasons for caring. *Journal of Applied Gerontology* 19 (2): 181–202.

Mason, S., and N. Linsk. 1999. Kin caregivers of HIV-affected children: Identifying services that support permanency. Report submitted to the Children and Family Research Center, Urbana, Illinois.

Melchior, L. A., M. De Veauuse, and G. J. Huba. 1998. Qualitative issues related to the transprofessional model of end-stage AIDS care. *Home Health Care Services Quarterly* 17 (1): 93–99.

Minkler, M., and K. M. Roe. 1993. *Grandmothers as Caregivers: Raising Children of the Crack Cocaine Epidemic.* Newbury Park, Calif.: Sage.

Montoya, I. D., J. W. Carlson, A. J. Richard, and W. A. Goodpastor. 1997. Managed care, cost-effectiveness, and rehabilitation: The case of HIV. *Rehabilitation Nursing* 22 (1): 7–19.

Moore, C. 2000. Personal communication.

Mullen, F. 2000. Grandparents and welfare reform. In C. Cox, ed., *To Grandmother's House We Go and Stay: Perspectives on Custodial Grandparents,* pp. 113–131. New York: Springer.

National Clearinghouse for Legal Services. 1996. The Federal welfare reform bill (1996). *Illinois Welfare News* 2 (4): 1–5, 10.

Osterbusch, S. E., S. M. Keigher, B. Miller, and N. L. Linsk. 1986. Community care policies and gender justice. *International Journal of Health Services Research* 17:217–232.

Pappas, G. 1998. Monitoring the health consequences of welfare reform. *International Journal of Health Services* 28 (4): 703–713.

Poindexter, C. C. 1997. Stigma and support as experienced by HIV-affected older minority caregivers. Ph.D. dissertation, University of Illinois at Chicago.

——. 1998. Promises in the plague: The Ryan White CARE Act as a case study for legislative action. *Health and Social Work* 24 (1): 35–41.

Poindexter, C. C., and N. L. Linsk. 1999. HIV-related stigma in a sample of HIV-affected older female African-American caregivers. *Social Work* 44:46–61.

Rutherford, G. W. 1998. Public health, communicable diseases, and managed care: Will managed care improve or weaken communicable disease control? *American Journal of Preventive Medicine* 14 (3S): 53–59.

Smith, K. 1996. Highlights of the impact of welfare reform legislation on children. *Pediatric Nursing* 22 (6): 564.

Stack, C. 1974. *All Our Kin: Strategies for Survival in a Black Community.* New York: Harper & Row.

Stein, T. 1991. *Child Welfare and the Law.* New York: Longman.

Strom-Gottfried, K. 1998. Is "ethical managed care" an oxymoron? *Families in Society* 79 (3): 297–307.

Taylor-Brown, S. 1991. The impact of AIDS on foster care: A family-centered approach to services in the United States. *Child Welfare* 70:193–209.

Testa, M. 1997. Kinship foster care in Illinois. *Child Welfare Research Review* 2:101–129.

Testa, M. F., K. L. Shook, L. S. Cohen, and M. G. Woods. (1996). Permanency planning options for children in formal kinship care. *Child Welfare* 75:451–470.

Thornton, J. L. 1991. Permanency planning for children in kinship foster homes. *Child Welfare* 70:593–601.

Wehr, E., and K. J. Rauch. 1998. Privatizing Medicaid: The implications for HIV prevention of privatizing government financing for health care services for low income populations. *International Conference on AIDS* 12:1061–1062.

Weissman, J. S., R. Witzburg, P. Linov, and E. G. Campbell. 1999. Termination from Medicaid: How does it affect access, continuity of care, and willingness to purchase insurance? *Journal of Health Care for the Poor and Underserved* 10 (1): 122–137.

White House Conference on Aging. 1996. *Final Report: 1995 White House Conference on Aging.* Washington, D.C.: U.S. Government Printing Office.

Wulczyn, F. H., and R.M. Goerge. 1992. Foster care in New York and Illinois: The challenge of rapid change. *Social Service Review* 66:278–294.

14

Global Implications

NAMPOSYA NAMPANYA-SERPELL

AIDS remains an unabated epidemic in many countries around the world. Data released by UNAIDS indicate that in 1999 an estimated 5.4 million adults and children became infected with the virus, bringing the worldwide total to an estimated 50 million since the disease was first recognized in 1981. Of that number, more than 34.3 million infected people are still alive. However, AIDS has killed 18.8 million, including 2.8 million who died in 1999 alone, a record level for any one year (UN AIDS Commission 2000).

The global and ecological catastrophe of this pandemic has given rise not only to personal tragedies for the individuals and families facing prolonged illness and premature deaths, but also to the increase in the number of orphans and HIV-affected children around the world, especially in sub-Saharan Africa, South and Southeast Asia, and the Caribbean. Parental deaths from HIV/AIDS have increased pressure on the elderly, particularly grandmothers, to care for these vulnerable children. Yet, at the family level, loss of breadwinners to AIDS, loss of income, impoverishment, loss of adult labor, changes in household and family structures, and grief and bereavement have all created an environment where it is much more difficult for the elderly to care adequately for orphaned children's needs as well as their own needs.

Global Epidemiology of HIV Disease

One of the most tragic results of AIDS-related premature parental deaths is the exponential rise in the number of orphaned and vulnerable children in diverse communities around the world. At the end of 1999, UNICEF estimated the number of children below fifteen years of age who had been orphaned by AIDS around the world to be approximately 10.4 million, with the majority (8.2 million) of those without a mother or both parents living in sub-Saharan Africa. Before AIDS, orphaning due to accidents, chronic diseases, wars, or natural disasters (e.g., floods, earthquakes, and fires) was a familiar phenomenon, at 1 percent of the child population in the industrialized world and just over 2 percent in sub-Saharan Africa. However, the rate at which orphaning is occurring due to the AIDS pandemic has reached alarming proportions. Estimates are staggering: 11 percent of children in Uganda; 9 percent in Zambia; 7 percent in Zimbabwe; and 6 percent in Malawi are now orphans because of AIDS (UNICEF 1999).

In Asia, it is estimated that the orphan population tripled between 1994 and 1999. Cambodia and Thailand are reported to have the highest proportion of AIDS orphans (one or both parents have died) in the Asian Pacific region. It is estimated that there are currently more than thirty thousand children under the age of fifteen orphaned by AIDS in Cambodia and that the number is likely to go up to 140,000 (approximately 3%) of all children under the age of fifteen by 2005 (Khmer HIV/AIDS NGO Alliance 2000). Another major concern of the UN AIDS Commission (UNAIDS) for Asia is the growing number of children living with an HIV-positive parent, which is far greater than the number of children already orphaned.

The global and systematic devastation of affected families and households by the AIDS pandemic is unprecedented in human history. Yet the impact of the disease on elderly caregivers of HIV/AIDS-infected or -affected children has not received much attention, either in research or action. Although there are data on the global epidemiology of HIV/AIDS, mother-to-child HIV transmission, and the growing number of orphaned children especially in sub-Saharan Africa, empirical research is lacking on the devastating impact of the epidemic on the lives of the elderly caregivers for those children at household level, and how the role of grandparenting has changed due to the AIDS pandemic.

The United Nations declared 1999 the International Year of Older Persons. In the briefing documents, strategy, and future policy development about the elderly, emphasis was placed on "two possible approaches to preparing long-term perspective plans on ageing. The first was to see older people (however defined) as a distinct group in society and to try to develop ways of improving their experience. The second was to try to improve the experiences of people generally, while at the same time dismantling the barriers that segregate older people from the rest of society." This was a welcome development. However, there is also need to pay attention to the impact of HIV/AIDS on grandparents or elderly caregivers for HIV/AIDS-infected/orphaned/affected (IOA) children as a distinct group in need of special attention worldwide.

In sub-Saharan Africa, grandparenting is viewed in the context of the social and cultural group process within the extended family, involving relationships and interdependence between three generations—mothers, grandmothers, and daughters. The issue of a skipped generation from grandmothers to grandchildren has not yet received adequate acknowledgment and/or research. There are however, a number of case studies and anecdotal accounts gathered about their status, especially the increased pressure on the elderly grandparents to take full responsibility for raising orphans in the wake of the HIV/AIDS pandemic. Some of this limited research on grandparents has revealed that most of these caregivers are elderly grandmothers over sixty years of age, are economically disadvantaged, and have been left with large numbers of orphans to care for (Serpell 1996; Barnett and Blaikie 1992; Foster et al. 1994; Hunter 1990). There has not yet been comprehensive research/surveys undertaken in sub-Saharan Africa and other parts of the world that focuses directly on the elderly caregivers of HIV/AIDS- infected/orphaned/affected children.

The aim of this chapter is to respond to the need for a global perspective on the impact of the AIDS pandemic on the elderly caregivers of the IOA children. The chapter will review how the AIDS pandemic has increased the number of sick and orphaned children around the world, thereby increasing the pressure on the elderly, especially grandmothers, to assume responsibility for these children; trends in HIV infection among women; current policy responses to the needs of elderly caregivers; and global policies and strategies that could be developed through the UN system to support elderly caregivers. Particular attention will be paid to sub-Saharan Africa because of the catastrophic loss of the parental generation and AIDS' being viewed as the "grandmother's disease."

HIV Infection in Women and Children

By the end of 1999, there were an estimated 15.7 million women living with HIV/AIDS globally; 7.7 million women have died since the beginning of the epidemic in the early 1980s. In 1999 alone, 2.3 million women worldwide were infected by HIV and 1.2 million died (UN AIDS Commission 2000). In Africa, the number of women with HIV now surpasses that of men. Of the 22.3 million adults in sub-Saharan Africa infected with HIV, 12.2 million, or 55 percent, are women; in North America 20 percent; in Western Europe 20 percent; in the Caribbean 35 percent; in Latin America 20 percent; in South and Southeast Asia 30 percent; in North Africa and the Middle East 20 percent; and in Australia and New Zealand 10 percent.

The UNAIDS report estimated that 620,000 children (age 0–15) were infected with HIV globally in 1999. Most of these children (530,000) lived in sub-Saharan Africa and became infected before or during birth or through breastfeeding. In contrast, fewer than 1,000 infants were reported infected in the whole of North America and Western Europe in the same year (UN AIDS Commission 2000).

Poverty, lack of health services, lack of preventive services, and lack of access to drug therapies accounted for some of this large global disparity. HIV-positive women in industrialized countries who become pregnant receive the antiretroviral drug Zidovudine (AZT) from the fourteenth week of pregnancy. The drug is also administered to infants for six weeks after birth. Access to Caesarian delivery and to safe artificial feeding also reduces the risk of mother-to-child transmission. These are very expensive regimes and are reported to account for a 5 percent or lower transmission rate in France and the United States. In developing countries, between 25 percent and 35 percent of children born to HIV-positive mothers acquire the disease during pregnancy or childbirth or through breastfeeding (UNICEF 1999).

In Asia, according to UNICEF, HIV prevalence among children is increasing in a number of countries that, until recently, had a relatively low incidence. For instance, in India, 48,000 children were infected with HIV at the end of 1997, triple the number infected in 1994. In China, Namibia, and Vietnam—countries that had maintained low levels of seroprevalence—the rate of infection among children quadrupled between 1994 and 1997.

Grandmothers as Surrogate Parents

Elderly caregivers are, according to Kreibick (1995), sometimes the forgotten casualties of the AIDS pandemic. Because AIDS affects young adults of childbearing age more often than not, grandparents have to raise not only their grandchildren but also their great-grandchildren because of HIV/AIDS. In a study of AIDS-orphaned children ages fifteen and younger in Zimbabwe, grandparents were the caregivers in 45 percent of the households. One-third of these grandparents were at least sixty years of age (Foster et al. 1996).

Limited data suggest that when a mother dies of AIDS in the United States, children most often go to live with a grandmother or aunt. In a pilot study in the New York City Division of AIDS Services, it was found that 58 percent of the children went to live with grandmothers or aunts, 16 percent of the caregivers were grandparents, and when a mother used injection drugs or lived alone, in a shelter, or with friends, almost 25 percent of all the children were cared for by their grandparents (Levine 1995).

In Cambodia, grandparents were found to be the favored option as caregivers of orphans because they were seen as having close blood ties to the children and would therefore be motivated to care for them. The children also felt that living with grandparents would reduce the stigma from their neighbors. The downside to this, according to another report, is that there are relatively few grandparents in Cambodia. Only 4 percent of the population is over sixty years compared to Singapore, which has 10 percent. "Quite often, those adults dying of AIDS were themselves adopted by these 'grandparents' after their own parents died during the Khmer Rouge era. Grandparents also have concerns of their own. Most will have given up work and will themselves be dependent on their extended family. Some are ill and infirm and find it difficult to have to start work again. Because of their age, they are usually denied credit, which makes it difficult for them to start small businesses. Very often, an older orphan will have to generate income for the grandparents and other siblings. Even despite this, grandparents as caregivers were seen to better provide for orphans socially, psychologically and physically than anyone else" (Khmer HIV/AIDS NGO Alliance 2000:26).

In addition to caring for orphans, grandparents have the added burden of caring for their HIV/AIDS-infected children, especially in developing countries. For instance, research undertaken in Thailand reveals extensive parental involvement in living and caretaking arrangements of adult children with HIV/AIDS. Thus, nearly two-thirds of adults who died of AIDS had lived during their illness with or next to a parent, and a similar proportion had been cared for by a parent. Among those living with a parent, these proportions exceeded three out of four. In half of the cases the mother was the main caregiver (Knodel and Van Landingham 2000). Studies done in sub-Saharan Africa have revealed similar patterns—that is, most persons with AIDS are eventually cared for by their parents or live with them shortly before they die

(Barnett and Blaikie 1992; Hunter 1991). The burden of care on elderly parents in Africa is exacerbated by the fact that in normal circumstances adult children are often the main source of support and care for parents in old age. Thus, given the length of illness and disability associated with HIV/AIDS, the impact of long-term care of adult sick children is particularly taxing for elderly parents.

The Grandmothers' Disease: Sub-Saharan Africa

In many parts of sub-Saharan Africa, AIDS is called the "grandmother's disease" because the burden of caring for the sick and surviving children falls on these mostly elderly women. Increased pressure on grandparents to look after AIDS orphaned children has been discussed in almost all the studies on orphaned children in Africa (Serpell 1998; Foster et al. 1994; Barnett and Blaikie 1992; Hunter 1991). Like Hunter and Barnett and Blaikie in their studies of Uganda, Foster and colleagues observed increasing reliance on grandparents as caretakers of AIDS-orphaned children in Zimbabwe. Most of these grandparents have neither the physical energy nor the financial resources to care adequately for those children. In fact, in normal circumstances these grandparents would themselves be dependents of their sons and daughters who are dying of AIDS.

The extent of the devastation of the AIDS pandemic on families, especially caregivers of AIDS orphans, cannot be sufficiently understood without putting an elderly, especially grandparent's, face on the situation.

To illustrate the point, the following two cases cited in surveys conducted on orphans in Uganda. The first is a story of a sixty-nine-year-old grandmother in Rakai district of Uganda, interviewed by Tom Masland and Rod Nordland (2000). According to UNICEF, Uganda has an estimated 1.1 million AIDS orphans.

The grandmother lives on a farm in Rakai district where 75,000 (32%) children under fifteen years old have been orphaned. Of the four daughters and nine sons, eleven have died, leaving her with many grandchildren to take care of. At first, there were twenty-two orphans living in a single hut. Her children didn't leave her with any means to look after the young ones. All they had was sold to help treat her sons and daughters. Overwhelmed, she took the children to the hut one day. "I told them to shut the door so we could all starve to death inside and join the others!" she said.

One of her surviving daughters returned home to help and an NGO-World Vision grant provided a three-bedroom house for the family.

Another grandmother interviewed in the same district was seventy years old, lost all eleven children, and was left with thirty-five grandchildren to take care of. "I was a woman struck with sorrow beyond tears!" she said.

These women are not alone. According to Uganda Women's Effort to Save Orphans (UWESO), one out of every four families in Uganda is now caring for an AIDS orphan. Elderly caregivers, especially grandparents, fear that they will not have the resources, energy, patience, or continued good health to cope with raising young children.

Household Impact:
What Happens to the Family when the Parents Die

Some factors that exacerbate the situation of elderly caregivers in sub-Saharan Africa include poverty (change in socioeconomic status [SES] of the caregiving family after breadwinners die), family displacement, old age, poor health, high fertility rates, higher HIV/AIDS-related deaths, and unprecedented higher numbers of vulnerable children due to HIV/AIDS. A survey of rural and urban HIV/AIDS-affected households in Zambia (Serpell 1996) revealed the following findings:

RELATIVE CHANGE IN THE SOCIOECONOMIC STATUS OF HIV/AIDS— AFFECTED FAMILIES   In the urban sample, 70 percent of deaths reported in AIDS-affected families were paternal; the majority of those were also the major breadwinners for those families as well as having been tenants of job related housing. These families were more likely to suffer economically than those households in which mothers died first. A review of the financial status of sixty families revealed a common pattern in which there was a considerable drop in the income level and/or family assets following the death of the father. The magnitude of this drop was dramatic, constituting a reduction of monthly disposable income by more than 80 percent for more than two-thirds of the families, and apparently rapid, such that the relative poverty profile of families within six months of the death of the breadwinner was very similar to that of families bereaved of their breadwinner as much as four years earlier.

FAMILY DISPLACEMENT   In the urban sample, the majority of HIV/AIDS–affected families (approximately 61%) had moved from their original home (which was provided by the deceased parents' employers) to cheaper housing on the outskirts of Lusaka. Most of them had also moved from relatively wealthy neighborhoods with good schools, electricity, and piped water supply to poorer site and service housing/compounds, sometimes without electricity and/or piped water. Thus, of the 141 households that had moved, 31 (approximately 22%) had lost electricity when they moved, and 55 (approximately 39%) of the households had lost piped water in their homes and had to draw water from the shared standpipes outside their houses. Some families did not have to move, either because their breadwinner (usually a father) was still alive and/or the family had built/bought their own home before the breadwinner died. Of the twenty-two families that did not move, eleven were now living in two rooms and renting out the rest of their rooms to earn some income. This resulted in overcrowding, with as many as five to eight children in one room.

Although family displacement was not a major issue in the rural sample because most of the families stayed in their original homesteads, labor loss was a critical issue. Most of the deceased fathers were subsistence farmers, so that on their deaths the food security of their surviving families became threatened, particularly because most of the heads of households were elderly maternal grandparents who lacked the energy to plow the fields or the financial resources to employ workers to help them grow more food. Fifty-seven percent of the caregivers in the rural sample were grandparents; 42 percent were maternal grandmothers; 38 percent of the grandparents were sixty years and older. More than 40 percent were classified in category five of the socioeconomic status (SES) scale, that is, as peasant farmers with insufficient food to last until the next rainy season.

Approximately 21 percent of females and 17 percent of males in the urban sample had dropped out of school, whereas over 8 percent of the girls and 6 percent of the boys in the rural sample dropped out of school after parental death.

Because of the high fertility rate in Zambia, estimated at 6.5 in 1992, a single HIV-infected mother directly affects the lives of four to ten children. The death of a father affects the standard of living and source of livelihood not only of his surviving children, but also of a wilder circle of the extended family. For instance, in the urban study indicated earlier, there were a number of families comprised of as many as ten to eighteen dependents, including orphans and grandparents living in the same household. Usually such families occupied very little living space (e.g., two small rooms). Thirty-five percent of AIDS-affected families in the rural sample had ten, 21 percent had twelve, and 5 percent had eighteen members living in the same house. Similar data have been reported for many sub-Saharan countries (e.g., Kenya, Malawi, Tanzania, and Uganda) (World Bank 1998; Hunter 1991).

In the United States, as noted, when a mother dies of AIDS her children go to live with a grandmother or aunt. Thus, for many young grandparents who are still in the labor market, providing childcare means that they are faced with long, taxing days. For those already retired, providing childcare means that they have less time to pursue other activities. Jendrek (1993) found that 80 percent of grandparents who cared for their grandchildren, either by becoming custodial guardians or providing daycare, had to alter routines and plans in order to care for their grandchildren, and 50 percent had less time for themselves and friends. However, on the upside, 55 percent of the grandparents reported that caring for their grandchildren gave them more purpose for living. Kornhaber (1996) cited one grandparent, who was interviewed in a grandparent study, describing the experience as "a new lease on life . . . although one I never expected. I never thought I would be good for much when I got old. But I was wrong. For Billy (his grandson), I'm his lifeline" (p. 136).

Clearly, providing childcare is a mixed blessing for grandparents. On one hand, they are able to help their grandchildren in time of need; on the other hand, grandparents recount the hardships of parenting during the time when there is an expectation that life should be getting easier (Burton and Bengston 1985), as is illustrated by the following case (from Levine 1995).

A fifty-one-year-old grandmother left with the responsibility of raising three HIV-infected grandchildren felt overwhelmed by the prospect of grandparenting sick children and had this to say: "I was only 51, but saw myself as a woman with no future."

In addition to the despair expressed by this young grandmother, grandparents rarely receive monetary compensation for childcare (Jendrek 1993), and when they do it is often below market prices (Presser 1989). Thus, apart from willingness of grandparents to provide care, critical issues that have to be addressed include not only their availability (especially working grandmothers), geographical location, and household structure, but also their ability to provide adequate care of grandchildren who are infected/orphaned/affected by HIV/AIDS.

In sub-Saharan Africa, the norm is for the elderly, and grandparents in particular, to be cared for by their sons and daughters. The distribution of wealth tends to be concentrated in the 25–55 age group, not in the elderly. The effect of this is that when the wage earners die due to AIDS, having spent most of their wealth and/or savings on expensive treatments and medical care, they leave very little or nothing at all for their surviving children and their own parents. Thus the elderly are becoming surrogate parents at a time when they do not have either the energy to work or the financial means to start raising children all over again. The high fertility rates in sub-Saharan Africa also contribute to the burden, due to the unprecedented number of orphans and vulnerable children who have to be taken care of by elderly grandparents.

Thus "many of the striking images of the HIV/AIDS epidemic around the world are of families, but of unfamiliar families: a grandparent surrounded by grandchildren, adolescent-headed families, often siblings and cousins bonded together, dying adults tended by their children and communities as families" (Reid 1995). These images are especially true of sub-Saharan Africa, a subcontinent that has been most severely ravaged by this silent war on humanity.

Grandparenting in a World with AIDS

As Guzman (1998) emphasizes, caring for a child is labor-intensive, time-consuming, and often quite challenging at the best of times when the children are healthy; however, if they are infected with HIV, the task is most daunting. Some of the unique challenges of AIDS-related deaths for children and their caregivers include the fact that the AIDS clinical course is often marked by characteristics that can be both disturbing and disruptive to children (Bauman and Wiener 1994)—marked physical changes such as dramatic wasting and disfiguring dermatological disorders; behavioral and cognitive changes such as AIDS encephalopathy and AIDS dementia complex, which can result in deterioration of short-term memory, mutism, loss of ability to walk, swallow, and void; and often severe debilitation. For many AIDS patients these physical and behavioral problems tend to result in loss of a job, income, and eventually a home.

No matter how devoted and willing grandparents are to look after their grandchildren, they are unable to bear the full burden of increased household-level illness, emotional disturbance, and the physically incapacitating nature of the disease, especially for those infected with HIV. In a New York study of black grandparents' health problems (Levine 1995) it was found that health problems such as diabetes, hypertension, back ailments, and low energy were ignored because the health needs of children were a higher priority in those families.

Community and National Responses

Despite the fact that AIDS is having a devastating impact on countries in sub-Saharan Africa, communities across the continent are rallying to react to the damage and to counter some of its worst effects on orphans and their caregivers. In 1991 the Malawi government set up a National Orphan Care Task Force. The government also supports community-based programs such as Community-based Options for Protection and Empowerment (COPE). This program, which is funded by USAID/Displaced Children and Orphans Fund (DCOF) and implemented by the Save the Children Federation, is a systematic approach to mobilizing community-based responses to the needs of orphans and all HIV/AIDS-affected families and households. The program includes identification and monitoring of orphans and other vulnerable individuals in the communities, community fundraising, providing material assistance to orphans and home-based care patients, developing community gardens, and forming youth anti-AIDS clubs.

In Zambia, which has the second largest number of AIDS orphans in the world after Uganda, nongovernmental organizations are working hard to provide food, clothing, and school fees to orphans and their families. USAID/DCOF has also funded an Orphans and Other Vulnerable Children (OVC) Program, which is a relatively low-cost/cost-effective community mobilization program to mitigate the impact of the AIDS epidemic on the lives and general welfare of HIV/AIDS-affected families and their children. The program provides support to communities so that they can help themselves in finding better and more sustainable ways of supporting orphans and vulnerable children. The OVC program strategy was premised on the observation that households were the front lines that were currently shouldering most of the weight of the problem of orphans and vulnerable children and that they needed to be targeted for capacity building. It was decided that Participatory Learning and Action (PLA) methodology would be utilized to raise awareness in the communities of the fact that the OVC problem was a community problem that required community action. The community identified the main needs of families with orphans and came up with action plans that would address those needs. The program strategy was therefore, to mobilize a community-owned, community-managed, and community-sustained response to the needs of orphans and vulnerable children at the community and district levels.

In Zimbabwe, where 7 percent of all children below fifteen years are orphaned by AIDS, a national policy on the care and protection of orphans was developed. The policy advocates that orphans should be placed in institutions only as a last resort and should be cared for by their families and communities whenever possible. A church-based NGO called Family, Orphans and Children Under Stress (FOCUS) was also established by volunteers in a rural community just outside Mutare in 1993. Volunteers in this program identify all orphaned children in each project's area and prioritize those households with the greatest needs. The volunteers then make visits to those families twice a month and provide those households with limited but essential material and in-kind support.

Janet Museveni, wife of President Yoweri Museveni, established the Uganda Women's Effort to Save Orphans (UWESO) in 1986 in the aftermath of the civil war. The organization assisted orphans in resettlement camps and returned them to their extended families. In the wake of the AIDS epidemic and its devastation in Uganda, the organization has shifted its emphasis to support AIDS orphans throughout the country.

National and International Responses

Policy responses to HIV/AIDS-infected/orphaned/affected children and their caregivers vary in different parts of the world, depending on the intensity of the epidemic and resource allocations in each country. The following is a brief overview of some policy responses that have been adopted in some countries around the world (European Forum on HIV/AIDS, Children and Families 1999:1–9).

Russian Federation

The Russian AIDS law is the first and possibly the most comprehensive law to address HIV-infected children and their families directly. Approved by the State Duma on February 24, 1995, Federal Law 38 reads as follows:

> Parents or guardians of children infected with HIV have the right to stay with their children under the age of fifteen years in the in-patient ward of an institution providing medical care and shall receive the following benefits for this period in accordance with government social insurance; free round-trip transportation shall be provided to the parent or another legal guardian accompanying an HIV-infected minor under the age of sixteen years to the place of treatment; one parent or other legal guardian granted leave from work to look after an HIV-infected minor under the age of eighteen years shall retain his or her work seniority provided she or he returns to work before the minor reaches some specified age, and the period of leave used to care for the HIV-infected minor shall be included in the individual's total length of service; priority provision of living accommodations in buildings of the state, municipal, or social housing fund in the event that they require better living conditions, if an HIV-infected minor under the age of eighteen years is living with them. The laws and other legal acts of the component jurisdictions of the Russian Federation may establish other measures for social protection of HIV-infected individuals and their family members.

France

In France, although there is no specific government policy, strategy, or provision of benefits for children affected by HIV/AIDS, there is a national policy for orphans, under which a host family of HIV/AIDS orphan(s) is entitled to receive about 550FF (approximately USD100) per month per child in government subsidies. However, a host family will not receive further funds for a child affected by HIV/AIDS without medical problems. If there are health problems, then the caregivers receive 1,000FF–5,500FF in benefits from the Special Education Allocation. The creation of specific services or programs for children affected by HIV/AIDS is still predominantly the work of NGOs.

Switzerland

Even though Switzerland is a small country where only one in a thousand pregnant women is thought to be HIV-infected, the government established a registry for children born to infected mothers in 1996. The Swiss Neonatal HIV study coordinates and collects prospective data of children born to HIV-positive mothers and their families. In 1997 a group of pediatricians caring for these children at different centers joined to form the Swiss Pediatric AIDS Group. The group coordinates care for the children, diagnostic procedures, follow-up, and therapy. It also formulates guidelines and recommendations that are released on a regular basis. This type of network and service provision is a good example of how strong national policies and strategies can positively influence all aspects of dealing with a rare disease in a small country.

Sweden

State and community support systems provide services to children and families affected by HIV in Sweden. Daycare and respite care for children, medical support to HIV-infected persons, home care, and domestic assistance are provided for those who need it. Thus, even if Sweden, like Switzerland, has only five hundred to a thousand HIV-affected families in a population of nine million, the government has responded in a timely manner to ensure that those few who are affected are provided with adequate services.

The Netherlands

In the Netherlands, funding for all AIDS-related activities is handled through AIDS Funds. Most of the infected women and children are immigrants and have not been officially designated as a "target group" for specific services. Therefore formal legislation is necessary to provide comprehensive services to all affected families. Nevertheless, the government has appointed home and case managers for families living with HIV/AIDS and nurses for infected/affected children. The main hospitals have also appointed social workers for HIV-affected children and families.

Global Perspective

In 1989 UNICEF initiated the UN Convention on the Rights of the Child, ratified by 187 countries. The 1999 UN International Year of Older Persons (IYOP), noted earlier, did not include any initiatives regarding the health and the rights of the world's elderly caregivers, who are facing major challenges as a result of the AIDS pandemic.

The Organization of African Unity (OAU), made the Tunis Declaration on AIDS and the Child in Africa in 1994, observing, "We must recognize that an effective response to the needs of AIDS affected children requires a multi-disciplinary, multisectoral response effectively coordinated. . . . We must recognize that the serious effect the AIDS epidemic is having on children must be seen as a national issue not just the concern of the communities most directly affected" (European Forum on HIV/AIDS 1999:9).

Specific targeting of caregivers as a special group is missing from the OAU declaration, just as it was from the UN IYOP charter. This calls for strong advocacy in such regional and global forums to ensure inclusion of clauses that focus on the impact of the AIDS epidemic on the lives of elderly caregivers of AIDS-AOI affected/orphaned children around the world.

Policy Recommendations

The global and systematic devastation of the lives of people affected by the AIDS pandemic is unprecedented in human history. It is now widely recognized that there is a substantial burden placed on the elderly members of our societies, especially grandparents taking care of HIV/AIDS-infected/orphaned/affected children. Hence some of the critical questions that need to be addressed at a global level especially through research and the UN system should include:

Is HIV/AIDS childcare the responsibility of the family or the state?

How are the needs of affected families assessed, that is, who is taking care of finding the balance between the health, social, legal, and educational needs of these children and their elderly caregivers?

At what point does the government's role stop? At what point does the role of nongovernmental organizations (NGOs) begin?

Who coordinates the care of elderly caregivers?

Where and how are the views of elderly caregivers and their rights to their own protection assessed?

Do the elderly caregivers participate in any way in decisions affecting their own lives and those of the children they are taking care of?

How do those decisions get incorporated into national/international and/or United Nations global HIV/AIDS policies and actions?

At the national level, policy development for a cause whose consequences are as far-reaching and of the magnitude of the AIDS pandemic requires a major political commitment. The governments' legislative authorities need to be made aware of the problems faced by elderly caregivers of HIV/AIDS-affected children, so that regulations can be put in place to protect their rights and to assist them to take adequate care of those children for whom they are responsible.

The following recommendations are drawn from governmental programs in those countries that have been the most successful in providing appropriate services.

Develop a strategy for improving and protecting the general welfare of HIV/AIDS-infected/orphaned/affected children and their caregivers (especially elderly grandparents). The first step toward developing this strategy is to carry out a situation analysis (needs assessment) of the elderly caregivers through national surveys and research that would include:

- number of children living in HIV/AIDS-affected families (if you cannot count them they do not exist)
- number, age, employment status, and gender of caregivers
- number of children and their caregivers who have access to state benefits
- number of children and their caregivers who have access to NGOs providing services to HIV/AIDS-affected children and families
- number of NGOs who receive help from the state to provide the services that they do.

Other strategies could include

- registering all categories of HIV/AIDS-infected/orphaned/affected children and have them classified under the disability act so that they can receive disability-related benefits, including the opportunity to have a legal caregiver/grandparent with a salary paid by the state
- organizing a national media system to provide information to those in need of services on "where and how to access those services"
- creating a comprehensive referral system including mobile home-care consultants to assist elderly caregivers
- developing legislation that addresses elderly caregivers of HIV/AIDS–infected/orphaned/affected children directly (e.g., regulations that allow free transportation, priority phone installation, housing, and free access to medical care by caregivers and the children they are looking after)
- providing resources to those nongovernmental and nonprofit organizations engaged in providing care to affected children and families, which need funding, adequate training, government support and supervision
- training a new cadre of HIV/AIDS–specialized social workers and nurses and placing them in every state hospital to deal with families and children with special HIV/AIDS–related needs.

Conclusion

This chapter has demonstrated that although the face of HIV/AIDS is global, the responses to the pandemic and the problems faced by infected, orphaned, and affected children and their elderly caregivers differ in nature and in scale in different parts of the world. An important difference between biomedical and sociocultural interventions lies in the degree of generalizability across populations. Whereas the course of HIV infection and AIDS is relatively constant for all those infected, the behavioral precursors of infection, and the social consequences for patients, their dependent children, and elderly caregivers, are embedded in sociocultural patterns that are highly variable from one social group to another. These differences call for research on the situation of elderly caregivers in different parts of the world, in order to understand the full range of societal responses to the epidemic and how those responses are conditioned not only by the HIV/AIDS prevalence levels, but also by the combination of culture, political, social, and economic systems in different parts of the globe. A concerted effort is needed to find lasting solutions to problems faced by children orphaned by AIDS. However, even more attention needs to be given to older caregivers of those children. After all, the health, educational, and developmental outcomes for AIDS orphans will depend on the medical, social, economic, and mental status of their elderly caregivers, the majority of whom are maternal grandparents. The UN needs to extend the protocol of the 1999 International Year of Older Persons to include treatment of HIV/AIDS-affected elderly caregivers as a special and distinct group in societies around the world in need of protection and care from their national governments. Orphaned children have to be taken care of until they are independent adults, normally around the age of twenty-one years. Thus, assistance to AIDS-related programs for the elderly caregivers should also be long-term.

References

Barnett, T., and P. Blaikie. 1992. *AIDS in Africa: Its Present and Future Impact.* London: Bellhaven Press.

Bauman, L., and L. Wiener, eds. 1994. *Journal of Developmental and Behavioural Pediatrics* 15 (3), June supplement.

Burton, L. M., and V. L. Bengston. 1985. Black grandmothers: Issues of timing and continuity. In V. L. Bengston and J. F. Robertson, eds., *Grandparenthood,* pp. 61–88. Beverly Hills, Calif.: Sage.

European Forum on HIV/AIDS, Children and Families. *Newsletter,* autumn 1999.

Foster, G., C. Makufa, R. Drew, S. Kambeu, and K. Saurombe. 1996. Supporting children in need through a community-based orphan visiting programme. *AIDS Care* 8:389–403.

Foster, G., F. Shakespeare, H. Chinemana, H. Jackson, S. Gregson, C. Marange, and S. Mashumba. 1994. Orphan prevalence in a peri-urban community in Zimbabwe. *AIDS Care* 6:3–18.

Guzman, L. 1998. The use of grandparents as child care providers. Center for Demography and Ecology *NSFH Working Paper No. 84,* University of Wisconsin, Madison.

Hunter, S. S. 1990. Orphans as a window on the AIDS epidemic in sub-Saharan Africa: Initial results and implications of a study in Uganda. *Social Science and Medicine* 31:681–690.

——. 1991. The impact of AIDS on children in sub-Saharan African urban centers. *African Urban Quarterly* 6 (1): 108–128.

Jendrek, M. P. 1993. Grandparents who parent their grandchildren: Effects on lifestyles. *Journal of Marriage and the Family* 55:609–621.

Khmer HIV/AIDS NGO Alliance. 2000. Children affected by HIV/AIDS: Appraisal of needs and resources in Cambodia. Unpublished report.

Knodel, J., and L. Van Landingham. 2000. Children and older persons: AIDs' unseen victims. *American Journal of Public Health* 90 (7): 1024–1025.

Kornhaber, A. 1996. *Contemporary Grandparenting.* Thousand Oaks, Calif.: Sage.

Kreibick, T. 1995. Caretakers' support group. In N. Body-Franklin, G. L. Steiner, and M. G. Boland, eds., *Children, Families, and HIV/AIDS: Psychosocial and Therapeutic Issues,* p. 167. London: Guilford Press.

Levine, C. 1995. Today's challenges, tomorrow's dilemmas. In S. Geballe, J. Gruendel, and W. Andiman, eds., *Forgotten Children of the AIDS Epidemic,* pp. 190–204. New Haven: Yale University Press.

Mann, J. D., J. M. Tarantola, and T. W. Netter, eds. 1992. *AIDS in the World: A Global Report.* Cambridge, Mass.: Harvard University Press.

Masland, T., and R. Nordland. 2000. Mapping the AIDS epidemic's hot zone: The orphans of AIDS. *Newsweek,* January 2000, pp. 37–49.

Michaels, D., and C. Levine. 1992. Estimates of the number of motherless youth orphaned by AIDS in the United States. *Journal of the American Medical Association* 268:3456–3461.

Preble, E. A. 1990a. Impact of HIV/AIDS on African children. *Social Science and Medicine* 31:671–680.

———. 1990b. Women, children and AIDS in Africa: An impending disaster. *New York University Journal of International Law and Politics* 12:959–972.

Presser, H. B. 1989. Some economic complexities of childcare provided by grandmothers. *Journal of Marriage and Family* 51:581–591.

Reid, E. 1995. *HIV and AIDS: The Global Interconnection.* New York: UNDP and Kumarian Press.

Serpell, R. 1992. African dimensions of child care and nurturance. In M. E. Lamb, K. J. Sternberg, C.-P. Hwang, and A. G. Broberg, eds., *Child Care in Context,* pp. 463–475. Mahwah, N.J.: Lawrence Erlbaum Associates.

———. 1996. Children of AIDS-affected Zambian families: Needs assessment and policy development. Unpublished report.

———. 1998. Children orphaned by HIV/AIDS in Zambia: Risk factors from premature parental death and policy implications. Ph.D. dissertation, University of Maryland.

UN AIDS Commission. 2000. Report on the global HIV/AIDS epidemic. Unpublished report.

UNICEF (United Nations Children's Fund). 1999. *UNICEF World AIDS Report.* New York: UNICEF.

World Bank. 1998. *Confronting AIDS: Public Priorities In A Global Epidemic.* New York: Oxford University Press.

World Health Organization. N.d. *Action for Children Affected by AIDS: Program Profiles and Lessons Learned.* Geneva: World Health Organization.

15

Conclusion

DAPHNE JOSLIN

As the twenty-first century opens, popular images of aging and HIV disease in the United States have evolved from dread and denial to optimism and hope. Pharmaceutical, nutritional, and holistic health advertisements portray vibrant, silver-haired elders and suntanned HIV-infected young adults. No longer victims of biological fate, both groups are presented as agents of their own lives whose physiological vulnerability can be effectively managed. "Successful aging" (Rowe and Kahn 1998) and "surviving AIDS' appear to be within the individuals' reach, dependent solely on personal determination and discipline. Both images presume tremendous control over one's life, where decisions affecting one's well-being can be approached with deliberateness and sufficient personal and material reserves.

The contributors to this book suggest that these cheerful images associated with healthy aging and living with HIV disease are far removed from the daily lives and concerns of older surrogate parents who are raising HIV-affected children and adolescents. Most of these caregivers have limited social and economic resources, mirrored by the paucity of community programs and public support. Around the world and within the United States, most AIDS orphans and their surrogate parents are from economically disadvantaged families and communities.

The contributors also describe the complex challenges HIV-affected surrogate parents face and suggest various programmatic responses as well as key areas for public policy reform. In this chapter I propose directions for practitioners and advocates from an empowerment perspective, viewing empowerment as a multilevel process through which individuals and communities "assume control and mastery over their lives in the context of their social and political environment" (Wallerstein 1992:198). The concept of empowerment has been successfully used in community organizing to challenge local structures of disenfranchisement and in community psychology to promote self-efficacy and group participation. As a health promotion and public health strategy, it has been applied in HIV prevention (Beeker, Guenther-Gray, and Raj 1998), where motivation and behavior are viewed not solely as being within the individual's complete and voluntary control but as resting on social and cultural pressures and opportunities (Beeker, Guenther-Gray, and Raj 1998). This perspective does not diminish the importance of fostering healthy individual behaviors but recognizes the inherent limitations of individually focused strategies for health promotion that fail to address familial and community circumstances under which individuals conduct their lives. As a broad concept, empowerment of elder surrogate parents proposes improved quality of life and social justice through greater individual and community efficacy and control. It implies a process of personal and social change that will enable individuals and communities to achieve improved health and well-being (Wallerstein 1992).

Caregiver Empowerment through Programs

Because of social isolation, reluctance to seek services, lack of education, and distrust and fear of formal institutions, elder caregivers may not obtain supportive services and financial benefits. Service barriers documented by research (Silverstein and Vehvilainen 2000) and reported by local and national grandparent advocacy coalitions are especially pronounced among HIV-affected caregivers because of disease-related caregiving demands and fear of stigmatization. Special outreach efforts are needed to address access barriers, especially among isolated caregivers (see chapters 3 and 10; see also Mullen 2000; Roe 2000). In-home visits are especially important to HIV-affected caregivers because of HIV stigma and the demands of HIV caregiving.

Broad community visibility is needed to promote the active education and support by family, friends, service providers, educators, and clergy who can encourage elder caregivers to seek services for themselves and provide contact information. Roe (2000) notes that because there will be continuous waves of grandparent caregivers, outreach and public information must be ongoing. In addition to active targeting of HIV affected caregivers, professionals need to encourage caregivers to seek services for themselves, noting that self-care through community services will help to ensure their ability to continue as parental surrogates (Joslin and Harrison 1998). Because caregivers often fear that making their own needs known will result in children's removal from their care (Joslin and Harrison 1998; Joslin and Brouard 1995; Minkler and Roe 1993), professional advocacy is needed so that caregivers will not avoid seeking services.

Increasingly, community interventions for grandparent and other elder-generation caregivers are promoting the active involvement of caregivers themselves. Caregivers serve on coalition advisory boards that advocate on behalf of grandparent and elder caregivers and conduct outreach, information and referral, peer education, counseling, and advocacy (Cox 2000; Roe 2000). In order to involve HIV-affected caregivers, organizers must be sensitive to and informed about the special problems of these older adults, including isolation, stigmatization, and stress associated with HIV disease and treatment management.

The families of older caregivers are clients of multiple public and private agencies including daycare, Head Start, schools, youth programs, HIV/AIDS medical and social services, pediatric clinics, mental health services, judicial and child-welfare systems, legal services, and income assistance programs. Like other custodial grandparents, HIV-affected elder caregivers are wedged between fragmented service systems, conflicting eligibility requirements, lack of accessible information, and inconsistent public policies. Moreover, few service systems make the elder caregiver the focus, making deliberate outreach, education, and service development necessary. Promoting caregiver help-seeking requires greater interagency coordination and professional networking so that institutions rather than caregivers assume the burden for navigating multiple service systems. Interagency collaboration in program development, client advocacy, and staff training can strengthen outreach and referral, improve client intake and assessment, and enhance client access to a broad spectrum of community resources.

Broad-based coalitions involving the HIV/AIDS, aging, child welfare, and human services networks (Joslin and Nazon 1996) are vehicles for building a social and geographical base from which professionals and caregivers can develop outreach, advocacy, training, and service models. One area for coalition-building is community-based long-term care. Lower AIDS mortality rates have been matched by reductions in Medicaid-funded in-home assistance (e.g., housekeeping, personal care), which in turn has increased the day-to-day burden of family care. In the absence of a public long-term care policy, HIV caregivers, like those caring for persons with Parkinson's disease, Alzheimer's disease, and other debilitating conditions, confront the vacuum of supportive services.

The empowerment perspective suggested by Cox (2000) reminds us that the vulnerability of custodial grandparents to stress, poorer health, and financial insecurity should not cast them as passive and helpless victims. At the same time, their resilience, sacrifice, and determination should not be taken as evidence that their caregiving responsibilities have no serious consequences. Dressel and Barnhill (1994) note that the elder surrogate parents "transcend the either-or dichotomies of being either needy or resourceful. They are both" (p. 688). The narratives in chapter 2 illustrate caregivers' strength and determination on one hand and their powerlessness and resignation on the other hand. Their devotion to children's care should be matched by a sense of entitlement and empowerment. Effective action on one's own behalf may be impeded by a lack of education in critical and abstract thinking, lack of access to relevant information (Cox 1998), the stress and fatigue of caregiving, and limited economic resources. Without advocacy skills, caregivers cannot challenge incorrect information or decisions on the part of family income assistance programs such as TANF or child welfare, educational, legal, housing, and other service systems.

Promoting skills, beliefs, and attitudes through caregiver groups is an effective model for building the self-efficacy of custodial grandparents (Cox 2000). Self-help capacity and diminished powerlessness can be achieved through the development of skills and competencies, opportunities for practice, tangible results, and practical knowledge (Staples 1990). Through an empowerment program model of peer supports, grandparent caregivers gain skills in advocacy, self-esteem building, communication, and problem-solving (Cox 2000). Strategies for caregiver health promotion can be developed from an empowerment perspective, inasmuch as there is clear evidence for the need to enhance self-care among custodial grandparents. The model of peer-based empowerment groups (Cox 2000) could be adapted within the health-education curriculum to provide participants with problem-solving skills and health information related to stress and chronic health problems.

Empowerment: Reframing the Gerontological Paradigm

Writing on behalf of grandmothers raising children of incarcerated mothers, Dressel and Barnhill (1994) challenge gerontological thought and practice to consider older adults within the social and economic structures of their families and communities. Their challenge is consistent with the empowerment perspective offered by this chapter, which proposes that caregiver well-being cannot be considered apart from families and communities of infected women. The reframing of research, practice, and policy proposed by Dressel and Barnhill in no way neglects elders who are alone, very old, or dependent in their daily activities. Rather, it recognizes the structural disadvantages of gender, social class, and race/ethnicity as much as age in determining the life chances of grandmothers raising the children of HIV-infected parents.

In the dominant gerontological research and practice paradigm, living alone and advanced age (i.e., seventy-five years and older) are the demographic criteria used to identify older adults at risk for poorer physical and mental health and diminished functional capacity. Evidence concerning the economic, physical, social, and psychological well-being of custodial grandparents indicates that parental surrogacy should also be considered a risk factor. A broadened gerontological paradigm would extend the concept of age as a basis of service and entitlement eligibility beyond chronological age to generational age, an extension that would recognize the risks associated with the role of familial or communal elder. For example, U.S. census data could be used to target services to communities with disproportionately high percentages of grandparent-headed households. Intergenerational collaboration in public policy advocacy is demonstrated by initiatives of Generations United and the Children's Defense Fund that recognize that the vulnerable, both young and old, often share the same family (Butts 2000). An empowerment policy agenda for HIV-affected elder caregivers would advocate for policies and programs that address the increasing infection rate among women, their lack of access to medical care and supportive services, and their diminished capacity for prevention and self-care.

Empowerment and Social Justice

Over the epidemic's two decades, HIV disease has been demographically and epidemiologically transformed in the United States and around the world. The incidence of new infections and greater risk of morbidity and mortality is increasingly interwoven with rural and urban poverty and with communities of color. In the United States, as a chronic disease and disease of poor and marginalized populations, HIV has "lost its salience as a public issue"

(Bayer 1999:1042). Like unemployment, family disorganization, violence, homelessness, and addiction, the epidemic is no longer perceived as a threat to the mainstream. Medical treatment of HIV disease has outpaced the social and political will to eliminate the social conditions that create greater risk of infection. The epidemic's entrenchment among the marginalized underclass reflects the convergence of two decades of social policies that have dismantled social welfare, housing, job training, education, and community programs. Notably, Mrs. N. and her family, whose narrative is presented in chapter 2, moved five months after the interview, unable to remain in dilapidated housing and unable to obtain section 8 housing because of a long waiting list. Mrs. N. now cares for her infected grandchild and eight other grandchildren in a public shelter.

Poor urban areas in the United States have become disproportionately burdened by HIV/AIDS. Economic and epidemiological evidence at the neighborhood level shows the geographical concentration of HIV disease among the poor and the role of economic deprivation in the spread of infection (Zierkler et al. 2000). The persistent increase in new female AIDS cases exposes the limits of individually focused HIV behavioral strategies that ignore the economic and cultural constraints in women's lives, which in turn limit their ability to reduce their risk unsafe sexual relations (Beeker, Guenther-Grey, and Raj 1998; Wingood and DeClemente 1996). The majority of HIV-affected elder caregivers in communities most affected by HIV have low incomes, limited education, inadequate housing, and chronic health problems. Like the caregivers profiled in chapter 2 and others living in poor urban and rural areas, their families may be severely disrupted by mental illness, substance abuse, homelessness, incarceration, and violence. As one HIV administrator noted, "HIV [disease] has become a part of the fabric of life in many poor families and communities. The tragedy is that children who are born to infected mothers escape infection as infants, through prophylactic medications, such as AZT but become infected as teen-agers" (Carol Mevi-Triano, personal communication, 2000).

The conditions that thrust mid-life and older women into the surrogate parental role are those that put women at risk of HIV infection and create barriers to self-care and medical treatment: poverty, lack of affordable housing, substance abuse, domestic violence, and inadequate education. The elder generation's well-being is inextricably linked to younger women's empowerment to govern their own health. Greater chronicity of HIV disease has contributed to the "Lazarus syndrome," in which those who were close to death acquire renewed health and vigor as a result of antiretroviral therapies. This can result in regression to addictive behaviors—a return to alcohol and drug use and sexual compulsion. Some elder caregivers cope with raising children of an infected, addicted mother who is intermittently involved in their lives but brings her addictive behaviors into the household. Lack of sufficient alcohol and drug treatment programs for women, especially infected mothers, is a major policy failure that harms the well-being of three generations—elder, adult child, and minor children. Recent legislation that removed substance abuse as a disabling condition that qualifies an infected person for HIV care (Levi and Kates 2000) has further removed medical and supportive services from addicted mothers.

The unprecedented number of children living in poverty in the United States is stark testimony to the erosion of the social contract with families (Henkin and Kingston 1998–1999). The failure to establish universal health insurance and the continued erosion of resources for housing, health, and educational programs represents "broken faith" (Reich 1999), an unraveling of the social compact that included social insurance such as Medicare and entitlement programs such as Aid to Families with Dependent Children. Significant in this erosion since the late 1970s is the decline of the premise, "It could happen to me" (Reich 1999). Those outside the margins of affluence and sustained productivity are viewed as socially dispensable, different, or suspect. Although images of grandparents raising grandchildren evoke sympathy, elder parental surrogates are the survivors of families and communities in which the younger generations have been lost to violence, drugs, chronic underemployment, incarceration, and HIV/AIDS.

Social historians note that American social welfare policies have long tried to distinguish the "deserving" from the "undeserving" poor (Abramowitz 1988). As elders in families whose social and economic needs often preceded parental surrogacy (Strawbridge et al. 1997), HIV-affected caregivers may be seen as "undeserving" older adults—not only economically marginal, but also failures in the societal project to age "successfully" and to leave the legacy of a functional "healthy" family. Caregivers themselves may succumb to this societal blame, believing that they are undeserving of public services and benefits because their children became infected through drug use or sexual relations with drug users or both. Their failure to protect their children from "the streets" may be seen as an individual failing, in their own and the public's eyes, not as the failure of society to ensure healthy communities that support families. From a social policy perspective, Braithwaite (1992) proposes that caregiving be considered as a societal burden rather than as a solely personal one. In this framework, elder parental surrogates to HIV-affected children have assumed responsibility for generation(s) neglected and abandoned by society, not just their own adult children and grandchildren. These caregivers are the parents of last resort whose own well-being may be sacrificed rather than supported.

Empowerment of these elders through the "reframing of gerontological thought and practice" (Dressel and Barnhill 1994) implies an intergenerational agenda of social justice that includes income support programs that are not means-tested (Schorr 1999); guaranteed economic security through a universal family or children's allowance (Abramowitz 1988); universal health insurance; affordable low- and middle-income housing; advocacy for sufficient drug treatment programs for women, especially mothers (Minkler and Roe 1993); and affordable in-home and community-support services for those with chronic illnesses. Caregiver empowerment must also include intergenerational public health strategies that target poor urban and rural communities and the invisible generation of elder parental surrogates who absorb the hidden costs of the epidemic. A multilevel approach would enhance individual health behaviors through supportive community networks, increase access to and quality of health care, and improve social and economic conditions underlying health behaviors and health risks (Freudenberg 2000).

As they care for children in the wake of HIV/AIDS, older parental surrogates embody the very response needed by society to this elder generation of caregivers and their families. It is the response of compassion and commitment. It asks, "What else could I do? They are my grandkids? Who else would care for them?' Their resilience and devotion challenge us as professionals, students, and advocates to create an imperative for personal and community empowerment, an imperative for social justice.

References

Abramowitz, M. 1989. *Regulating the Lives of Women: Social Welfare Policy from Colonial Times to the Present.* Boston, Mass.: South End Press.

Bayer, R. 1999. Clinical progress and the future of HIV exceptionalism. *Archives of Internal Medicine* 159 (10): 1042–1048.

Beeker, C., C. Guenther-Gray, and A. Raj. 1998. Community empowerment, paradigm drift and the primary prevention of HIV/AIDS. *Social Science and Medicine* 46 (7): 831–842.

Braithwaite, V. 1992. Caregiving burden: Making the concept scientifically useful and policy relevant. *Research on Aging* 14 (1): 3—27.

Butts, D. M. 2000. Organizational advocacy as a factor in public policy regarding custodial grandparenting. In B. Hayslip and R. Goldberg-Glen, eds., *Grandparents Raising Grandchildren: Theoretical, Empirical, and Clinical Perspectives*, pp. 350–361. New York: Springer.

Cox, C. 1998. Empowerment interventions in aging. *Social Work with Groups* 11:111–125.

——. 2000. Empowering grandparents raising grandchildren. In C. Cox, ed., *To Grandmother's House We Go and Stay: Perspectives on Custodial Grandparents*, pp. 253–267. New York: Springer.

Dressel, P. L., and S. K. Barnhill. 1994. Reframing gerontological thought and practice: The case of grandmothers with daughters in prison. *The Gerontologist* 34 (5): 685–691.

Freudenberg, N. 2000. Time for a national agenda to improve the health of urban populations. *American Journal of Public Health* 90:837–840.

Henkin, N., and E. Kingston. 1998–1999. Keeping the promise. *Generations* 22 (4): 6–9.

Joslin, D., and A. Brouard. 1995. The prevalence of grandmothers as primary caregivers in a poor pediatric population. *Journal of Community Health* 20 (5): 383–402.

Joslin, D., and M. Nazon. 1996. HIV/AIDS and aging networks. In Kathleen Nokes, ed., *HIV/AIDS and the Older Adult*, pp. 129–140. Washington, D.C.: Taylor & Francis.

Joslin, D., and R. Harrison. 1998. The "hidden patient": Older relatives raising children orphaned by HIV disease. *Journal of the American Medical Women's Association* 53:65–71.

Levi, J., and J. Kates. 2000. HIV: Challenging the health care delivery system. *American Journal of Public Health* 90:1033–1036.

Minkler, M., and K. Roe. 1993. *Grandmothers as Caregivers: Raising Children of the Crack Cocaine Epidemic*. Newbury Park, Calif.: Sage.

Mullen, F. 2000. Grandparents and welfare reform. In C. Cox, ed., *To Grandmother's House We Go and Stay: Perspectives on Custodial Grandparents*, pp. 113–131. New York: Springer.

Reich, R. B. 1999. Broken faith: Why we need to renew the social compact. *Generations* 22 (4): 19–24.

Roe, K. M. 2000. Community interventions to support grandparent caregivers: Lessons learned from the field. In C. Cox, ed., *To Grandmother's House We Go and Stay: Perspectives on Custodial Grandparents*, pp. 283–304. New York: Springer.

Rowe, J. W., and R. L. Kahn. 1998. *Successful Aging*. New York: Pantheon.

Schorr, A. 1999. Income supports across the life course. *Generations* 22 (4): 64–67.

Silverstein, N. M., and L. Vehvilainen. 2000. Grandparents and schools: Issues and potential challenges. In C. Cox, ed., *To Grandmother's House We Go and Stay: Perspectives on Custodial Grandparents*, pp. 268–282. New York: Springer.

Staples, L. 1990. Powerful ideas about empowerment. *Administration in Social Work* 14:29–42.

Strawbridge, W. J., M. I. Wallhagen, S. J. Shema, and G. A. Kaplan. 1997. New burdens or more of the same? Comparing grandparent, spouse and adult-child caregivers. *The Gerontologist* 37:505–510.

Wallerstein, N. 1992. Powerlessness, empowerment and health: implications for health promotion programs. *American Journal of Health Promotion* 6:197–205.

Wingood, G., and R. DeClemente. 1996. HIV sexual risk reduction interventions for women: A review. *American Journal of Preventive Medicine* 12:209–217.

Zierkler, S., N. Krieger, Y. Tang, W. Coady, E. Siegfried, A. DeMaria, and J. Auerbach. 2000. Economic deprivation and AIDS incidence in Massachusetts. *American Journal of Public Health* 90:1064–1073.